Verlauf der wichtigsten Knochen- und Gelenkerkrankungen im Röntgenbilde

Eine anschauliche Prognostik

von

Privatdozent Dr. med. Victor Hoffmann

Oberarzt der Chirurgischen Universitätsklinik
im Augusta-Hospital zu Köln

Mit deutschem und englischem Text

In 156 Serien mit 584 Abbildungen

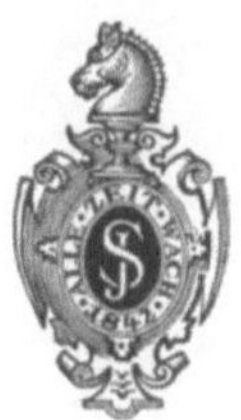

Berlin
Verlag von Julius Springer
1931

ISBN-13: 978-3-642-98555-3   e-ISBN-13: 978-3-642-99370-1
DOI: 10.1007/978-3-642-99370-1

In Dankbarkeit und Verehrung
dem Gedächtnis
PAUL FRANGENHEIMs
gewidmet

Vorwort.

In diesem Buch sind die wichtigsten Knochen- und Gelenkerkrankungen in ihrem Verlauf dargestellt. Benutzt ist dazu das Röntgenbild. Ist es doch der Erkenntnisweg, der den Werdegang dieser Krankheitsgruppe am besten zur Anschauung bringt und zugleich nächst dem histologischen Schnitt am tiefsten vordringt. Wesentliches, was im Röntgenbild nicht zum Ausdruck kommt, ergänzen die beigefügten klinischen Daten, so daß die Ganzheit des Krankheitsvorganges gewahrt ist. *Immer wird der gleiche Fall in seinem Ablauf gezeigt,* nicht etwa verschiedene Stadien einer Krankheit an verschiedenen Objekten. Dadurch erhält die Darstellung eine konkrete Präzision wie wir sie im täglichen Leben, wenigstens hinsichtlich des ganzen Verlaufes so oft nicht sehen. Sodann treten uns gerade die Knochen- und Gelenkerkrankungen in markanten Typen vor Augen. Findet man doch bei der Durchsicht eines Archives oder beim Durchblättern verschiedener Bücher der Röntgenkunde außerordentlich ähnliche und oft gleiche pathologische Befunde im Bilde, obgleich diese doch von ganz verschiedenen Menschen stammen. Wir dürfen also sicherer als bei vielen anderen Krankheiten aus einer Anzahl besonderer Beispiele auf andere der gleichen Gruppe schließen. Es ist daher mein Plan gewesen, in dem Buch für die wichtigsten Knochen- und Gelenkerkrankungen *eine in der Praxis brauchbare Anschauung der Prognose zu schaffen.*

Die Auswahl ist so getroffen, daß die einzelnen Fälle gewissermaßen das ganze breite Gebiet beleuchten. Sie zeigen die inneren Wesenszüge, die wir aus aller Vielgestaltigkeit herausfinden und die uns orientieren. Berücksichtigt sind in erster Linie die häufigen Krankheiten. Von den seltener vorkommenden sind solche, die in der Krankheitslehre grundsätzliche Bedeutung haben, wie die Ostitis fibrosa oder die Wachstumsstörung der Hüfte, mehrfach belegt; auf die Darstellung ganz seltener habe ich verzichtet. Aber auch bei den häufigen Krankheiten war eine Beschränkung notwendig. Könnte man doch einzelne Abschnitte, z. B. das Kapitel Verletzungen oder Tuberkulose wegen der großen praktischen Bedeutung zu selbständigen Monographien erweitern.

Soweit ich sehe, ist ein gleiches Werk in der Weltliteratur bisher nicht vorhanden. Es finden sich Bilderserien in Monographien über ein ganz spezielles Thema oder einzelne Bilderreihen in neueren Lehrbüchern der Röntgenkunde. Seit Jahren habe ich an unserer Klinik derartige Röntgenbilderserien des Krankheitsverlaufes als Wandtafeln hergerichtet und für den Unterricht benutzt. Aus diesem Grundstock ist die in diesem Buch vorliegende Sammlung entstanden.

Das Buch ist für den Arzt und für den Studierenden bestimmt. Ihm vermag es auf einem umgrenzten Gebiet der Pathologie das Wesen der Krankheiten — ihre Eigenart und ihre Auswirkung — durch die Anschauung leichtfaßlich propädeutisch zu vermitteln. Der Arzt wird eine solche Anschauung in weiterer Auswirkung brauchen können. Wenn er in einem Fall des Buches den „gesetzmäßigen" Ablauf einer Krankheit vom Anfang bis zum Ende betrachtet, wird er sein Auge schärfen für die ersten kleinen Anfänge des Prozesses, leichter die Richtung der Fortentwicklung erkennen und somit für die Praxis Nutzen ziehen. Oder er wird einer glatten Narbe leichter ansehen, daß sie der Endzustand eines langdauernden, mit Lebensgefahr oder anderen Komplikationen verbundenen Prozesses ist, z. B. bei der Osteomyelitis. Für den ärztlichen Gutachter ist dieses besonders wichtig. Sodann erscheint mir das Studium des Krankheitsverlaufes geradezu als ein Praktikum der Differentialdiagnose. Ich habe deshalb ein Stichwortverzeichnis am Schluß angefügt.

Alles ist so abgestimmt, daß Worte zurücktreten und die Anschauung lehrt. Mir schwebte dabei vor, eine wirkliche Erfahrung hinzustellen, die für die Aufgaben der Praxis ein Maßstab sein kann. Besteht doch in der heutigen Zeit für die ärztliche Praxis in erhöhtem Maße die Gefahr, daß wir das Wesentliche nicht schauen, die Heilkraft der Natur nicht bedenken, statt dessen Vieltuerei üben, ein sicheres Urteil und Handeln nicht finden. Wenn aber die anatomische Betrachtungsweise, die diesem Buche zugrunde liegt, in der Klinik heute vielfach als überwunden gilt, so kann das in Wirklichkeit nur für eine einseitig deskriptive Art berechtigt sein. Vielmehr ist aus dem anatomischen Bild, insbesondere einer Bilderreihe, ein lebender Werdegang ablesbar. Wir sehen mit der Form die Art des Prozesses und aus dem Nebeneinander verschiedener Stadien bereits Hinweise seiner Entwicklungsrichtung. Aber wie wir erst mit zunehmender Schulung mehr und mehr Einzelheiten feststellen, so lernen wir auch erst durch Übung mehr und mehr im Bild den Körper sehen, in einer Phase den Verlauf schauen. Ich selbst denke dankbar zurück an den Unterricht der pathologischen Anatomie, in dem uns P. ERNST in Heidelberg eine solche Schulung zuteil werden ließ.

Die Verwirklichung dieses Buches war mir möglich, weil in der Klinik FRANGENHEIMS, der ich seit Jahren angehöre, den Knochen- und Gelenkerkrankungen infolge des persönlichen Interesses des Leiters, besondere Aufmerksamkeit geschenkt wird. Über einem eigenen, groß angelegten Werk hat ihn in diesen Tagen auf der Höhe seines Lebens der Tod ereilt. Dem großen Kenner auf diesem Gebiete zum Gedächtnis seien diese Blätter in dankbarer Verehrung gewidmet.

Die Beobachtungsreihen stammen hauptsächlich aus der chirurgischen Universitätsklinik im Augusta-Hospital (Prof. Dr. FRANGENHEIM †), einzelne aus der unter gleicher Leitung stehenden chirurgischen Klinik im Bürgerhospital, woselbst die Röntgenaufnahmen in dem Zentralinstitut (Prof. Dr. GRAESSNER †, Prof. Dr. GRASHEY) angefertigt worden sind. Da aber das hier zur Darstellung gebrachte Material auch aus dem Archiv einer großen Klinik allein nicht gewonnen werden konnte, habe ich manche Bilderserien aus fremden Instituten beschafft: aus der chirurgisch-orthopädischen Klinik des Eduardushauses Köln (Chefarzt Dr. WIEMERS) die Serien 31, 45, 109, 110, 153, aus der Hautklinik der Universität Köln (Prof. Dr. ZINSSER) die Serien 55 u. 58, aus der Kinderklinik der Universität Köln (Geheimrat Prof. Dr. SIEGERT) die Serien 51, 52, 75, 79, 98 u. 103, aus der Orthopädischen Klinik der Universität Köln (Professor Dr. HACKENBROCH) die Serien 101 u. 155, aus dem Strahleninstitut der Allgemeinen Ortskrankenkasse Köln (Chefarzt Dr. TESCHENDORF) die Serien 42, 64 u. 65, aus dem Kantonhospital Aarau (Chefarzt Dr. BIRCHER) die Serie 80.

Von vielen Seiten bin ich unterstützt worden und ich danke allen, die mir geholfen haben, von Herzen, nicht zuletzt dem Herrn Verleger für das große Entgegenkommen.

Das Buch ist in deutscher und in englischer Sprache verfaßt; es begleitet meine Hoffnung, daß es dadurch zur Förderung gemeinsamer wissenschaftlicher Arbeit unter den verschiedenen Nationen zu seinem Teil beitragen möge.

Köln (Augusta-Hospital), im Oktober 1930.

VICTOR HOFFMANN.

Preface.

The object of this book is to demonstrate the most important bone and joint diseases and their subsequent course. X-ray photographs have been used because by them, it is possible to show the various stages and general course of this disease group, and because, after histological representation, they leave the most profound impression.

The accompanying clinical dates are essential since they allow the disease to be followed throughout its course. The various stages which are shown, belong to one and the same case and are not the different stages of a disease in different patients. In this way, the entire course is accurately presented in a way that is rarely possible to see in daily life and the striking types of bone and joint diseases are shown in a manner which is particularly easy to understand.

If one looks through collected works or turns the leaves of various books of radiology, he will find extraordinarily similar, indeed often pathologically identical conditions presented, even though the photographs are of totally different people. It has therefore been my plan to produce a work that would show the course and the prognosis of the most important bone and joint diseases in the same patient.

These cases are chosen so that they may be representative of the whole subject. They show the inside pecularities that we find among the manifold varieties and help us in our orientation.

It is the more frequent diseases that are chiefly taken into consideration. Those that are less common, such as osteitis fibrosa or growth disturbance of the hip, but which have a fundamental influence on medical teaching, are also repeatedly illustrated. It has of course, been necessary to limit the presentation of some of the commoner conditions, since some chapters such as those relating to injuries or tuberculosis, on account of their tremendous practical importance, could be presented as independant monographs.

As far as I know, no book such as this has, as yet, been published. Series of pictures exist in monographs dealing with one special subject and also a few pictures in modern text-books of radiology. For many years I have arranged series of X-ray photographs portraying the course of a disease on a board in the clinic and these have been used for instruction. It is from this collection that most of the pictures here presented, are taken.

This book is intended for the physician and the student. In the limited sphere of pathology, the pictures will help to establish the nature of the disease, its peculiarities and its effects. To the physician, this is a great advantage. If he follows the entire course of a disease from beginning to end, he should be able to recognize the first slight signs at the onset of the process and more easily identify the direction of its course. He will be able to see that a smooth scar is the final result of a lengthy process, such as osteomyelitis, which has been a danger to life. This is of great importance to the medical expert. The study of the course of a disease seems to me, to be a training in differential diagnosis and I have therefore arranged a differential diagnostic index at the end of the book.

The pictures are intended to take precedence over the text. One should learn by contemplation. My intention was to submit actual experience that could be used in practice. At the present time, there exists in the medical profession an increasing tendency to overlook the essential fact — that is, the healing power of nature; taking instead, small unimportant things into account and failing to make either the correct diagnosis or treatment. If the anatomical examination method, on which this book is based, is sometimes looked upon as out of date in some of our clinics, this is really only justified when related to a one-sided descriptive form. From an anatomical picture — more particularly from a series, the development of a process in the living subject may be understood. By its form, we recognize the type of pathological process and by following it throughout its various stages, we can identify the direction of its progression. In the same way that we are able, with our ever increasing knowledge, to verify more and more detail, so by practice, do we learn to visualise the body and by observing one aspect, to follow its further course. I myself, look back with gratitude to the lectures of pathological anatomy which were given by P. ERNST. He stressed the importance of tbis method.

The publishing of this book was possible, because in FRANGENHEIM's clinic, to which I have been attached for many years, exceptional attention was paid to joint and bone diseases by the principal himself. He was engaged upon an extensive work on this subject when he died a few days ago, in the prime of his life. These pages are gratefully dedicated to the memory of this great scientist.

The series of pictures are taken chiefly from the surgical University-Clinic of the Augusta-Hospital (Prof. Dr. FRANGENHEIM †), some are taken from the surgical clinic of the Bürger-Hospital which is under the same management as the former. The Röntgen photographs from both hospitals were taken in the Central-Institute. (Prof. Dr. GRAESSNER †, Prof. Dr. GRASHEY.) As it was not possible to acquire all the material for this book in one clinic alone, I have taken some series of pictures from other institutes. It is made up as follows: Surgical-Orthopaedic clinic of Eduardushausen, Cologne (Chief Dr. WIEMERS) series 31, 45, 109, 110, 153. Skin clinic of the Cologne university (Prof. Dr. ZINSSER) series 55 and 58. Childrens clinic of the Cologne university (Geheimrat Prof. Dr. SIEGERT) series 51, 52, 75, 79, 98 and 103. Orthopaedic clinic of the Cologne university (Prof. Dr. HACKENBROCH) series 101 and 155. Radiation institute of the Allgemeine Ortskrankenkasse (Local Insurance Hospital), Cologne (Chief Dr. TESCHENDORF) series 42, 64 and 65. Canton hospital Aarau (Chief Dr. BIRCHER) series 80.

I wish to offer my gratitude to all who have assisted me, and to my publisher in particular.

This book is written in German and English language and I sincerely hope that this fact will be benefitial to mutual scientific work between the different nations.

Cologne (Augusta-Hospital), October 1930.

VICTOR HOFFMANN.

Inhaltsverzeichnis.

I. Kapitel.
Akute Entzündungen.

Seite

A. Hämatogene (Serie 1—13), dentale (Serie 14—16) und traumatische (Serie 17—19) Osteomyelitis   1
B. Akute spezifische (Serie 20—22) und unspezifische (Serie 23—25) Arthritiden 34

II. Kapitel.
Chronische spezifische Entzündungen.

A. Tuberkulose (Serie 26—50) 45
B. Angeborene und erworbene Syphilis der Knochen und Gelenke (Serie 51—58) 88

III. Kapitel.
Geschwülste.

Primäre und sekundäre Knochengeschwülste (Serie 59—70 c) 105
Anhang: Exostose, Hyperplasie (Serie 71—73) 125

IV. Kapitel.
Wachstums-, Zirkulations- und Stoffwechselstörungen.

A. Chondrodystrophie, Osteogenesis imperfecta, Osteopsathyrosis, Mißbildung (Serie 74—78) . . 128
B. Myxödem, Kretinismus (Serie 79 und 80) 135
C. 1. Aseptische Epiphysennekrosen: Osteoarthritis def. juvenilis (Serie 81—85), Coxa vara adulescentium (Serie 86 und 87), SCHLATTERsche, KÖHLERsche Krankheit, Epiphysenstörung der Wirbelsäule (Serie 88—90) 139
   2. Ostitis fibrosa (Serie 91—95), Osteochondritis dissecans (Serie 96 und 97) 154
D. Rachitis, BARLOWsche Krankheit (Serie 98—103). — Gicht und Kalkgicht (Serie 104 und 105) 168

V. Kapitel.
Chronische unspezifische Gelenkleiden.

A. Progressiver Gelenkrheumatismus (Serie 106—110) 184
B. Arthritis deformans (Serie 111—116) und tabische Arthropathie (Serie 117—120) — Blutergelenk (Serie 121) 194

VI. Kapitel.
Verletzungen.

A. Heilung des Knochenbruches (Serie 122—128), Pseudarthrose (Serie 129 und 130), Epiphysenverletzung (Serie 131—134), Gelenkbruch (Serie 135—140) 208
B. Myositis ossificans, traumatische Knochenatrophie, ischämische Muskelkontraktur (Serie 141 bis 147) 238

VII. Kapitel.
Knochentransplantation und Gelenkbildung.

A. Freie Auto- und Heterotransplantation (Serie 148—151) 246
B. Gelenkplastik und Nearthrose (Serie 152—156) 255

Sachverzeichnis 263

Index.

Chapter I.
Acute Inflammations.

Page

A. Haematogenous (Series 1—13), dental (Series 14—16) and traumatic (Series 17—19) Osteomyelitis   2
B. Acute specific (Series 20—22) and unspecific (Series 23—25) Arthritieds 34

Chapter II.
Chronic Specific Inflammations.

A. Tuberculosis (Series 26—50) 46
B. Congenital and Acquired Syphilis of bones and joints (Series 51—58) 89

Chapter III.
Tumours.

Primary and secondary bone tumours (Series 59—70 c) 106
Supplement: Exostoses, Hyperplàsia (Series 71—73) 125

Chapter IV.
Growths-Metabolic and Nutritional disturbances.

A. Chondrodystrophia, Osteogenesis Imperfecta, Osteopsyarthrosis, Malformations (Series 74—78) . 128
B. Myxoedema, Cretinism (Series 79 and 80) 135
C. 1. Aseptic epiphyseal necroses: Osteoarthritis def. of juveniles (Series 81—85), Coxa Vara of
       adolescents (Series 86 and 87), SCHLATTERS and KÖHLERS disease, Epiphyseal disturbance
       of the spine (Series 88—90) 139
   2. Osteitis fibrosa (Series 91—95), Osteochondritis dissecans (Series 96 and 97) 155
D. Rickets, BARLOWS disease (Series 98—103). — Gout and Chalk gout (Series 104 and 105) . . 169

Chapter V.
Chronic Unspecific Joint Diseases.

A. Progressive joint rheumatism (Series 106—110) 184
B. Arthritis deformans (Series 111—116), Tabetic arthropathy (Series 117—120) 194

Chapter VI.
Injuries.

A. Healing of bone fractures (Series 122—128), Pseudarthrosis (Series 129 and 130), Epiphyseal
   injuries (Series 131—134), Joint fracture (Series 135—140) 208
B. Myositis ossificans, Traumatic bone atrophy, Ischaemic muscle-contraction (Series 141—147) . 238

Chapter VII.
Bone Transplantations and Joint Formation.

A. Free auto and hetero transplantation (Series 148—151) 246
B. Joint plasty and Nearthrosis (Series 152—156) 255
Index 263

I. Kapitel.

Akute Entzündungen der Knochen und Gelenke.

A. Hämatogene, dentale und traumatische Osteomyelitis.

Die eitrige Entzündung der Knochen ist eine gewaltige Erkrankung. Die septische Allgemeininfektion, deren Metastase sie ist, bedroht das Leben; an Ort und Stelle vernichtet der Prozeß das feste Knochengewebe, aber er setzt zugleich auch den Anreiz zur Wiederherstellung. Ist einmal die Entscheidung über Leben und Tod gefallen, so steht der örtliche Vorgang im Knochen im Vordergrund; er ist gekennzeichnet durch das *Nebeneinander von Zerstörung und Wiederaufbau*. In den mittleren Wachstumsjahren erfolgt die Knochenzerstörung häufig mit einem großen Schlage; eine ganze Diaphyse stirbt ab und wird aus dem lebendigen Zusammenhang gelöst. Dann aber entspricht der Zerstörung auch die Großartigkeit der Regeneration. Nicht die Ausnahme, sondern *die Regel ist es,* daß ein ganzer Radius (Serie 4), eine ganze Tibia (Serie 1 u. 2) oder der lange Femur (Serie 3) ganz oder fast *vollwertig wiederhergestellt werden.* Ist der betroffene Bezirk im Knochen kleiner — vielleicht infolge einer abgeschwächten Infektion, besonderer Lokalisation und öfter um das Ende des Wachstumsalters — so gehen Zerstörung und Ersatz noch mehr ineinander über. Der Umbau ist dann eine Auflösung des Knochengewebes ohne nennenswerte Sequesterbildung und ein schrittweiser Ersatz. Wir sehen einen solchen Ablauf bei der Osteomyelitis der Wirbelsäule (Serie 7) und auch an den langen Extremitätenknochen, bei denen auch wieder die geschlossene Röhre gebildet wird. Wie das Ausmaß und das Tempo der Zerstörung sein mag, auf alle Fälle dürfen wir mit einer großen Regenerationskraft rechnen. So geschah bei der 26jährigen Frau (Serie 8) schließlich doch die Wiederherstellung des Röhrenknochens. Oft möchte man als Gutachter nach Jahren gar nicht die schwere Zerstörung annehmen, weil der Wiederaufbau in großartiger Weise erfolgt ist. Nicht so günstig ist die Prognose der *Komplikationen. Hier herrscht die Defektheilung vor.* Zwar reicht die eitrige Entzündung oft bis hart an eine oder beide Wachstumsfugen heran, so daß man ihre Schädigung befürchten muß; doch nehmen sie gewöhnlich keinen Schaden. Auch eine leichtere Alteration, wie sie in Serie 4 besteht, braucht keine Hemmung des Längenwachstums zur Folge zu haben. Kommt es aber zu einer Epiphysenlösung (Serie 11), so ist der angerichtete Schaden unwiederbringlich. Ebenso zu werten ist ein Übergreifen des Prozesses auf benachbarte Gelenke. Entsprechend ihrer Heftigkeit führt die Entzündung leicht zu einer Zerstörung des Knorpelüberzuges und zu einer knöchernen Verwachsung der Gelenkenden, wie das am Ellenbogen (Serie 10) und am Knie (Serie 8) geschehen ist. Dagegen ist die Dehnungsverrenkung durch einen einfachen sympathischen Erguß prognostisch günstig; nach der Einrichtung ist eine Restitutio ad integrum zu erwarten (Serie 9).

Grundsätzlich das Gleiche wie bei der hämatogenen Osteomyelitis gilt prognostisch für die dentale (Serie 14—16) und die traumatische (Serie 17 u. 18); der betroffene Bezirk wird zerstört und erneuert, nur ist er gewöhnlich umschriebener. Auch hier bedingen Komplikationen an der Wachstumsfuge und an den Gelenken Defektheilungen.

Chapter I.

Acute Inflammation of Bones and Joints.

A. Haematogenous, Dental and Traumatic Osteomyelitis.

Pyogenic inflammation of bones is a serious condition, because it is a metastasis of a septic general infection which is a menace to life. The affection destroys the firm bony tissue, but at the same time it incites regeneration. Once the danger to life has passed, the local bone process is of prime importance and is characterised by destruction and reconstruction occurring side by side. As a rule, bone destruction usually takes place about the middle of the growing years. An entire diaphysis dies and separates from the living whole, but then the wonderful regenerative process keeps pace with the destruction. It is the rule rather than the exception, that an entire radius (Series 4), an entire tibia (Series 1 and 2) or the long femur (Series 3) are almost, or entirely, completely reconstructed. If there is a special localisation, or if the affected area in the bone is small (possibly caused by a debilitating infection and usually occurring towards the end of the growth period), destruction and restoration will go still more hand in hand. The reconstruction is then rather a dissolving of the bone tissue without any sequestrum formation worth mentioning and a gradual step by step substitution. We see just such a process in the osteomyelitis of the spine (Series 7) and also in the long bones of the extremities, in which the closed tubes were again reconstructed. Whatever may be the extent and speed of destruction, we can rely on the regenerative faculty. In the case of the 26 year old woman (Series 8), the hollow bone was finally reconstructed in this way. It often happens that even an expert cannot judge the severity of the previous disturbance after a considerable lapse of time, because the reconstruction has been so complete.

The prognosis of complications is not so favourable, because in most cases defective healing results. Although septic inflammation often reaches very close to one or both epiphyses, thus causing grave anxiety, it is only rarely that they are injured. A slight change, such as may be seen in Series 4, is also not necessarily detrimental to growth. If however, it progresses as far as the loosening of an epiphysis (Series 11), then the injury is irreparable. The same may be said of an involvement of the neighbouring joints. Corresponding to the severity, the inflammation easily leads to destruction of the cartilage covering and a bony union of the joint ends, results. This may be seen in the elbow (Series 10) and in the knee (Series 8). On the other hand, the prognosis of an expansion sprain caused by a simple sympathetic effusion is favourable and complete recovery may be expected after setting (Series 9).

The prognosis of dental (Series 14—16) and traumatic (Series 17 and 18) osteomyelitis is fundamentally identical with that of haematogenous osteomyelitis. The area attacked is destroyed and then renewed. Generally speaking however, it is more circumscribed. Here also complications at the epiphysis or joint involvement will result in defective healing.

Serie 1.
Osteomyelitis der Tibia.

Die Krankheit des 8 jährigen Knaben begann hochfieberhaft und verlief längere Zeit septisch. Am 4. Tage wurde
eine ausgedehnte Markphlegmone der Tibia breit aufgemeißelt (im Eiter: hämolytische Staphylokokken), in
der 5. Woche ein großer Sequester entfernt und mehrfach
Weichteilabscesse incidiert. Ohne stärkere Totenlade
bildete sich aus dem Inneren heraus das Regenerat.

Series 1.
Osteomyelitis of the tibia.

An eight years old boy's illness began with high fever and
ran a protracted septic course. On the fourth day, an
extensive marrow-phlegmon was chiselled open (in pus:
haemolyt. staphylococci). In the fifth week a large sequestrum was removed and several abscesses in the soft
parts were opened. Regeneration took place from the
inside without any great periosteal growth.

$^6/_{10}$ n. Gr.   1.   2.   3.

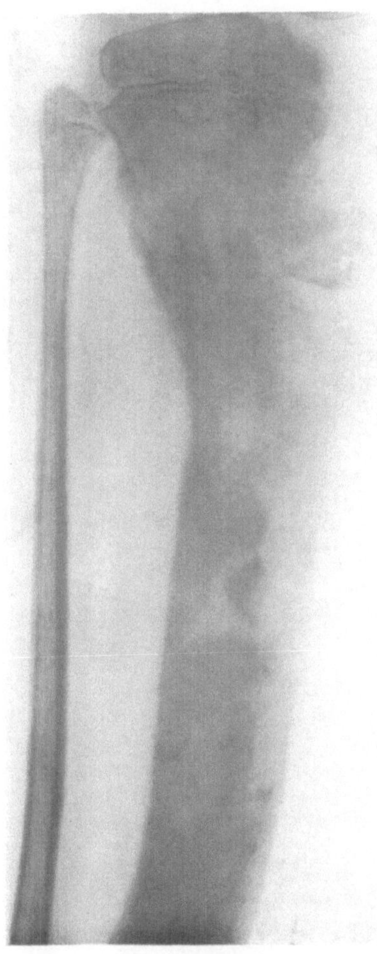

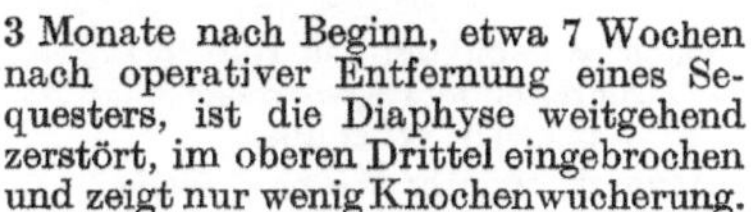

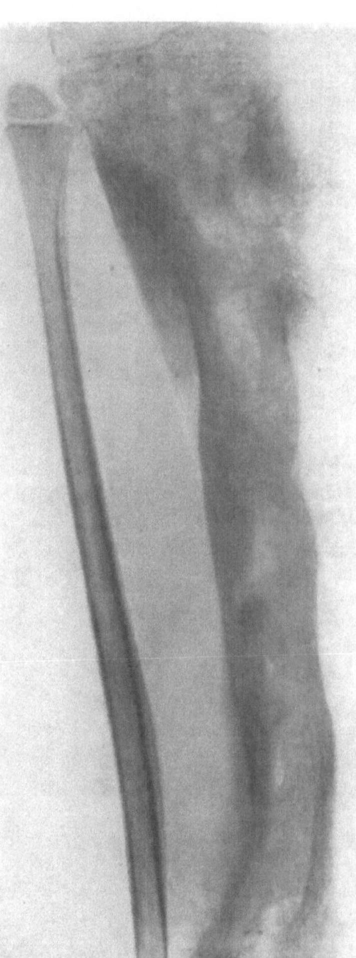

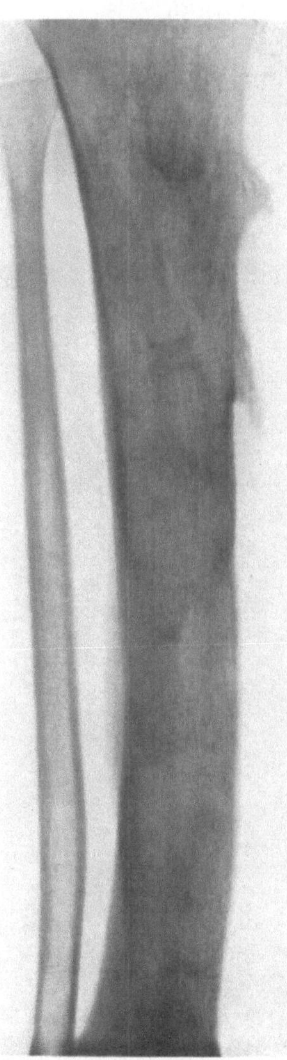

3 Monate nach Beginn, etwa 7 Wochen
nach operativer Entfernung eines Sequesters, ist die Diaphyse weitgehend
zerstört, im oberen Drittel eingebrochen
und zeigt nur wenig Knochenwucherung.

Three months after commencement,
about seven weeks after the removal of
sequestrum by operation, the diaphysis
is extensively destroyed, the upper third
fallen in and showing very little bone
growth.

Nach 4$^1/_2$ Monaten ist der Knochenschaft
zwar noch mehrfach durchlöchert, läßt
aber schon Rindenschicht und Markraum hervortreten.

After four months and a half the bone-
shaft shows several holes but the cortex
and marrow space are prominent.

Nach 3 Jahren ist ein kräftiger
Knochen gebildet, der normales
Längenwachstum zeigt und nur an
kleinen Unregelmäßigkeiten der
Umrisse bzw. der inneren Struktur
den überstandenen schweren
Krankheitsprozeß vermuten läßt.

After three years a strong bone has formed. The longitudinal growth
is normal and only by slight irregularities of the outlines and of
the interior structure can the severity of the past illness be imagined.

Serie 2.

Osteomyelitis der Tibia.

Bei dem 8jährigen Knaben entstand unter stürmischen Erscheinungen die Knochenmarkentzündung des Schienbeins. Unter konservativen Maßnahmen kam es zum spontanen Eiterdurchbruch und zum Absterben fast der ganzen Diaphyse. Nach 8 Wochen wurde der eingebrochene große Sequester entfernt (Eiter: Staph. pyog. aureus); wenige Monate später war die Tibia wieder aufgebaut und entfaltete von da ab auch ein normales Längenwachstum.

Series 2.

Osteomyelitis of the Tibia.

An eight year old boy became ill with violent symtoms of bone-marrow inflammation of the tibia. Conservative measures were taken, resulting in spontaneous discharge of pus and in decay of almost the entire diaphysis. Eight weeks later the large sequestrum was removed (pus: staph. pyog. aureus). A few months later the tibia was again renewed and from that time longitudinal growth was normal.

$^6/_{10}$ n. Gr.   1.   2.   3.

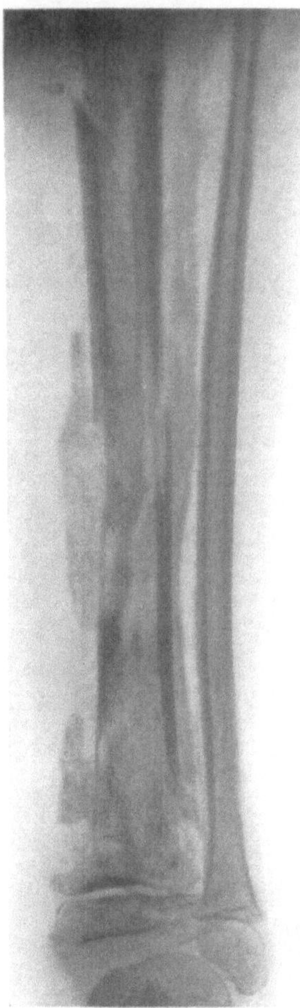 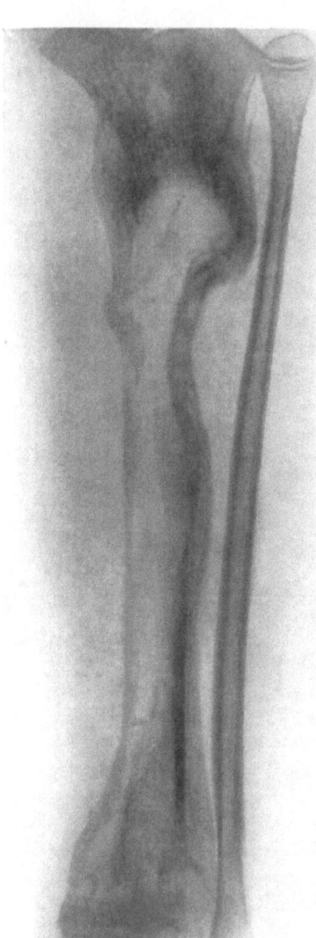 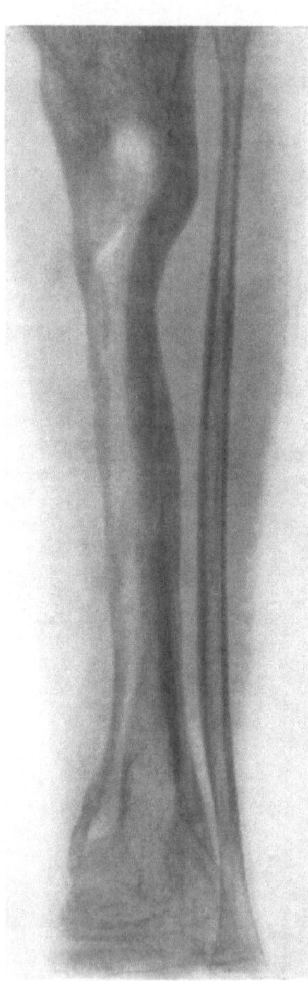

8 Wochen nach Beginn besteht eine ausgedehnte Zerstörung mit Fraktur und Sequestrierung nahezu des ganzen Schienbeins; Totenladenbildung ist deutlich im Gang.

Eigth weeks after commencement: Extensive destruction with fracture and beginning sequestration of almost the entire tibia. Formation of "coffin" distinctly taking place.

Nach 5 Monaten, nachdem der große Sequester vor 10 Wochen entfernt ist, hat die Bildung des neuen Knochenschaftes begonnen.

After five months. The large sequestrum had been removed ten weeks before and the rebuilding of the bone-shaft has begun.

Nach 6 Monaten ist die fortschreitende Regeneration deutlich erkennbar.

After six months the progressive regeneration is plainly recognizable.

Serie 2.

4.

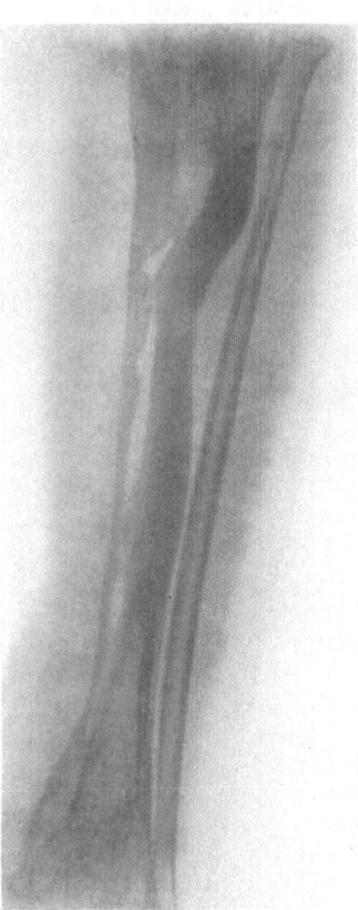

Nach 8 Monaten hat die Knochenbildung weiter zugenommen, so daß der
Kranke im Gipsverband gehfähig ist.

After eight months the bone formation
has increased to such an extent that
the patient can walk with a plaster
of Paris bandage.

Nach 4 Jahren ist die Tibia normal
gebildet, abgesehen von einer kleinen
Unregelmäßigkeit fein struktuiert und
hat ein unvermindertes Längenwachstum
entfaltet.

After four years the tibia has become
normal and delicately structured with
the exception of a slight irregularity;
the longitudinal growth was unimpaired.

5.

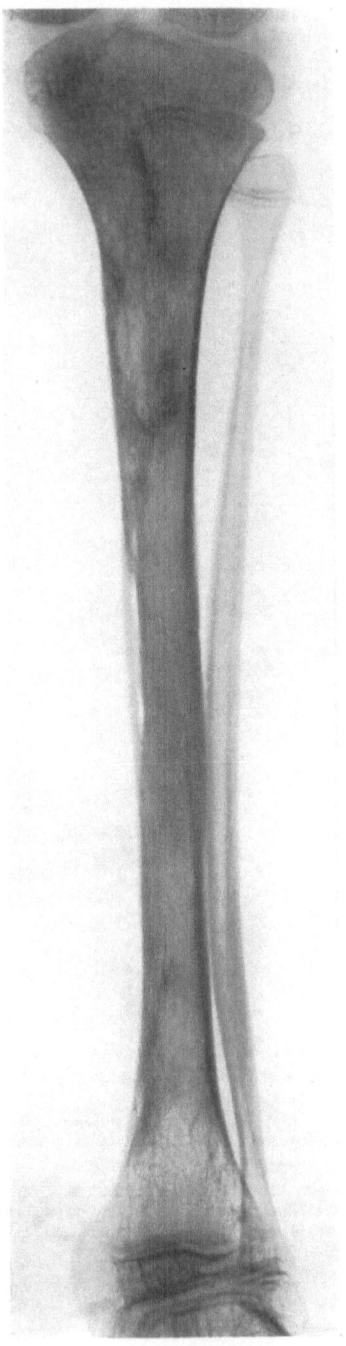

Serie 3.

Osteomyelitis des Femur.

Als der 12jährige Knabe hochakut erkrankte, wurde die Markphlegmone des Femur sofort aufgemeißelt (Eiter: Staph. pyogen. aureus). Die Krankheit hatte einen längeren septischen Verlauf, führte zur Bildung eines nahezu totalen Sequesters, der nach 5 Monaten operativ entfernt wurde, und heilte mit einem wachstumsfähigen Regenerat.

$^{1}/_{2}$ n. Gr.   1.

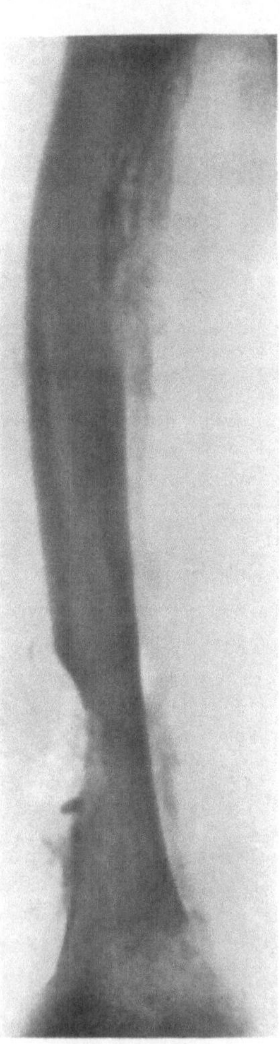

3 Wochen nach Beginn zeigt der angemeißelte Knochen vor allem in der oberen Hälfte Auflösung und periostale Wucherung.

Three weeks after commencement the chiselled bone has loosened, principally in the upper half and there is abundance of periosteal growth.

Series 3.

Osteomyelitis of the Femur.

A twelve year old boy became very ill and the marrow-phlegmon was immediately chiselled open (pus: staph. pyogen. aureus). The illness was of long septic duration and led to the formation of what was almost a total sequestrum. This was removed five months later by operation. Regeneration with growth-ability followed.

2.

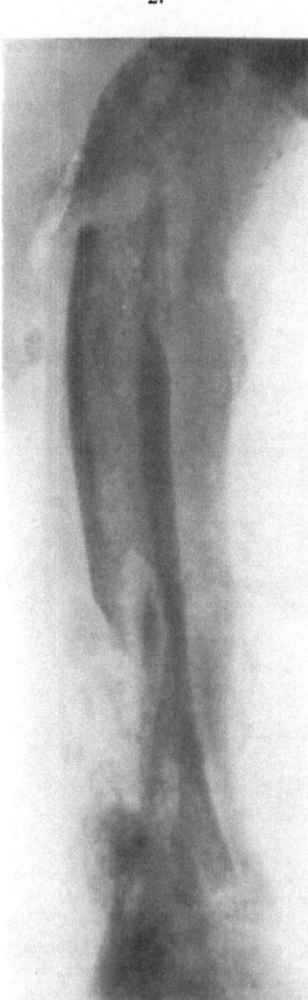

Nach 3 Monaten ist die Totenladenbildung deutlich im Gang und der größte Teil des Schaftes als Sequester gelöst.

After three months the shaping of the "coffin" is clearly taking place and the largest part of the shaft is sequestrated and loosened.

Serie 3.

3.

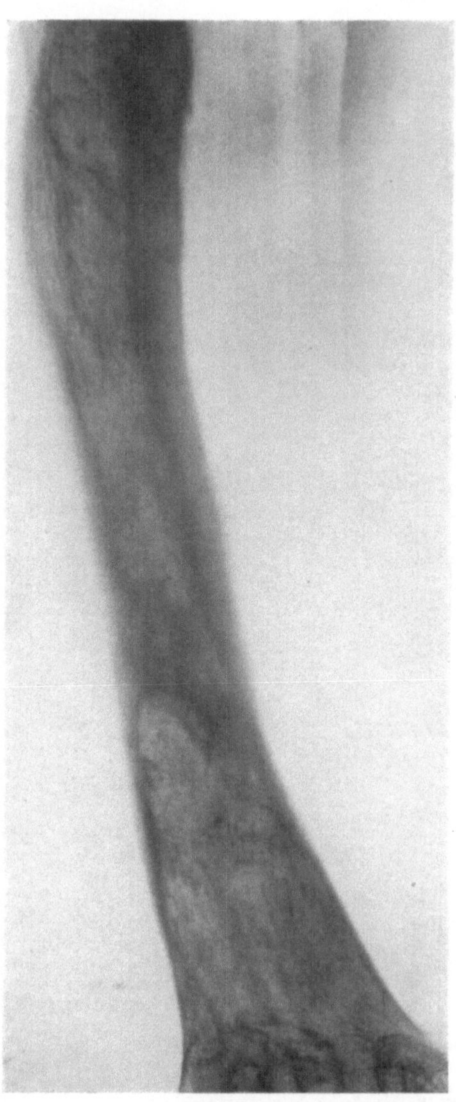

12 Jahre später ist der Femur ein massiver Knochen, hat aber eine regelmäßige Strukturzeichnung
nicht erreicht.
Twelve years later. The femur is now a massive bone but has not attained a regular structure.

Serie 4.

Osteomyelitis des Radius.

Der 3jährige Knabe erkrankte im direkten Anschluß an Masern mit einer sehr schmerzhaften Anschwellung des Unterarmes. 14 Tage später geschah die Absceß- incision (in dem Eiter: Staph. pyogen. aureus), wobei man auf rauhen Knochen stieß. Es bildete sich ein Totalsequester des betroffenen Radius, nach dessen operativer Entfernung eine vollwertige Regeneration des Röhrenknochens zustande kam.

Series 4.

Osteomyelitis of the Radius.

A three year old boy had just recovered from measles when he had a very painful swelling of the forearm. The abscess was incised a fortnight later and the bone was discovered to be rough. A total sequestrum of the affected radius was formed, and after removal by operation, the hollow-bone was absolutely regenerated.
(In pus: Staph. pyogen. aureus.)

²/₃ n. Gr. 1.   2.   3.

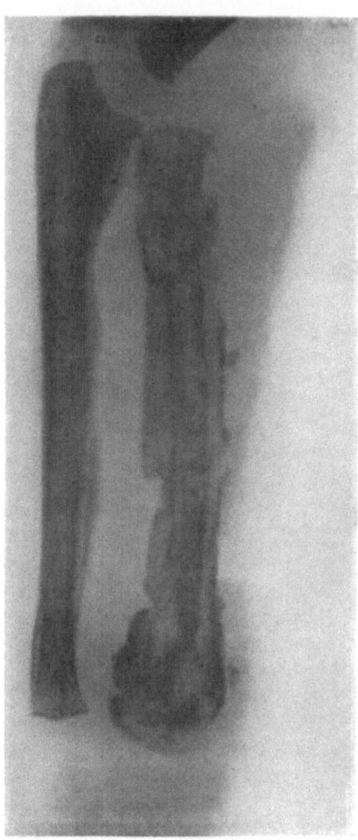 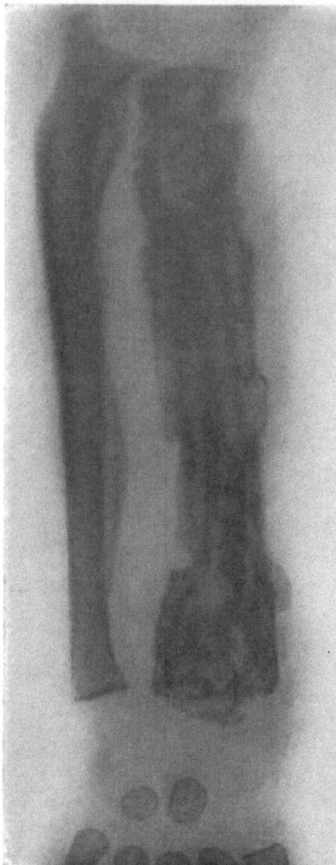 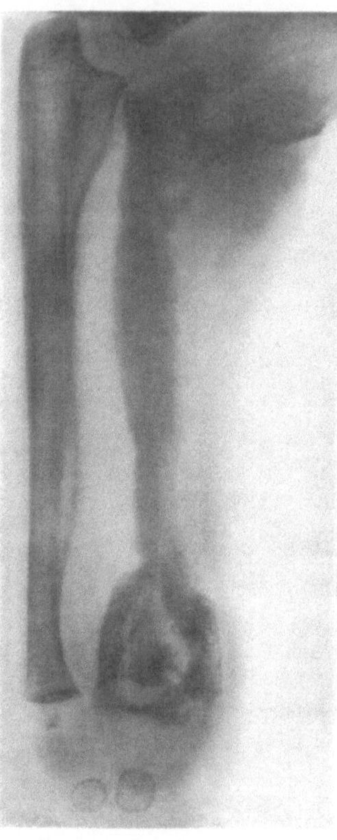

6 Wochen nach Beginn, 4 Wochen nach der Absceßincision ist der Radius in ganzer Länge abgestorben und bereits von einer ausgiebigen Totenlade umgeben.

Six weeks after commencement and four weeks after incision of abscess. The radius throughout its entire length has died and is already surrounded by an ample "coffin".

Nach 10 Wochen hat die regeneratorische Periostwucherung noch zugenommen.

After ten weeks. There has been abundant increase of periosteal growth.

Nach 18 Wochen — 20 Tage nach der Entfernung des Totalsequesters — hat die einstige Totenlade bereits die Form eines Knochenschaftes angenommen. (Der kleine Sequester hat sich später ausgestoßen.)

After eighteen weeks. Twenty days after the removal of total sequestrum by operation, the former "coffin" has already taken on the shape of the bone-shaft. (The small sequestrum was expelled later.)

Serie 4.

4.

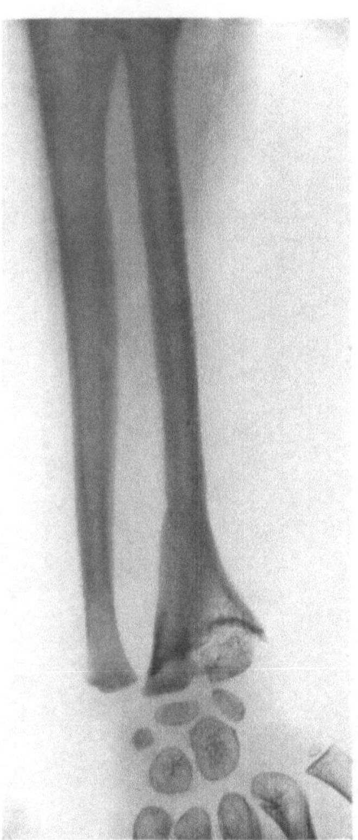

Nach 2 Jahren ist — abgesehen
von einer Unregelmäßigkeit an der
distalen Wachstumsfuge — ein
regelmäßiger Röhrenknochen
regeneriert.

After two years. With the exception of a slight irregularity at the
distal epiphysis, a normal hollow
bone has been formed.

5.

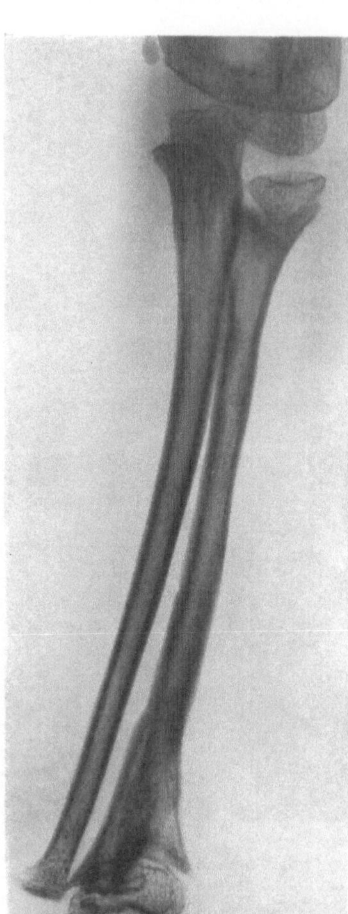

Nach 6 Jahren ist dieser Radius in
dem gleichen Maße wie der der anderen
Seite gewachsen.

After six years. The growth of this
radius has kept pace with that of the
other side.

Serie 5.

Osteomyelitis des Femur.

Das 8jährige Mädchen erkrankte im Anschluß an eine Lungenentzündung an einer metastatischen umschriebenen Markphlegmone des Femur. Nach der Aufmeißelung am 4. Tag (im Eiter: Pneumokokken) vollzog sich die langsame Reinigung des Krankheitsherdes unter ·Ausstoßung mehrerer kleiner Sequester, während gleichzeitig eine gute regenerative Knochenwucherung vor sich ging. Nach etwa 1¹/₂ Jahren hatte der Knochen nahezu wieder normale Gestalt.
Die nahe Wachstumsfuge erfuhr keine Schädigung.

Series 5.

Osteomyelitis of the Femur.

An eight year old girl was affected with metastatic circumscribed marrow-phlegmon of the thigh following inflammation of the lungs. It was chiselled open on the fourth day (in pus: pneumococcus) and gradually the infected area became clean, several small sequestra being expelled. At the same time a good regeneration of bone took place. About a year and a half later the bone had almost regained its normal shape.
The neighbouring epiphysis was not injured.

1.   2.   3.

⁶/₁₀ n. Gr.

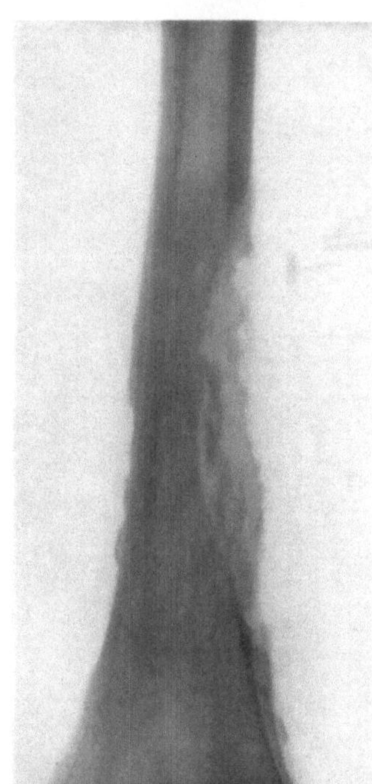 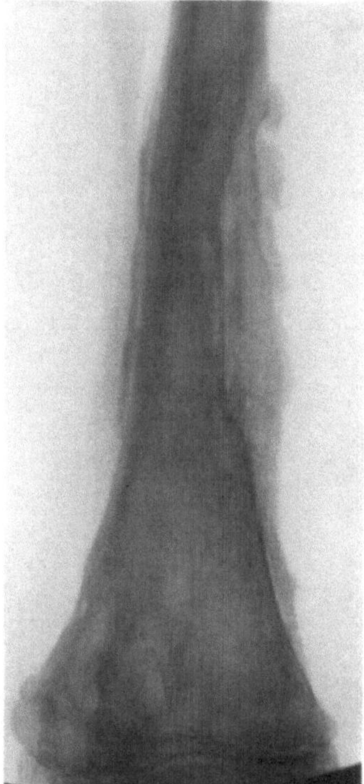 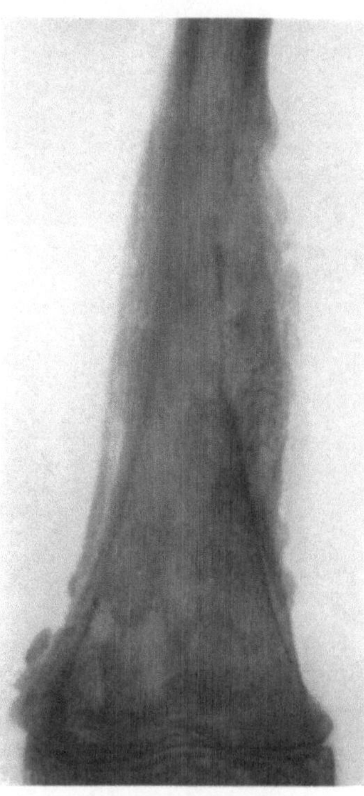

Nach 11 Wochen zeigt der angemeißelte Knochen kleine Sequester und deutliche Knochenneubildung.

After eleven weeks the chiselled bone shows small sequestra and distinct new bone formation.

Nach 19 Wochen.

After nineteen weeks.

Nach 24 Wochen.

After twenty-four weeks.

Mehr und mehr zunehmende Regeneration.

Continued increasing regeneration.

Serie 5.

4.

5.

6.

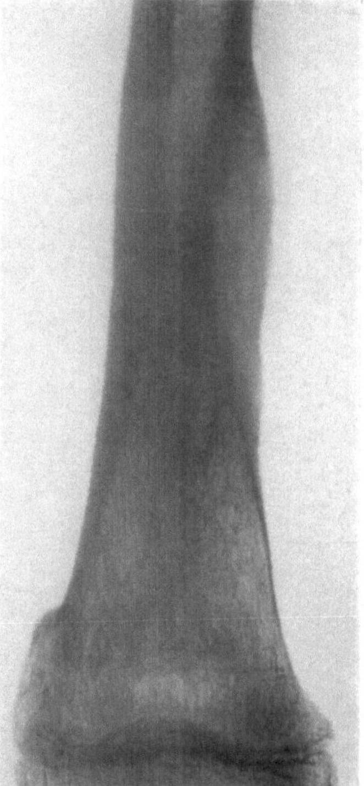

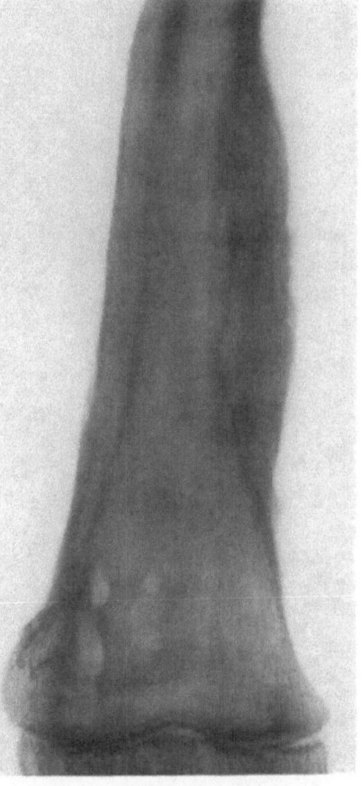

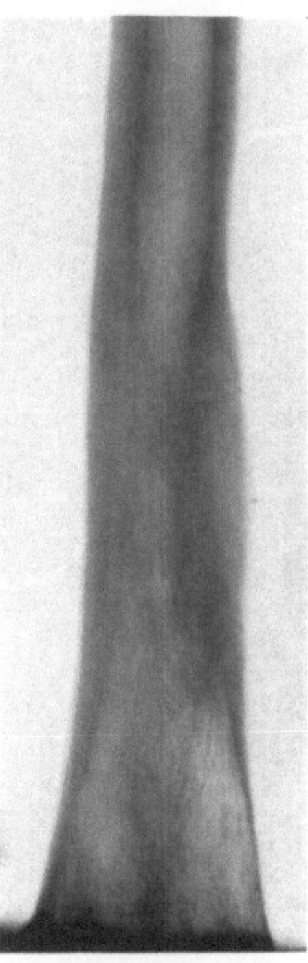

Nach 11 Monaten ist der Defekt
weitgehend ergänzt. Es ist noch ein
kleiner Sequester vorhanden,
der entfernt wird.

After eleven months, the defect is
considerably regenerated. A small
sequestrum was removed.

Nach 16 Monaten besteht sogar ein
Überschuß des Regenerates.

After sixteen months. There is even a
superfluity of regenerating material.

Nach 19 Monaten ist der
Wulst zurückgebildet, so-
daß eine fast gleichmäßige
Form des Knochens
erreicht ist.

After nineteen months.
The thickness has decrea-
sed and an almost regular
shape of the bone has been
attained.

Serie 6.

Osteomyelitis des Femur.

Als der 15 jährige Knabe hochfieberhaft erkrankt war, wurde die umschriebene Markphlegmone im oberen Drittel des Femur am 4. Krankheitstag aufgemeißelt. In dem Eiter fanden sich hämolytische Staphylokokken. Unter wochenlang anhaltendem hohen Fieber und erheblicher Eiterung geschah die zunehmende Reinigung und der Umbau des Knochens, ohne daß auch nur ein etwas größerer Sequester ausgestoßen wurde.

Series 6.

Osteomyelitis of the Femur.

A boy of fifteen became ill with high fever. Four days .later the circumscribed marrow-phlegmon in the upper third of the femur was chiselled open. Haemolytic staph. were found in the pus. The high fever lasted many weeks and the quantity of pus was considerable. The purification and rebuilding of the bone proceeded without the expulsion of any sequestra worth mentioning.

$^3/_7$ n. Gr.   1.   2.   3.

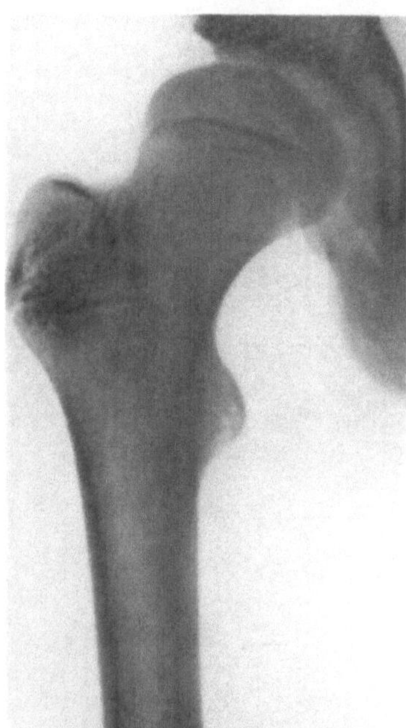 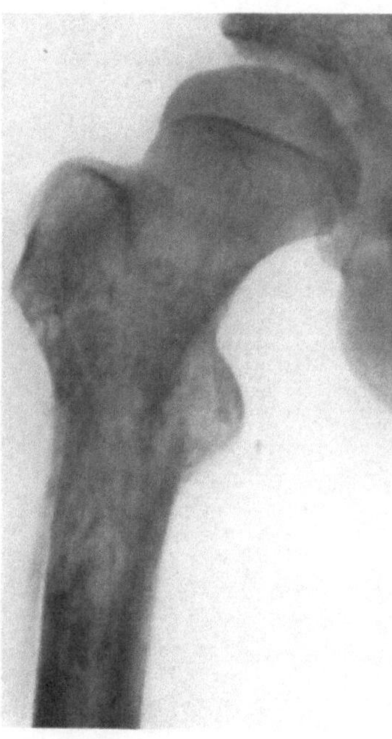 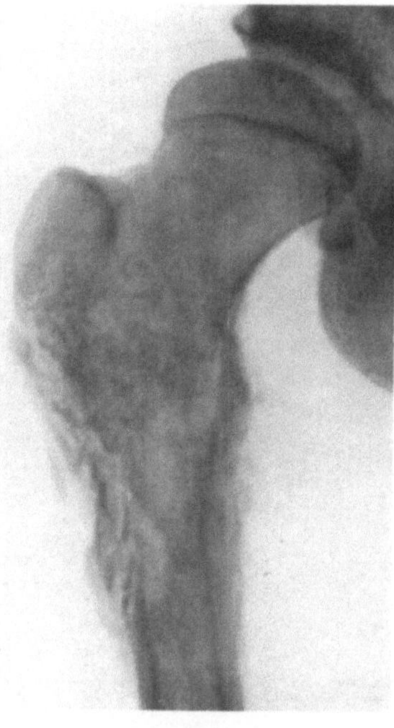

Am 4. Krankheitstag waren noch keine Knochenveränderungen erkennbar.

On the fourth day after commencement no bony changes could be seen.

4 Wochen später zeigt der angemeißelte Knochen einen Auflösungsprozeß und geringe Periostwucherung.

Four weeks later. The chiselled open bone shows a dissolving process and slight growth of periosteum.

Nach 8 Wochen überwiegt noch die Auflösung bzw. Resorption.

After eight weeks. The dissolving process predominates over the resorption.

Serie 6.

4.

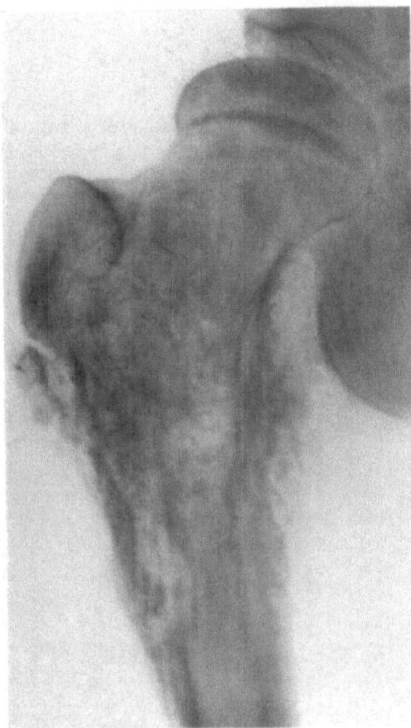

Ebenso nach 4 Monaten überwiegt
noch die Auflösung bzw. Resorption.

After four months.

5.

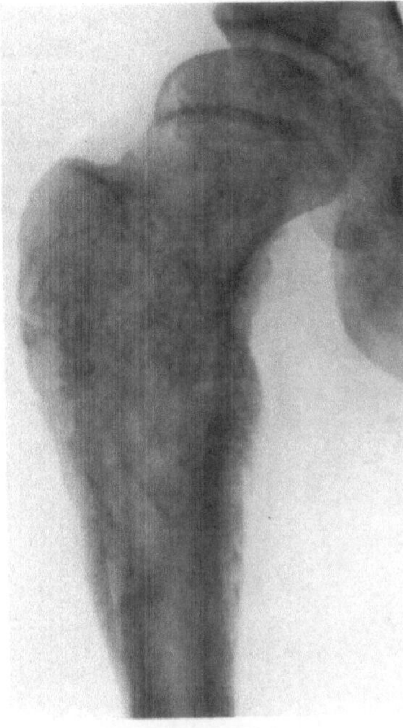

Nach 5½ Monaten
nimmt die Apposition zu.

After five months and a half.
Predominence of bone apposition.

6.

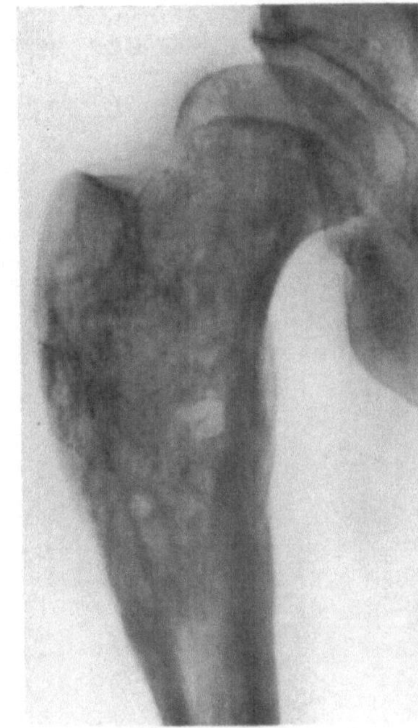

Nach 10 Monaten

After ten months the same.

7.

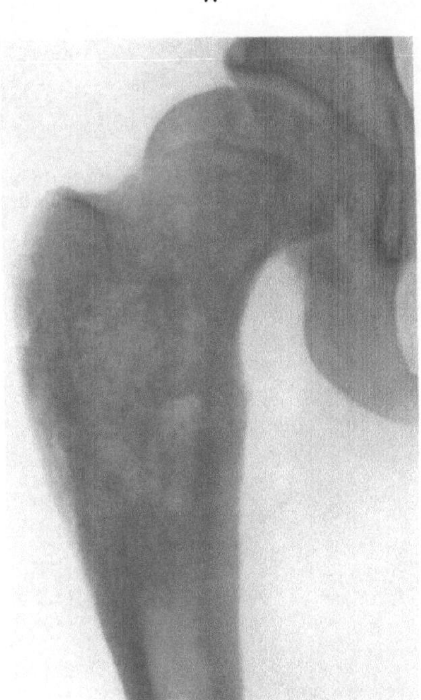

Nach 1 Jahr ist die Wiederherstellung weitgehend,
aber noch nicht ganz erfolgt; Rindenschicht und
Markraum treten wieder hervor.

After one year. Regeneration has advanced but is
not quite completed. Cortex and marrow-space are
again to be seen.

Serie 7.

Osteomyelitis der Wirbelsäule.

Im Verlaufe einer schweren Allgemeininfektion durch den (im Blut nachgewiesenen) Staphylococcus pyogen. aureus entstand bei dem 13 jährigen Mädchen als erste Knochenmetastase die Osteomyelitis des 3. Lendenwirbels. Diese heilte unter konservativer Therapie, indem die eitrige Entzündung den Knochen zerstörte, aber noch während des Zerstörungsprozesses wieder aufbaute; dabei wurden die statisch schwachen Stellen abgestützt. Schon vor Ablauf eines Jahres war das Kind von seiten der Wirbelsäule beschwerdefrei.

Series 7.

Osteomyelitis of the Spine.

The first bony metastasis, which appeared during the course of a severe general infection occurred in the third lumbar vertebra. (Staph. pyog. aureus were found in the blood of the patient who was a thirteen year old girl.) This healed with conservative treatment. While the destructive process caused by the septic inflammation was progressing, it was being renewed and the weak statical parts supported. As far as the spine was concerned, the child was free from complaint in less than one year.

$^7/_{10}$ n. Gr.   1.   2.   3.

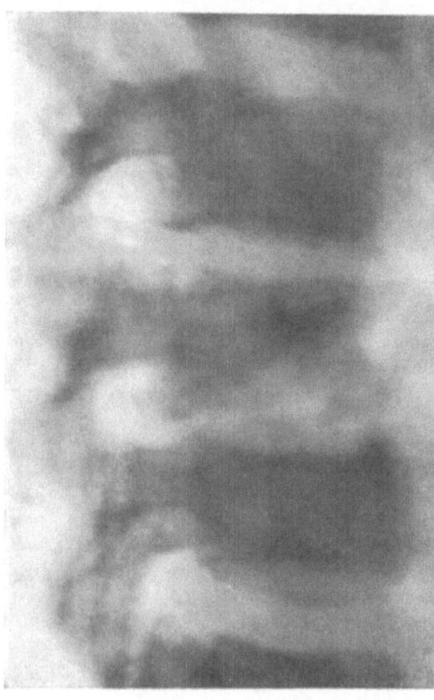 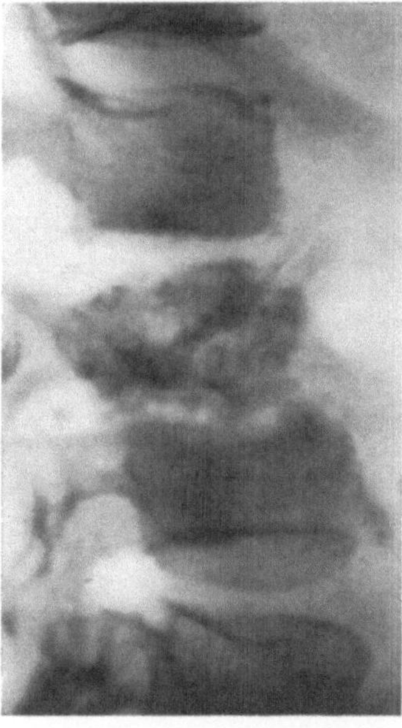 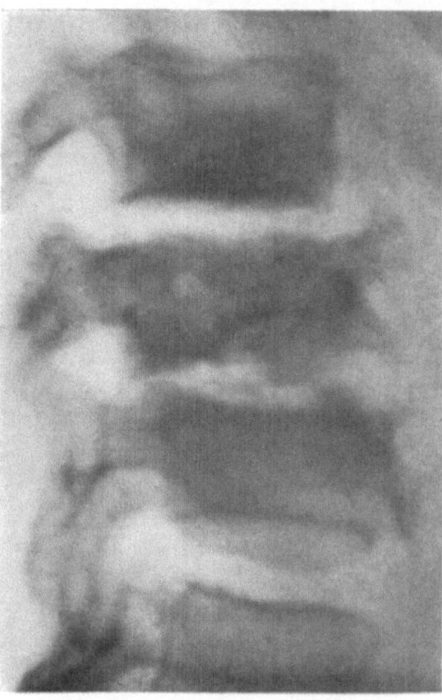

2 Monate nach Beginn ist der 3. Lendenwirbel fleckig gezeichnet und zum Teil unregelmäßig begrenzt.

Two months after commencement. The third lumbar vertebra has a speckled appearance and the outline in parts is irregular.

Nach 6 Monaten hat die Zerstörung den Höhepunkt erreicht: der Wirbel ist vollständig „zerfressen".

After six months, the destruction has reached its height, the vertebra is completely eroded.

Nach 9 Monaten ist der Wirbelkörper weitgehend wiederhergestellt.

After nine months, the vertebral body is to a great extent reconstructed.

Serie 7.

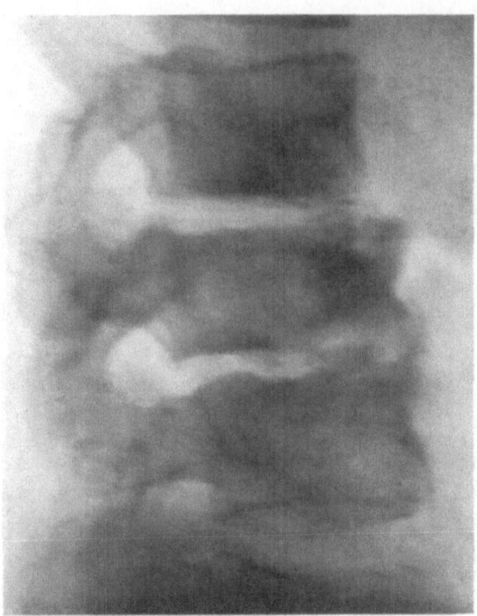

4.

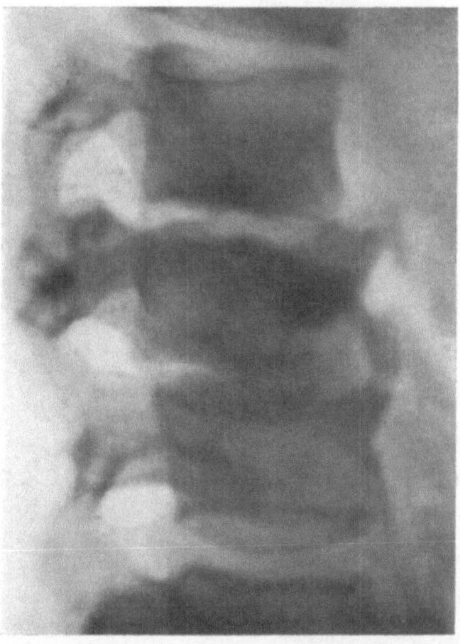

5.

Nach 2¹/₄ Jahren ist der Wirbelkörper zwar im Wachstum zurückgeblieben, ist aber zum größten Teil wieder gleichmäßig gebaut; nur die vordere Kante ist an den Ecken noch nicht ausgeglichen.

After two years and three months, although the growth of vertebral body is retarded, it is for the most part regular in outline. Only the front edge is not yet regular.

Nach 3 Jahren ist die Knochenstruktur noch dichter, die vordere untere Ecke durch eine feste Knochenspange abgestützt.

After three years, the bone-structure is more compact and the front lower corner is supported by a firm bridge of bone.

Serie 8.
Osteomyelitis des Femur.

Das bereits 26 jähriges Mädchen erkrankte 2 Monate nach einem septischen Abort schleichend an der Knochenmarkentzündung des Oberschenkels, dessen Erreger hämolytische Staphylokokken waren. Die Regeneration war erstaunlich schwach, so daß es noch nach Monaten zur Spontanfraktur des angemeißelten Knochens kam, die sehr langsam konsolidierte. Zudem griff die Entzündung auf das Kniegelenk über, was eine knöcherne Ankylose zur Folge hatte. Erst nach 1¹/₂ Jahren begann die Wiederherstellung des Röhrenknochens.

Series 8.
Osteomyelitis of the Femur.

A girl of twenty-six years had a septic abortion. Two months later she became ill with marrow inflammation of the femur, caused by haemolytic staphylococcus. Regeneration was astonishingly weak and months after the bone had been chiselled open, a spontaneours fracture occurred which consolidated very slowly. The inflamation spread to the knee-joint and caused bony ankylosis, the actual regeneration of the marrow-bone only beginning a year and a half later.

⁶/₁₀ n. Gr.   1.   2.   3.

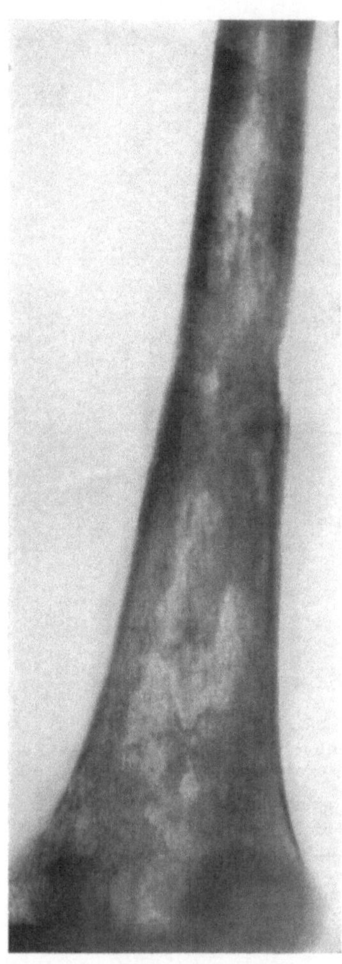 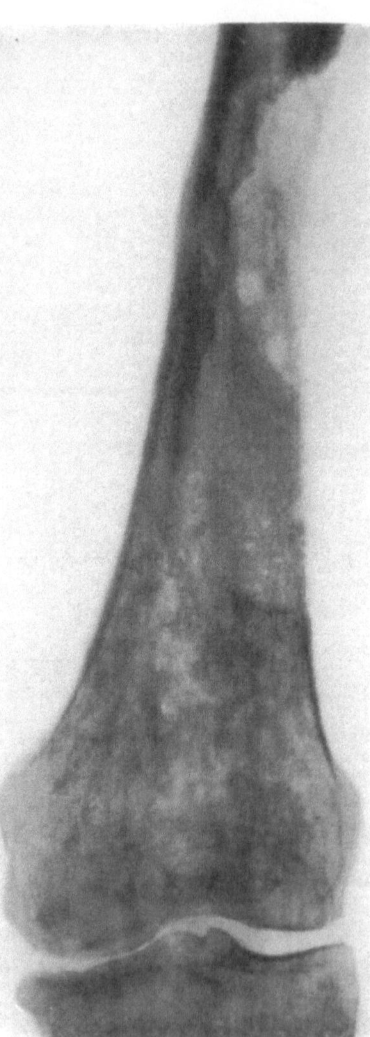 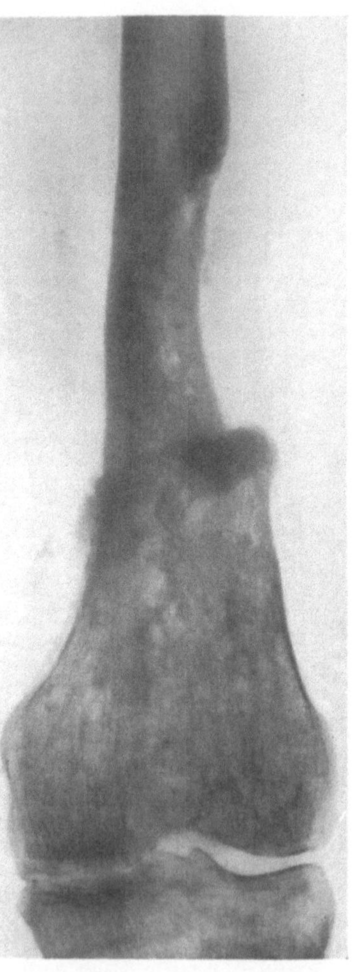

3 Monate nach Beginn ist der Femur in seinen unteren zwei Dritteln hochgradig zerfressen, ohne daß es zu einer reaktiven Knochenwucherung gekommen ist.

Three months after onset. The lower two thirds of femur are extensively eroded but there is no reactive bone growth.

Nach 5 Monaten — 5 Wochen nach der operativen Aufmeißelung — ist der Femur noch mehr kalkverarmt. Das versteifte Kniegelenk zeigt medial eine Verschmälerung des Gelenkspaltes.

After five months. Five weeks after the operation, the decalcification of femur has increased. The stiff knee-joint shows a decrease of the joint'-cleft on the medial side.

Nach 10 Monaten ist der Knochen wohl kalkreicher, aber die vor 10 Wochen entstandene Spontanfraktur zeigt noch keinen Callus. Die medialen Kniegelenkflächen sind usuriert und miteinander verwachsen.

After ten months. The bone is somewhat richer in chalk but the spontaneous fracture which had occurred ten weeks before, still shows no callus. The medial surfaces of the knee-joint are eroded and have united.

Serie 8.

4.   5.   6.

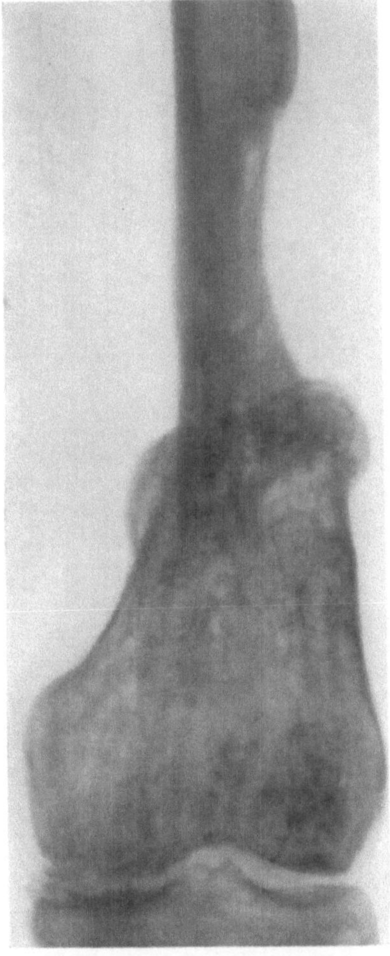 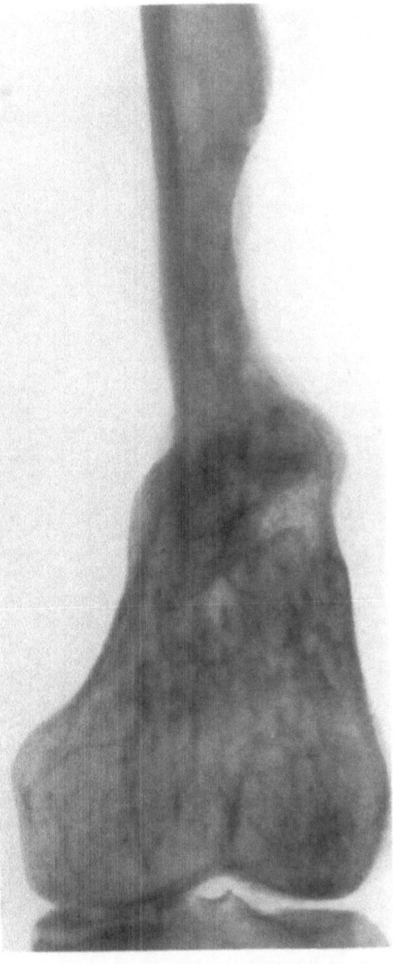 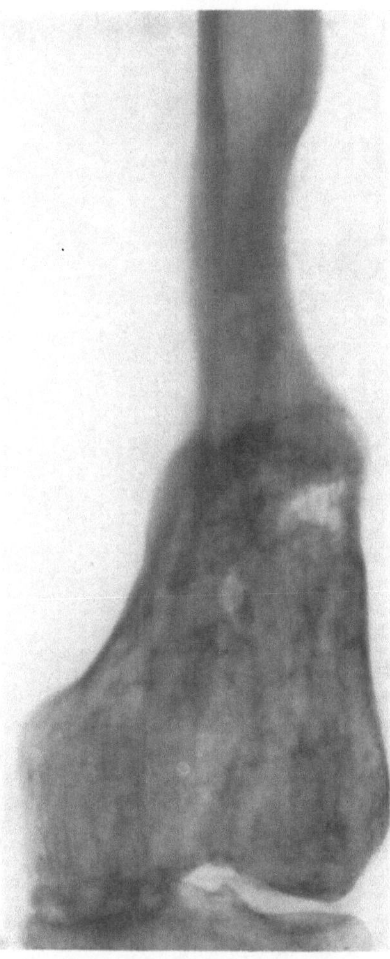

1 Jahr nach Krankheitsbeginn ist der Meißeldefekt etwas ausgeglichen und die Fraktur zeigt eine geringe Calluswucherung.

One year after commencement of disease. The chisel defect is more regular and there is a slight amount of callus at site of fracture.

Nach 16 Monaten ist der Knochen im ganzen etwas dichter.

After sixteen months. The bone in general is more compact.

Nach 19 Monaten ist die Frakturstelle etwas abgeflacht; im Bereich der Meißelstelle ist die Markhöhle geschlossen und eine kompakte Rindenschicht wird gebildet. Die knöcherne Verwachsung der medialen Knieseite ist noch dichter.

After nineteen months. The fractured part is more level, the marrow-cavity in the neighbourhood of the chiselled part has closed, and a thick cortex is forming. The bony growth of the medial side of the knee has become more dense.

Serie 9.

Osteomyelitis der Beckenschaufel.

Das 4 jährige Mädchen erkrankte unter septischen Erscheinungen an einer hämatogenen Osteomyelitis des Darmbeins, die im weiteren Verlauf mit Spontanluxation der Hüfte — infolge Gelenkergusses — kompliziert war. Operative Freilegung bzw. Aufmeißelung des Knochens und später unblutige Einrichtung der Hüfte führten in etwa $1^1/_2$ Jahren Ausheilung und völlige Wiederherstellung der Gelenkfunktion herbei; auch anatomisch geschah eine weitgehende Restitutio.

$^2/_8$ n. Gr.   1.

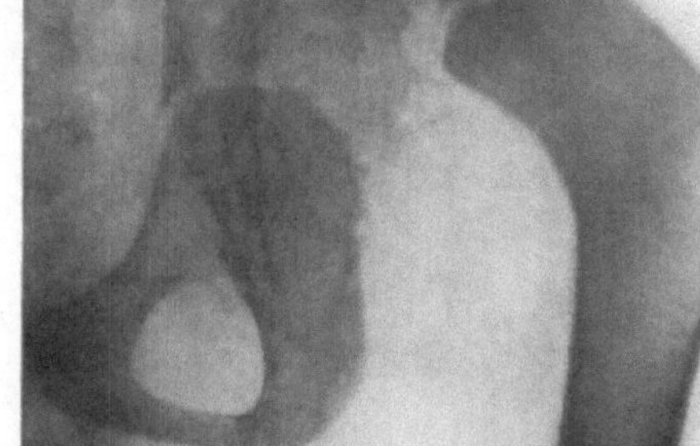

$^1/_4$ Jahr nach Beginn der Krankheit zeigt die Darmbeinschaufel neben dem Meißeldefekt reichliche periostale Wucherungen. Das Hüftgelenk ist ganz unscharf konturiert und der *Oberschenkelkopf ist aus der Pfanne getreten.*

Three months after commencement of illness. Beside the chisel defect, the hip-bone shows prolific periosteal growth. The outline of hip-joint is indistinct and the femoral head is outside the joint socket.

Series 9.

Osteomyelitis of the Ilium.

The four year old girl was attacked by haematogenous osteomyelitis of the ilium. It was later rendered more complicated by a spontaneous luxation of the hip caused by a joint effusion. The bone was chiselled open and later the hip was set bloodlessly. In about one and a half years, it had healed with entire restoration of the jointfunction. Extensive anatomical restitution.

2.

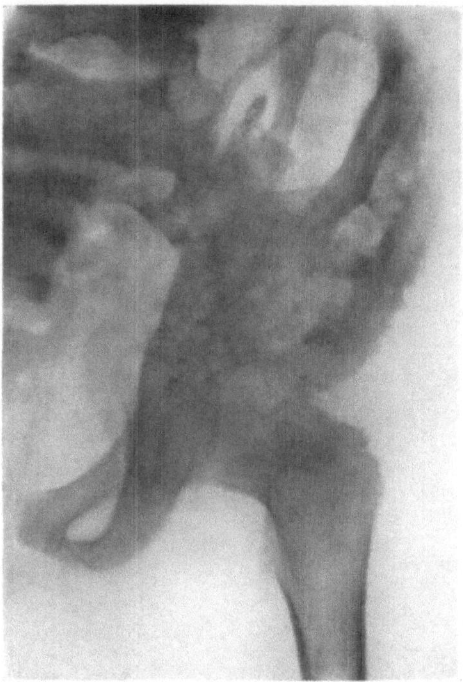

Nach $^1/_2$ Jahr ist die Luxation beseitigt; die Knochenbildung hat noch zugenommen.

After six months, the dislocation has been remedied and the bone growth is increasing.

Serie 9.

3.

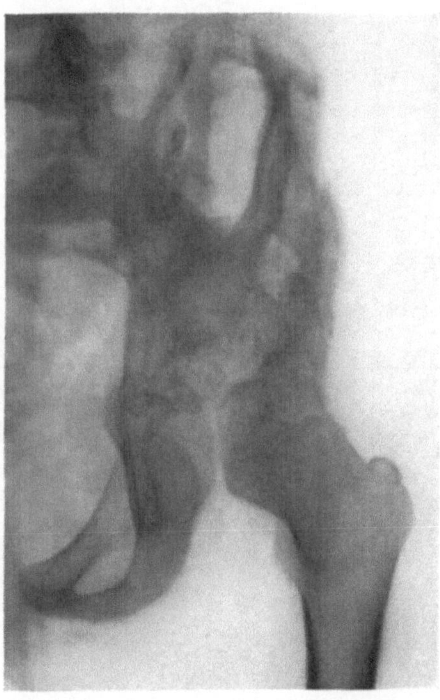

Nach 7 Monaten hat sich die frische Wucherung verdichtet und beginnt sich zu formen.

After seven months, the new growth has become more compact and is taking shape.

4.

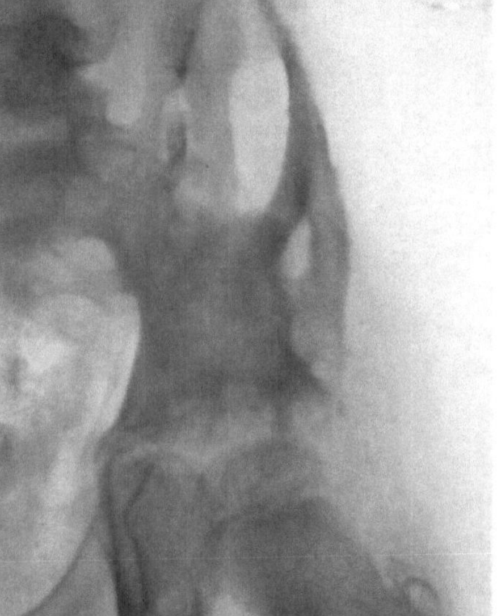

Nach 1¹/₂ Jahren ist die Struktur des regene-
rierten Darmbeins schon viel gleichmäßiger und
seine Form abgerundet. Das Hüftgelenk — besonders das Pfannendach — treten wieder deutlich konturiert hervor. (Nach 2¹/₂ Jahren war
der Knochenbefund im Röntgenbild nahezu
der gleiche.)

After one year and a half, the structure of the
regenerated ilium is more proportionate and
the shape rounded. The hip-joint, particularly
the acetabular roof shows distinct outlines again.
(After 2¹/₂ years when another X-ray picture was
taken, hardly any alteration had taken place.)

Serie 10.

Osteomyelitis des Humerus.

Bei dem 16jährigen Knaben trat die Osteomyelitis des Oberarmes schleichend in Erscheinung und heilte nach operativer Aufmeißelung sowie späterer Sequesterentfernung nur langsam. Vor allem aber trat als Komplikation die Zerstörung und Verwachsung des Ellenbogengelenkes ein.

Series 10.

Osteomyelitis of the Humerus.

The osteomyelitis commenced slowly in a boy of sixteen. The humerus had to be chiselled open and later a sequestrum was removed. Healing also took place very slowly and was complicated by destruction and ankylosis of elbow-joint.

$^6/_{10}$ n. Gr.　　　　1.　　　　　　　　　　2.　　　　　　　　　　3.

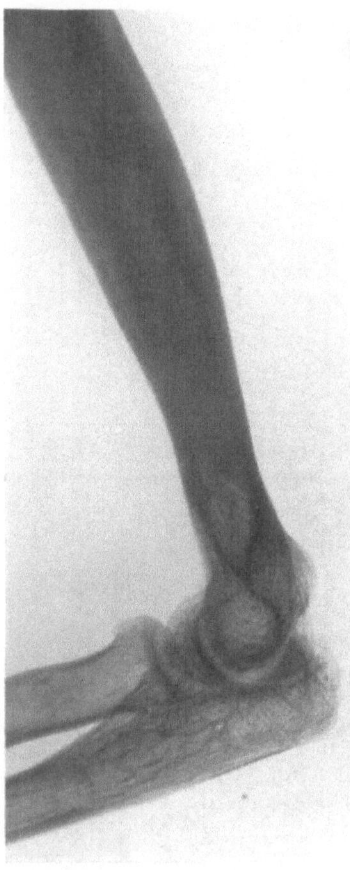

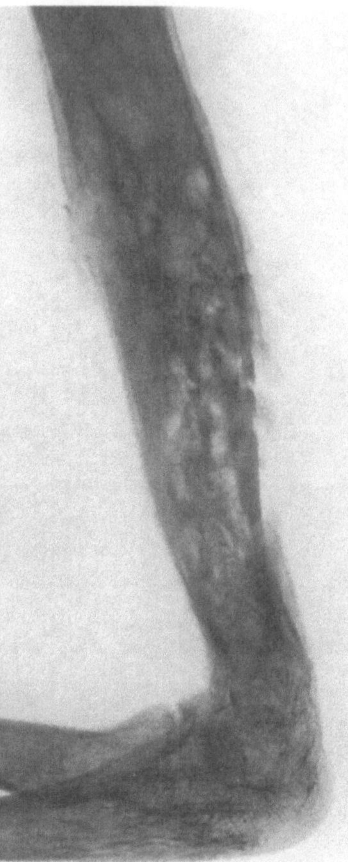

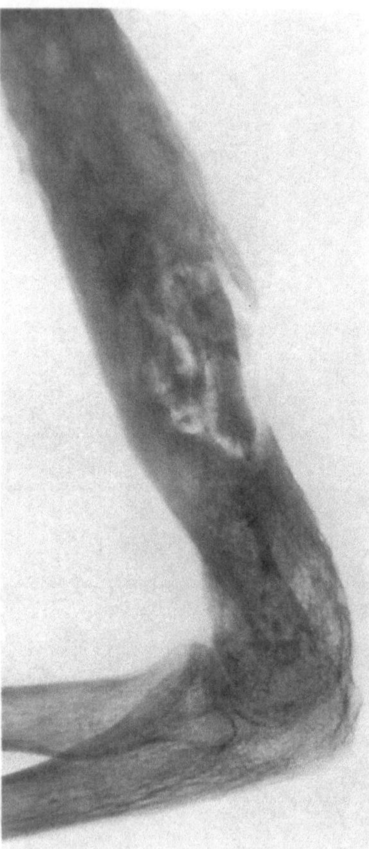

Nach etwa 4 Wochen ist der Humerus etwas aufgetrieben und läßt jede Strukturzeichnung vermissen.

After about four weeks the humerus is somewhat dilated and the structure is not visible.

Nach 4 Monaten — $^1/_4$ Jahr nach der Aufmeißelung — ist der Humerus allenthalben zernagt. Ein Sequester befindet sich in Lösung und geringe periostale Wucherungen haben sich gebildet. — Das Ellenbogengelenk läßt einen Gelenkspalt nicht erkennen.

After four months. Three months after the operation the humerus is eroded throughout. A sequestrum is about to become loosened and but very little periosteal-growth has formed. No joint cleft can be seen at the elbow-joint.

Nach einem halben Jahr ist der Sequester gelöst und der Knochen im Inneren stellenweise ergänzt.

After six months. The sequestrum is loosened and the bone interior is here and there renewed.

Serie 10.

4.

5.

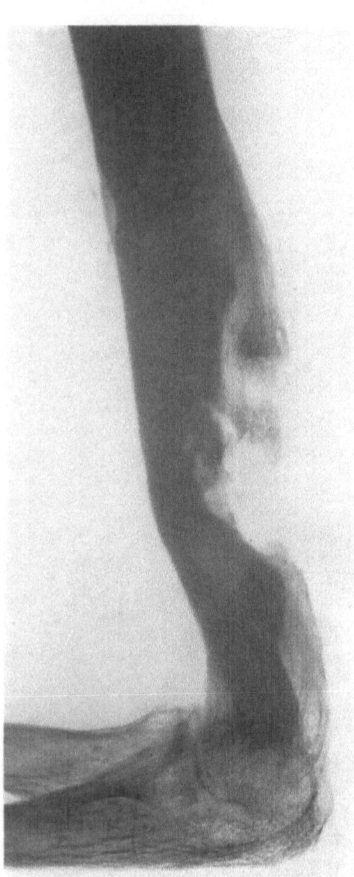

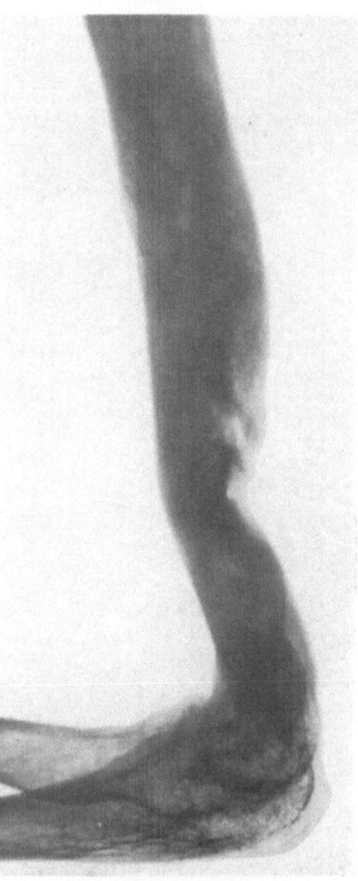

Nach 7 Monaten ist der größere Sequester entfernt und ein kleinerer liegt noch in der offenen und glatten Höhle. Der Knochen hat sich zunehmend verdichtet. Die Struktur des Ellenbogengelenkes zeigt die knöcherne Verwachsung.

After seven months. The larger sequestrum has been removed but a smaller one still lies in the smooth open hollow. The bone has become increasingly compact. The structure of the elbow-joint shows the bony growth.

Nach 10 Monaten ist eine weitere Regeneration des Defektes festzustellen.

After ten months. The further regeneration of the defect is confirmed.

Serie 11.

Osteomyelitis des Femur.

Die hämatogene Osteomyelitis des 7jährigen Knaben war in der proximalen Hälfte des Femur lokalisiert und kompliziert durch die Lösung der Schenkelkopfepiphyse. Der Femurstumpf fand eine Arretierung in der Gegend des oberen Pfannenrandes.

Series 11.

Osteomyelitis of the Femur.

A seven year old boy had a long septic illness. The haematogenous osteomyelitis affected the proximal half of femur and was complicated by the dissolving of the epiphysis of the femurhead. The femur stump was arrested in the neighbourhood of the upper acetabular edge.

$^6/_{10}$ n. Gr.　　　1.

2.

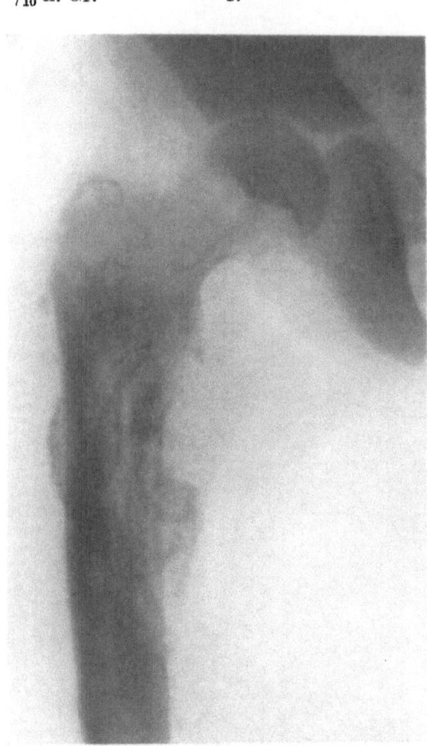

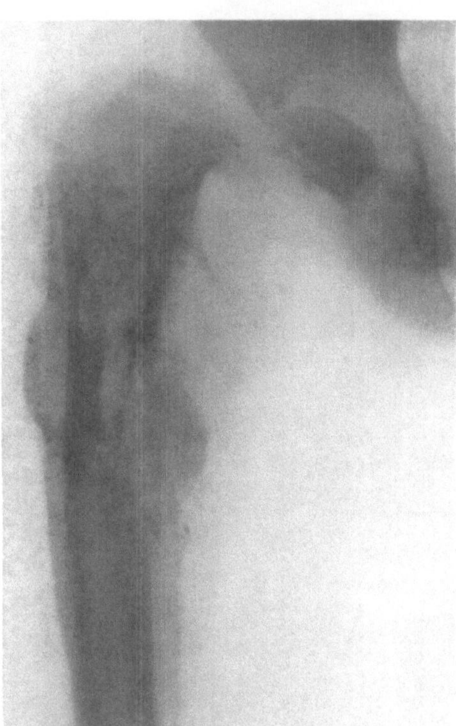

8 Wochen nach Beginn besteht eine ausgedehnte Knochenauflösung, welche auch in der Wachstumsfuge erkennbar ist außerdem reichliche periostale Wucherung.

Eight weeks after commencement. An extensive dissolving of bone is also recognizable in the epiphysis, in addition to which there is profuse periosteal growth.

Nach 15 Wochen ist der Schenkelkopf gelöst und der Femur hochgetreten. Die Knochenregeneration hat zugenommen.

After fifteen weeks. The femoral head has become loosened and the femur is drawn upwards. Bone regeneration has increased.

Serie 11.

3.

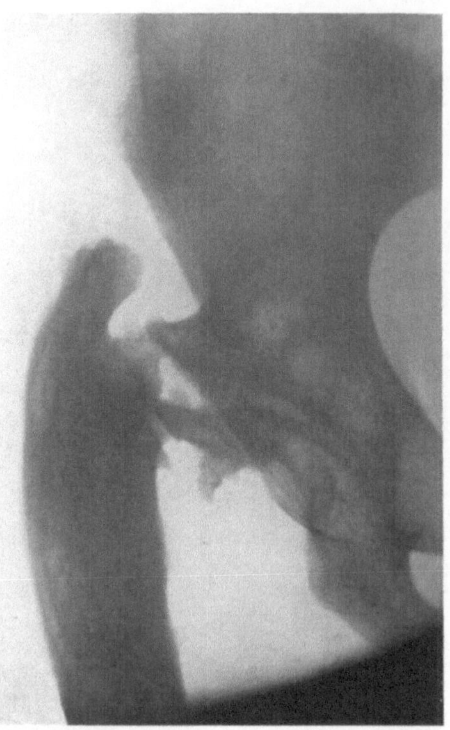

Nach 10 Jahren sind Reste des Schenkelkopfes in der flachen Pfanne noch erkennbar. Der Femurschaft ist solide wieder hergestellt und mit seinem zackigen oberen Ende im Pfannenrand verwachsen.

After ten years. The remains of the femur head are recognizable in the levelled acetabulum. The femur shaft has become solid again and the notched ends have united with the acetabular edge.

Serie 12.

Osteomyelitis des Humerus (Säugling).

Von der infizierten Nabelwunde kam es bei dem 14 Tage alten Säugling zu einer septischen Metastase in der oberen Metaphyse des Humerus und somit zur hämatogenen Osteomyelitis, hervorgerufen durch hämolytische Staphylokokken. Der Absceß wurde eröffnet, und der Prozeß heilte ab. Aber die Wachstumsfuge und die Kopfepiphyse waren ihm zum Opfer gefallen, noch bevor ihre Ossification begonnen hatte.

Series 12.

Osteomyelitis of the Humerus (Infant).

Through an infected umbilical wound, a baby, only fourteen days old, contracted a septic metastasis in the upper metaphysis of the humerus and consequently haematogenous osteomyelitis was caused by haemolytic staphylococci. The abscess was opened and the process healed, but the epiphyseal line and head epiphysis were sacrificed before their ossification had commenced.

$^9/_{10}$ n. Gr.   1.   2.   3.

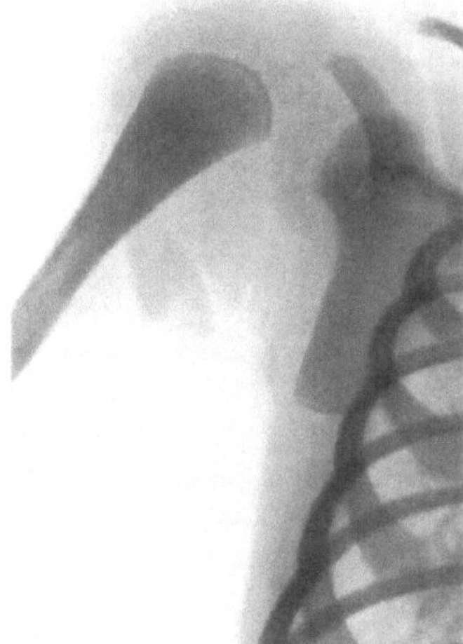 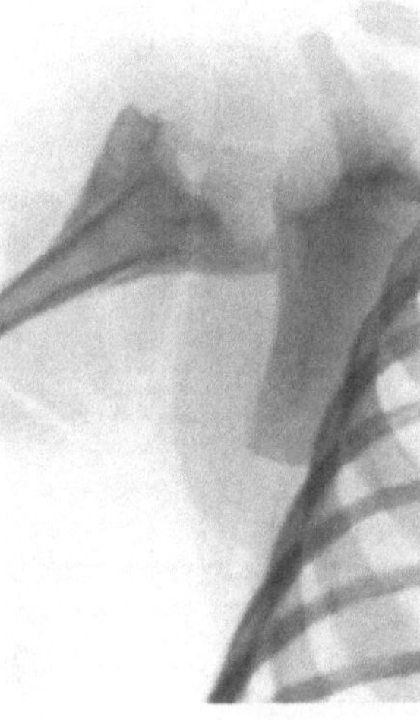 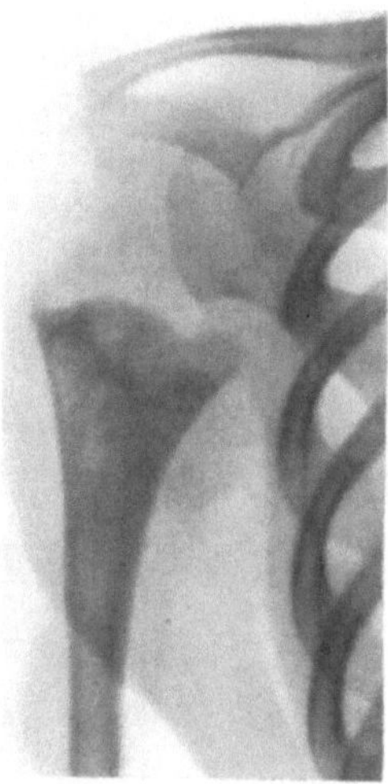

Lebensalter: 14 Tage.
Ein aufgehellter Streifen der Metaphyse verrät die beginnende Zerstörung.

Fourteen days old. A light stripe in the metaphysis shows the commencing destruction.

3 Monate.
Eine kräftige reaktive Periostwucherung hat sich um die Zone der destruierenden Entzündung gebildet.

A vigorous reaction of periosteal growth has formed round the area of destructive inflammation.

6 Monate.
Die Wundfläche des oberen Humerusendes hat begonnen sich zu glätten und sich zu schließen. Aber der (normalerweise auf der anderen Seite im 3. Monat aufgetretene) obere *Epiphysenkern fehlt.*

The wound surface of the upper end humerus of the has begun to close and has become smooth, but the upper epiphyseal centre, which normally appears in the third month, is missing.

Serie 13.

Knochenabsceß der Tibia.

Der *Brodie*sche Knochenabsceß wurde kurz nach einem Stoß gegen das Knie, auf den die Schmerzen zurückgeführt wurden, festgestellt und dann über 3 Jahre lang konservativ (ruhigstellende Verbände, Diathermie usw.) behandelt. Die für diese Erkrankung charakteristischen Symptome — intermittierender Gelenkerguß und Schmerzen — häuften und verschlimmerten sich aber mehr und mehr, so daß der Staphylokokkenabsceß schließlich aufgemeißelt wurde.

Series 13.

Bone-Abscess of Tibia.

The Brodie abscess was discovered shortly after a knock against the knee and pain was attributed to this. For three years conservative treatment was carried out (bandage preventing movement, Diathermy). The characteristic symptoms of this complaint — intermittent joint effusion and pain — grew more frequent and increased in severity, necessitating the chiseling open of the staphylococcal abscess.

⁴/₅ n. Gr.   1.   2.

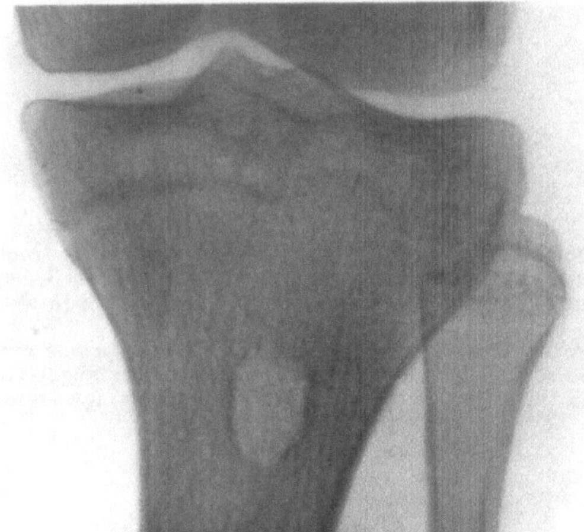 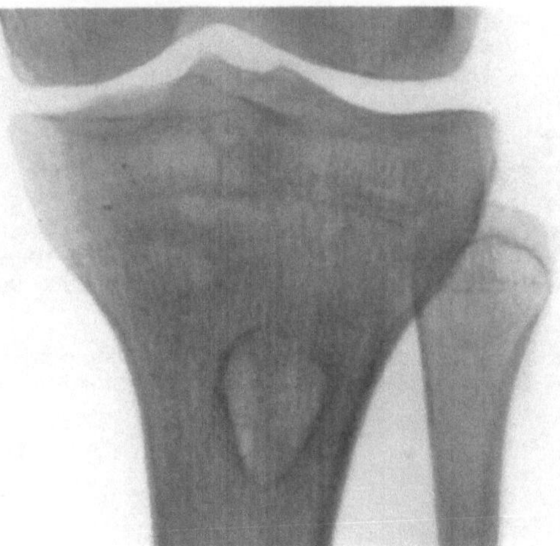

Die glattwandige Knochenhöhle an bevorzugter Stelle.

The smooth sided bone cavity at site of predilection.

Die Absceßhöhle ist nach über *3 Jahren* zwar deutlich größer, jedoch im Verhältnis zu der langen Zeit nur wenig gewachsen. — Die Abgrenzung durch eine wallartige Knochenverdichtung ist noch auffälliger.

More than *three years* later the abscess cavity is distinctly larger but, considering the length of time, has not grown to any great extent. The margin has become more distinct by the increase of compact bone.

Serie 14.

Osteomyelitis des Unterkiefers.

Bei dem 19 jähr. Mann ging von einer cariösen Zahnwurzel
eine Unterkiefer-Osteomyelitis aus, die nach Entfernung
eines größeren Sequesters mit der Regeneration des Kiefers
heilte.

$^2/_3$ n. Gr.   1.

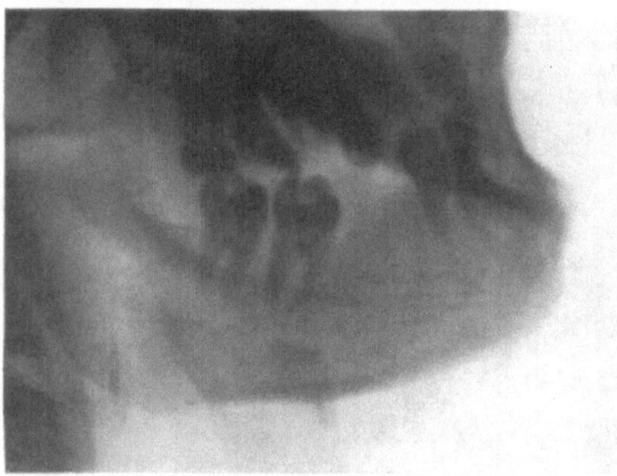

4 Tage nach Beginn der Anschwellung bzw. der Wurzel-
extraktion ist am Knochen ein krankhafter Befund nicht
nachzuweisen.

Four days after the appearance of the swelling caused by
the extraction of tooth, no sign of disease is visible.

Series 14.

Osteomyelitis of Lower Jaw.

A young man of nineteen had osteomyelitis of the lower
jaw which was caused. After the removal of a large
sequestrum it healed with entire regeneration of the
bone.

2.

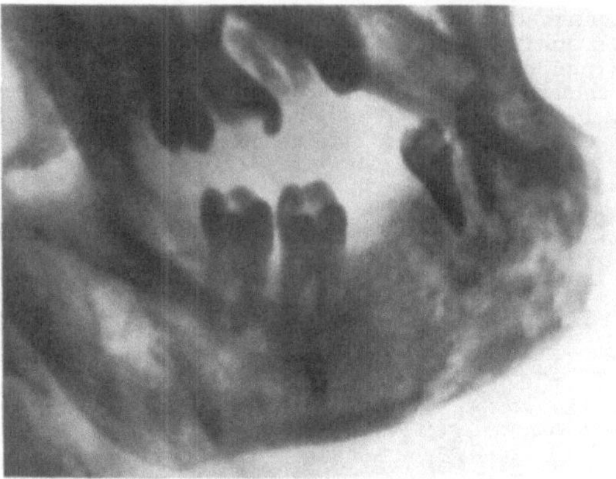

Nach 18 Tagen ist der Unterkieferast hochgradig atrophisch.
weist im Bereich der erkrankten Alveole einen Bruchspalt
und einen größeren in Lösung begriffenen Sequester auf.

After eighteen days the ramus of lower jaw is atrophic
to a high degree. There is a cleft in the neighbourhood
of the affected alveolar and a large dissolving sequestrum.

Serie 14.

3.

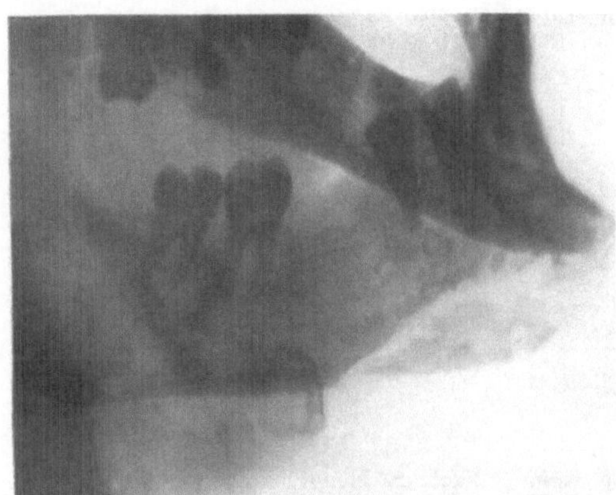

Nach 36 Tagen ist der Sequester vollständig gelöst,
im übrigen der Unterkiefer wieder kalkreicher.

After thirty-six days the sequestrum is entirely dissolved
and the lower jaw contains more chalk.

4.

Nach 78 Tagen besteht noch der Knochendefekt.

After seventy-eight days the bone defect is still present.

5.

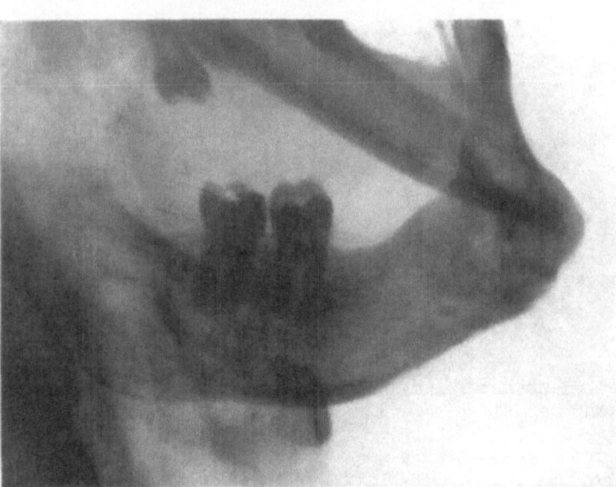

Nach 6 Monaten ist der Unterkiefer wieder gleichmäßig regeneriert.

After six months. The bone is again restored to normal.

Serie 15.

Sequestrierende
Zahnkeimentzündung.

Bei dem 6jährigen Knaben wurden wegen einer „Zahnfleischeiterung" die zwei prämolaren Milchzähne extrahiert. Die paradontitische Entzündung hatte aber bereits auf den Kieferknochen übergegriffen und der osteomyelitische Prozeß heilte erst nach Ausstoßung der entsprechenden Zahnkeime des bleibenden Gebisses.

Series 15.

Sequestral Inflammation
of Tooth Germ.

A 6 year old boy had the two premolar milk teeth extracted on account of a pyorrheal condition. The paradontic inflammation had already spread to the jaw-bone and the osteomyelitic process only healed after the expulsion of the germs of the corresponding second teeth.

$\frac{1}{1}$ n. Gr.   1.

2.

3.

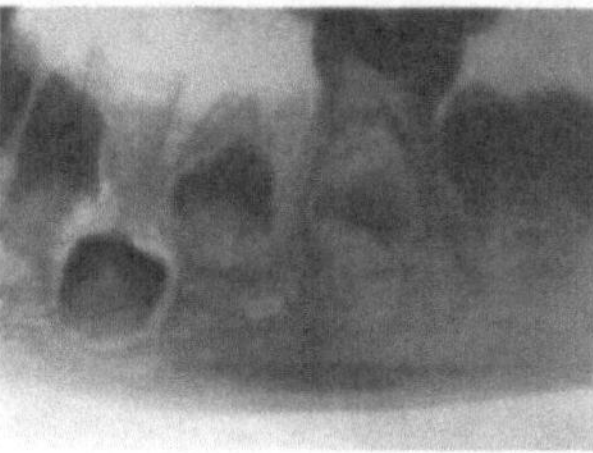

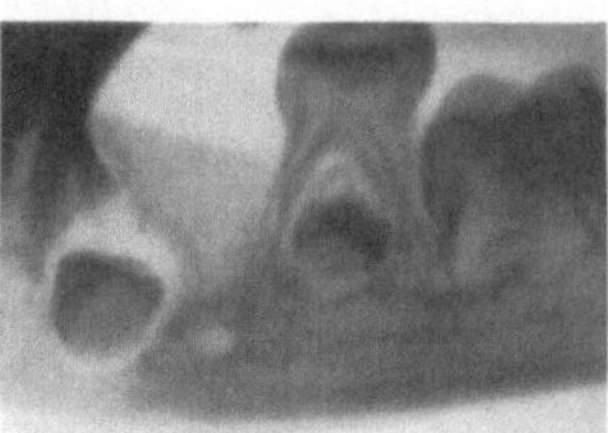

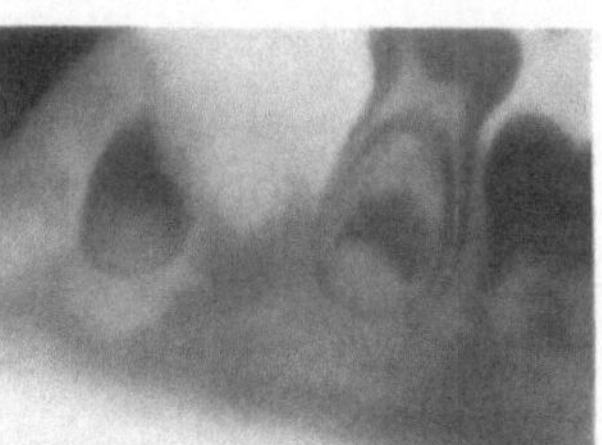

Bei der Extraktion der Milchzähne war die Eiterung bereits in die Knochenhöhle des 1. prämolaren Zahnkeimes vorgedrungen.

At the time of the extraction of the milk teeth, the pus had already penetrated into the bone cavity of the first premolar.

Nach 1 Monat: der eine Keim ist bereits ausgestoßen, der andere in der Knochenhöhle „sequestriert".

After 1 month. One germ has been expelled, the other is „sequestered" in bone-cavity.

Nach 2 Monaten: der zweite Zahnkeim ist in Ausstoßung begriffen.

After 2 months: the expulsion of the second tooth-germ is taking place.

4.

5.

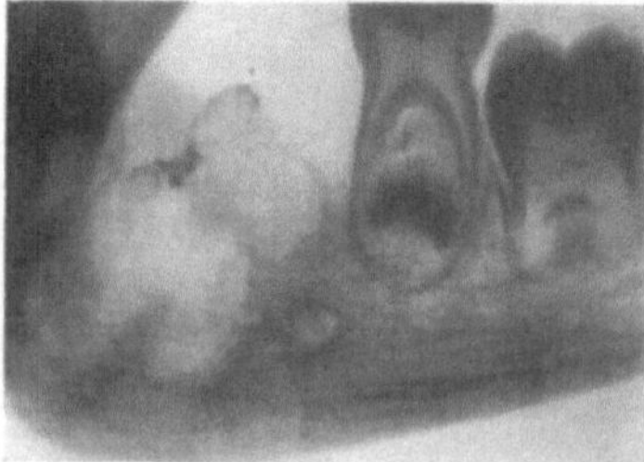

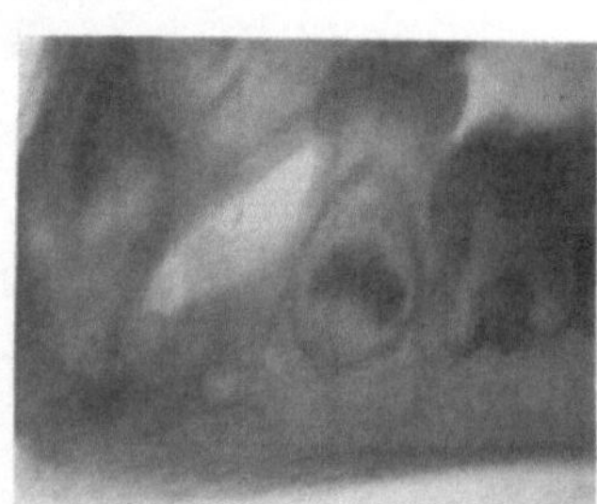

Nach 3 Monaten: die leeren Knochenhöhlen sind noch erkennbar.

After 3 months: the empty bone-cavities are still recognisable.

Ein weiteres Vierteljahr später: der Kiefer ist ausgeglichen.

3 months later the jaw is uniform.

Serie 16.

Paradentitis apicalis.

Die chronische granulierende Paradentitis — eine dentale Ostitis — heilte nach Eröffnung und Wurzelspitzenresektion mit Regeneration des Oberkieferdefektes aus.

Series 16.

Paradentitis apicalis.

The chronic granular paradentitis — a dental osteitis — was cured after laying open and the resecting root-point. The defect of the upper jaw regenerated.

$^1/_1$ n. Gr.   1.

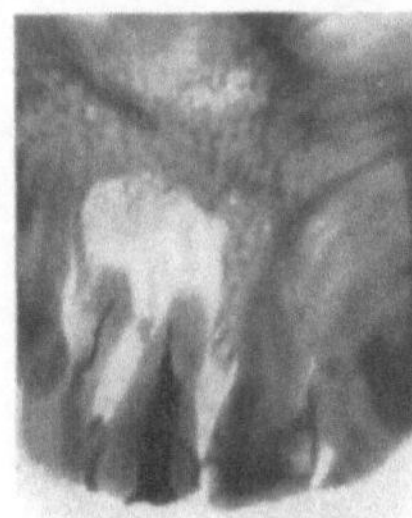

Knochendefekt 14 Tage nach einer nicht ganz vollständig durchgeführten Wurzelspitzenresektion.

Fourteen days after an incomplete root apex resection.

2.

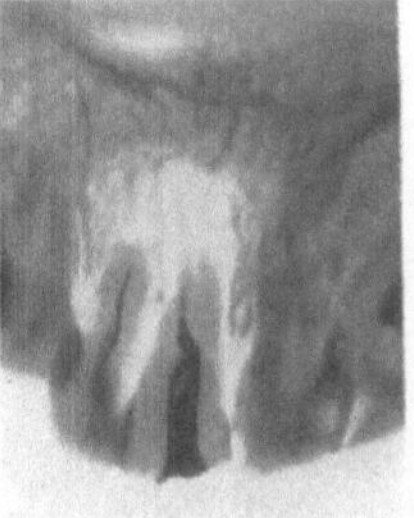

Nach 5 Monaten sind erst Anfänge der Knochenregeneration vorhanden.

After five months, the bone regeneration is just commencing.

3.

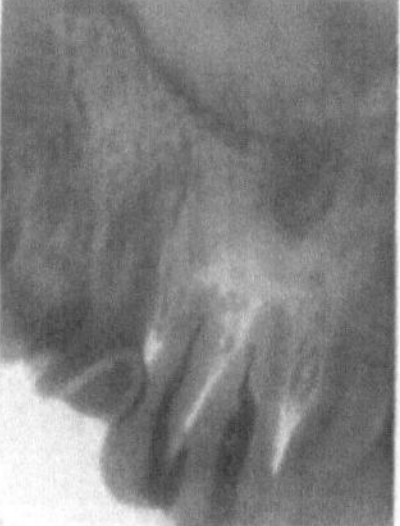

Nach 1 Jahr ist die Höhle knöchern ausgefüllt.

After one year, the cavity is filled with bone.

Serie 17.

Panaritium ossale.

Der 6jährige Knabe erlitt eine offene Fingerverletzung; diese traumatische Osteomyelitis führte — ebenso wie die hämatogene — unter Eiterung und Sequesterausstoßung zur Regeneration der Phalangen, war aber auch von charakteristischen Komplikationen — Epiphysenschädigung, Gelenkverödung — begleitet.

Series 17.

Panaritium Ossale.

A boy six years of age had an open wound on his finger. Traumatic osteomyelitis resulted and led (just as the haematogenous type does) to regeneration of the phalanx which was accompanied by the formation of pus and expulsion of the sequestrum. It was accompanied however, by the characteristic complications — epiphyseal injury and joint destruction.

⁴/₅ n. Gr.   1.   2.   3.

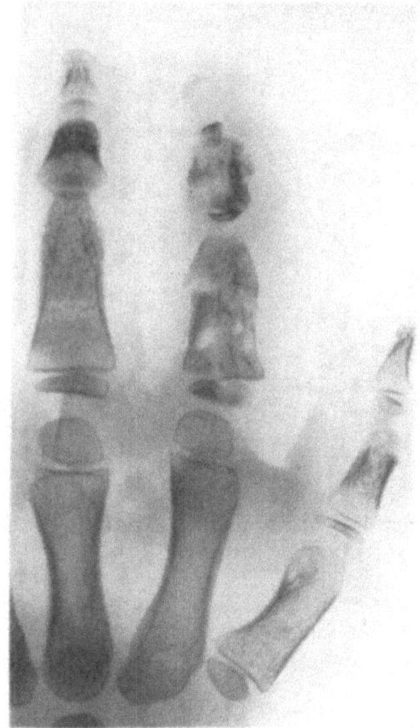 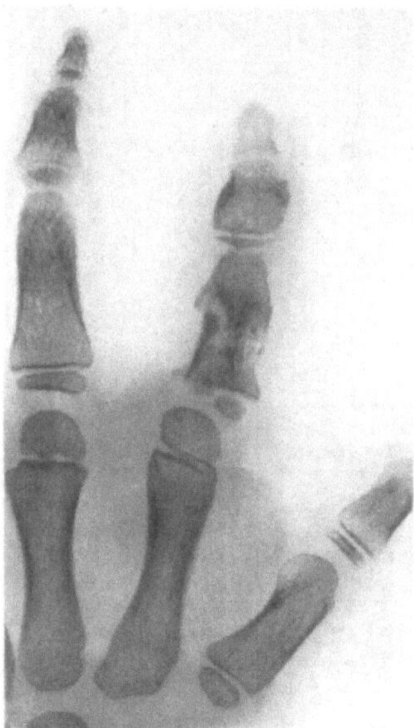 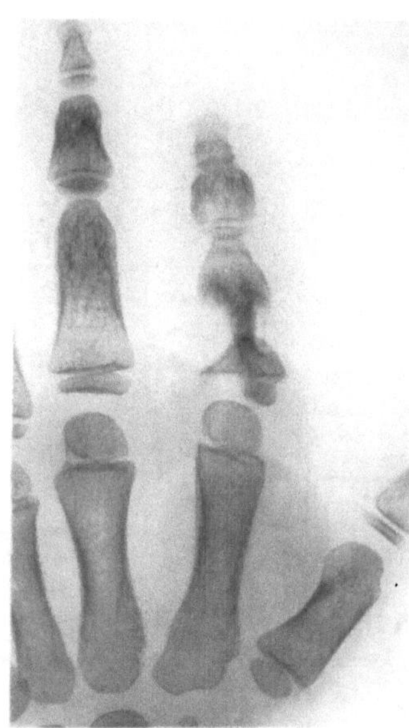

16 Tage nach der Verletzung besteht eine ausgedehnte osteomyelitische Knochenzerstörung am Zeigefinger.

Sixteen days after the accident extensive osteomyelitic destruction exists in the first finger.

Nach 25 Tagen ist eine Demarkierung kleiner Sequester in der Epi- sowie Diaphyse der Grundphalanx II erkennbar.

After twenty-five days demarkation of small sequestra in the epiphysis and diaphysis of the basal phalanx II is recognizable.

Nach 6 Wochen sind die Sequester ausgestoßen.

After six weeks the sequestra have been expelled.

Serie 17.

4.

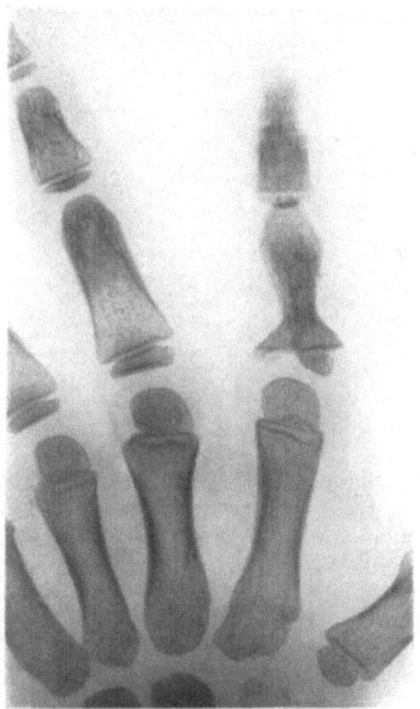

Nach 12 Wochen ist die Phalange weitgehend regeneriert, aber das Endgelenk und die Epiphysenfuge des Grundgliedes sind knöchern verwachsen.

After twelve weeks the phalanx is greatly regenerated but the joint-end and the epiphyseal line have become ossified.

5.

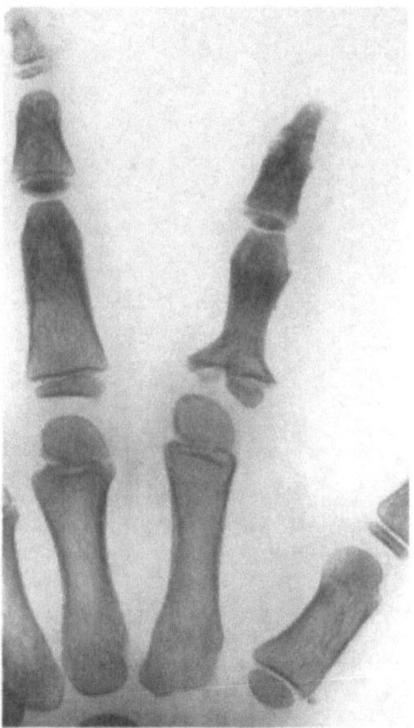

Nach 6 Monaten ist der Phalangenschaft noch mehr ersetzt, seine Epiphyse jedoch läßt die bleibende Schädigung — teilweise Zerstörung und vorzeitige Verknöcherung der Wachstumsfuge — erkennen. — Nach einem weiteren Jahr wurde der gleiche Befund erhoben.

After six months the regeneration of shaft of phalanx has advanced further but the epiphysis shows the permanent damage — partial destruction and premature ossification of epiphysis. One year later the condition was found to be unaltered.

Serie 18.
Komplizierte Fußfraktur.

Die komplizierte Mittelfußfraktur des 8 jährigen
Knaben — eine Überfahrungsverletzung — heilte
auf dem Umwege der traumatischen Osteomyelitis:
Regeneration mit Ausstoßung der Totalsequester,
Epiphysenschädigung mit nachfolgender
Wachstumshemmung.

Series 18.
Complicated Fracture of Foot.

A boy eight years of age, by being run over,
sustained a complicated fracture of the middle
foot which healed in the roundabout way of
traumatic osteomyelitis. Regeneration occurred
after total sequestration, epiphyseal injury and
subsequent stunting of growth ensued.

²/₃ n. Gr.   1.   2.

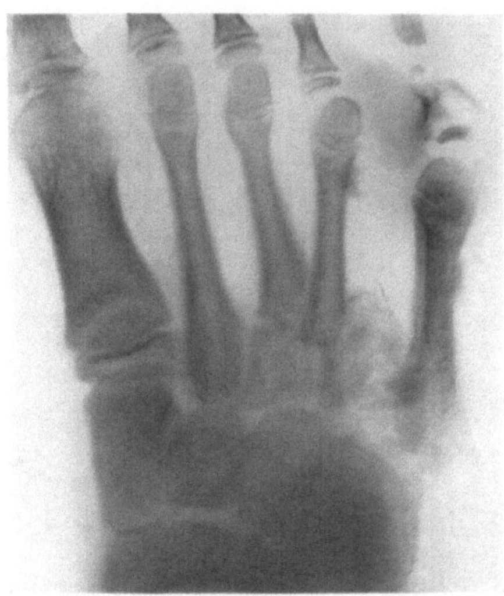
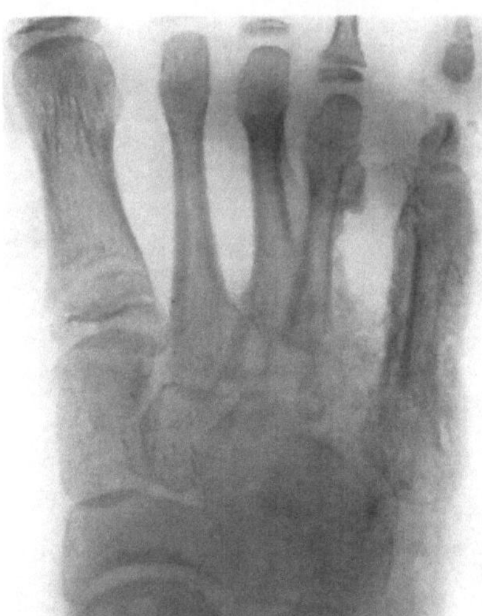

4 Wochen nach der Verletzung — Querfraktur
an der Basis des Metatarsus III—V — ist die
traumatische Osteomyelitis an der periostalen
Knochenwucherung erkennbar.

Four weeks after accident — Diagonal fracture at
the base of metatarsus III—V — the traumatic
osteomyelitis is recognizable by the periosteal
growth of bone.

Nach 8 Wochen besteht am Metatarsus V eine dichte
Totenlade um den Totalsequester; am IV. Mittelfußknochen ist der gleiche Prozeß im Gange.

After eight weeks there is a sharply outlined
sequestrum-bed in the fifth metatarsal. The
same process is taking place around the total
sequestration of the fourth tarsal bone.

3.

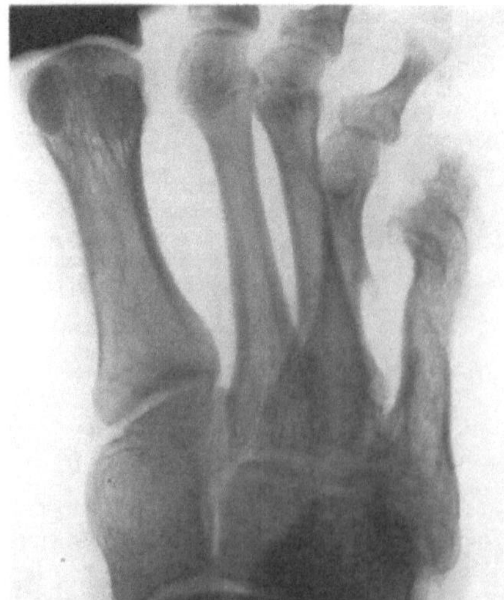

Nach 6 Jahren verraten Unregelmäßigkeiten der Konturen und eine geringe Verkürzung des 4. und
5. Mittelfußknochens die überstandene Osteomyelitis.

After six years, irregularities of contour and a slight shortening of the fourth and fifth tarsal bones
betray the osteomyelitis, which has been overcome.

Anhang.

Serie 19.

Sekundäre Periostitis.

Die Periostreizung ging von einer eitrigen Phlegmone der Ober-
schenkelmuskulatur aus und führte — gemäß der dem Periost
eigenen Fähigkeit — zur Bildung eines Knochensaumes,
eine *sympathische, unspezifische* Entzündung.

Supplement.

Series 19.

Secondary Periostitis.

A suppurating phlegmon of the muscles of upper-leg caused
an irritation of the periosteum which led, in accordance with
the faculty of periosteum, to the formation of a bone-edge —
a *sympathetic, non-specific* inflammation.

$^2/_3$ n. Gr.　　1.　　　　　　2.　　　　　　3.　　　　　　4.

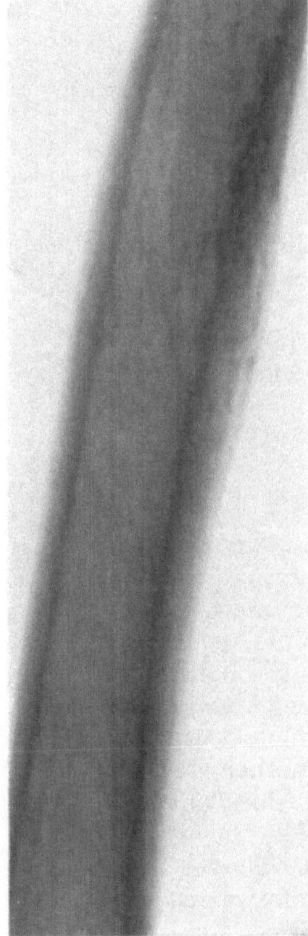 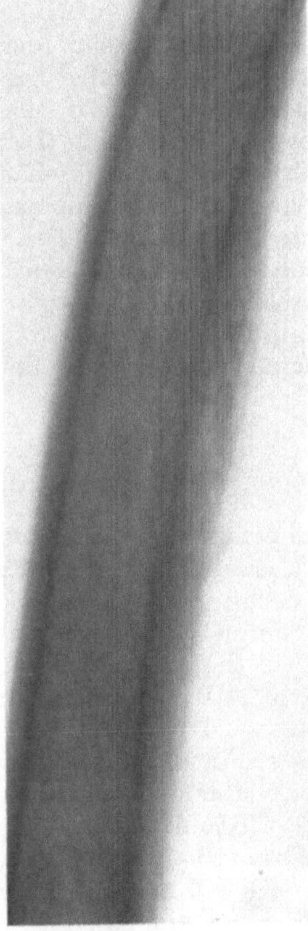 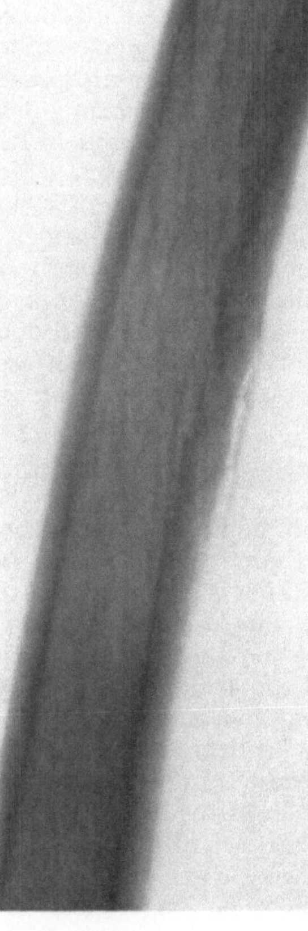 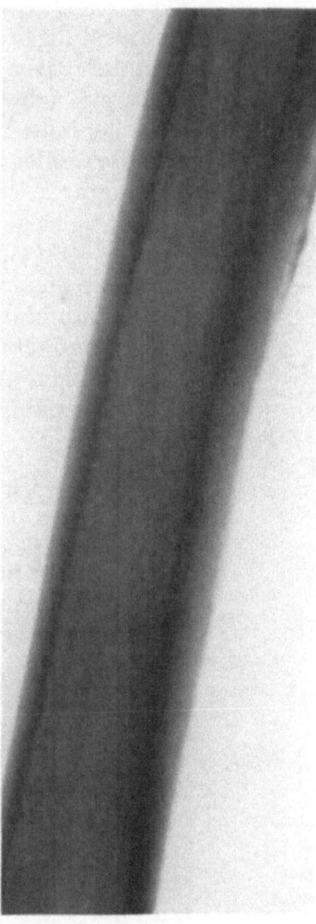

Etwa 6 Wochen nach Auf-
treten der Weichteilschwellung findet sich eine Periost-
auflockerung.

About six weeks after ap-
pearance of swelling of the
fleshy parts, there is a
loosening of the periosteum.

3 Wochen später — nach
der Incision — ist bereits
Rückbildung der Periostitis
eingetreten.

Three weeks later. After
incision, the periostitis is
already retrogressing.

Nach 4 Monaten hebt sich
aus der im ganzen zurückge-
gangenen Periostverdickung
ein feiner Knochensaum ab.

After four months. A fine bone-
edge may be seen from out
of the regressing thickness of
the periosteum.

Dieser Saum ist nach Abheilung
des Weichteilprozesses noch
dichter geworden und $1^1/_2$ Jahre
später als dauerndes Residuum
erkennbar.

This edge has become more
compact since the healing of
the process in the fleshy parts
and a year and a half later is
recognized as having become
permanent.

B. Akute, spezifische und unspezifische Gelenkentzündungen.

Die Prognose der akuten Gelenkerkrankungen ist *abhängig von der destruktiven Komponente des Entzündungsprozesses*. Das gilt in gleicher Weise für die spezifischen Entzündungen, deren wichtigste die gonorrhoische ist, als auch für die unspezifischen mannigfaltiger Ursache. Eiterungen veröden das Gelenk mehr oder weniger, auch wenn sie ursprünglich reine Kapselprozesse sind; gehen sie aber primär von einem Knochenherd aus, so ist die Zerstörung des Gelenkes sicher. Wir sehen die Ankylose bei der phlegmonösen gonorrhoischen Kniegelenksentzündung (Serie 20) wie bei der metastatischen Koxitis (Serie 25). Alle Grade der Gelenkschädigung ereignen sich in gleicher Weise bei den spezifischen als auch bei den unspezifischen Infektionen. Solange nicht die Gelenkenden nach Zerstörung des Knorpelüberzuges geradezu zu einem einzigen Knochenstab verwachsen, wird nach dem akuten Stadium der Entzündung eine Wiederherstellung des Gelenkes, d. h. geglätteter Knochenenden und eines Gelenkspaltes unter dem Einfluß der Funktion mehr (Serie 21) oder weniger (Serie 23) erfolgen, auch wenn eine nennenswerte Beweglichkeit und Gebrauchsfähigkeit nicht mehr erreicht wird.

B. Acute Specific and Unspecific Joint Inflammations.

The progress of acute joint conditions depends upon the destructive power of the inflammatory process. The same may be said of specific inflammations; the most important of which is gonorrhoea — in addition to the unspecific inflammations of different origin. Pus usually partially or completely destroys the joints, even if it was originally a pure capsular process. When the primary cause is in the bone, then destruction of the joint will certainly occur. We see this in the phlegmonous gonorrhoeal inflammation of the knee-joint (Series 20) as well as in the metastatic coxitis (Series 25). All degrees of joint injuries occur in the same way whether the inflammation is specific or non-specific. If bony union of the joint ends does not occur after destruction of the cartilage covering, the joint will be more or less reconstructed by functional use, after the acute inflammatory stage has passed. That is the bone ends will become smooth and a joint cleft will result even when movemen and normal function is no longer possible (Series 21 and 23).

Serie 20.

Gonorrhoische Kniegelenkentzündung.

Wenige Wochen nach einer Eierstockoperation erkrankte die 30 jährige Frau an der sehr schmerzhaften phlegmonösen Kniegelenkentzündung, die allen therapeutischen — auch intraartikulären — Maßnahmen zum Trotz zur Zerstörung des Gelenkes führte und mit knöcherner Verwachsung heilte.

$^2/_3$ n. Gr.

Series 20.

Gonorrhoeal Inflammation of Knee-Joint.

A woman of thirty years had been ill for many months with an ovarian complaint for which she underwent an operation. A few weeks afterwards she complained of great pain in the knee and was found to be suffering with phlegmonous knee-joint inflammation: Despite all treatment (including intra-articular treatment), the joint was destroyed an became ankylosed.

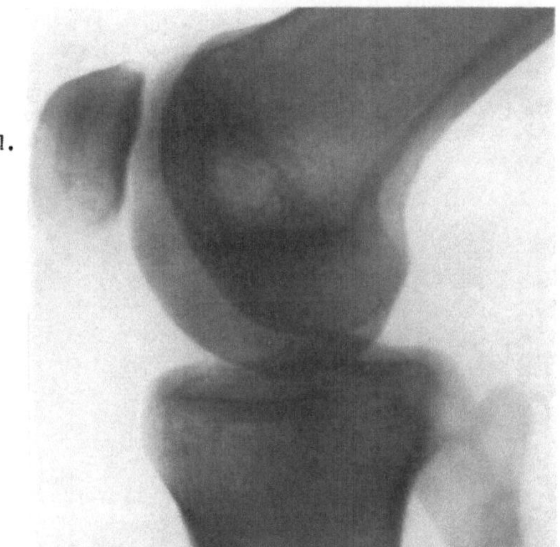

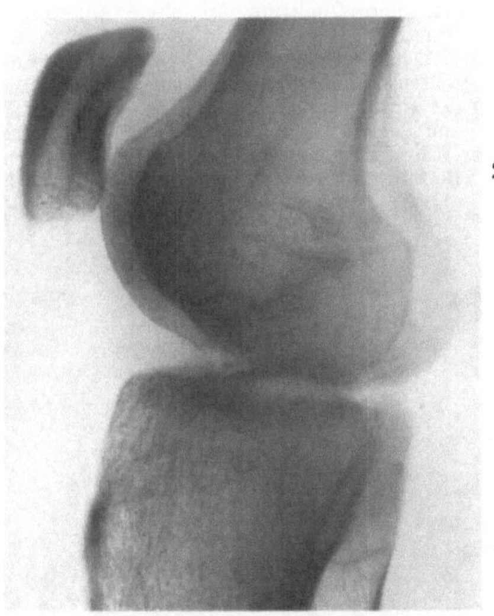

1.

2.

3 Wochen nach Beginn noch keine erkennbaren Knochenveränderungen, trotz der schweren Kapselphlegmone mit Empyem.

Three weeks after onset no alteration of the bone is noticeable in spite of the severe capsular phlegmon with empyema.

Nach 13 Wochen sind die Gelenkflächen usuriert und durch eine schmale Knochenbrücke bereits verwachsen.

After thirteen weeks, the joint surfaces are destroyed and already attached to one another by a small bone bridge.

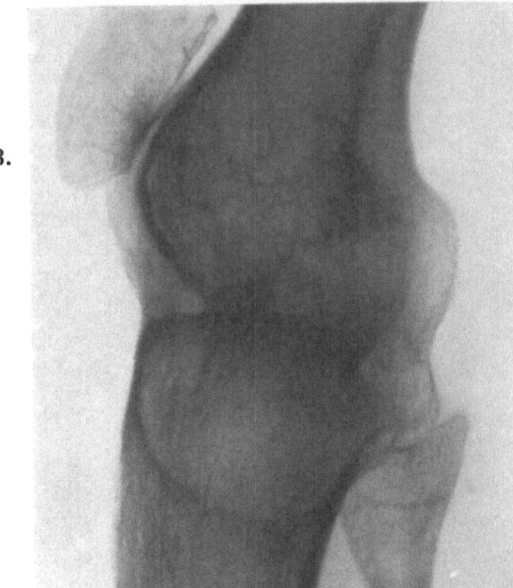

3.

Nach 2 Jahren sind Femur und Tibia in ganzer Breite zusammengewachsen und geradezu ein Knochen geworden.

After two years, femur and tibia have completely united.

Serie 21.

Gonorrhoische Hüftgelenkentzündung.

Das 26 jähr. Mädchen erkrankte 7 Wochen nach der genitalen Infektion an einer außerordentlich schmerzhaften Hüftgelenkentzündung. Es bestand lange Zeit hohes Fieber, eine sehr starke Anschwellung und völlige Unbeweglichkeit der Hüfte. Nach Rückgang der Entzündung, die eine starke Kalkverarmung des dem Gelenk angehörigen Knochens verursacht hatte, führte eine konsequente Bewegungsbehandlung rasch den normalen Zustand und volle Funktion herbei.

$^6/_{10}$ n. Gr.   1.

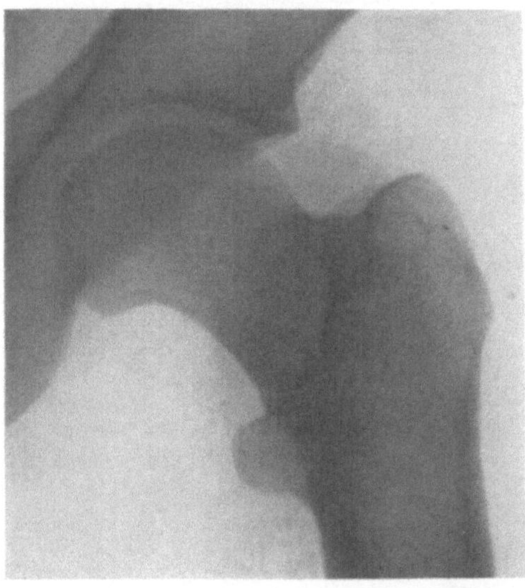

Am 4. Tag der Krankheit sind die Gelenkkonturen unverändert und der Gelenkspalt ist durch das Exsudat verbreitert.

On the fourth day of illness, the joint outlines are unaltered and the joint cleft is widened by the exudation.

Series 21.

Gonorrhoeal Inflammation of Hip-joint.

Seven weeks after the genital infection, the twenty six year old girl was taken ill with an extremely painful inflammation of the hip-joint. For a long time she had high fever, a large swelling and complete immobility of the hip. After the inflammation, which had caused considerable chalk-impoverishment in the bone appertaining to the joint, had subsided, the normal state and full function was achieved by logical exercise.

2.

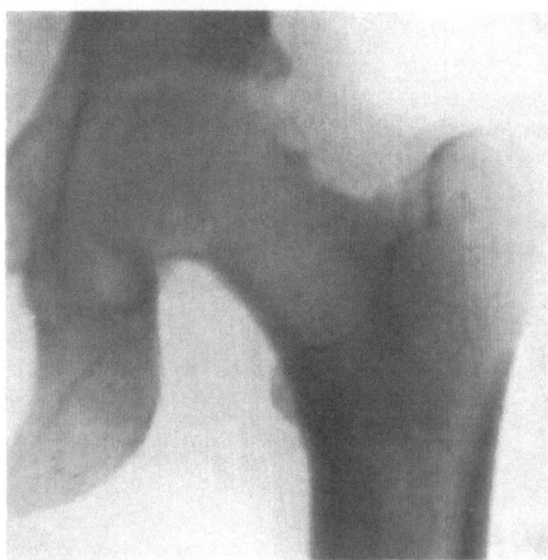

8 Wochen später hat die Entzündung zu einer Kalkverarmung des knöchernen Gelenkteiles geführt.

Eight weeks later the inflammation had caused chalk-impoverishment to the bony part of joint.

Serie 21.

3.

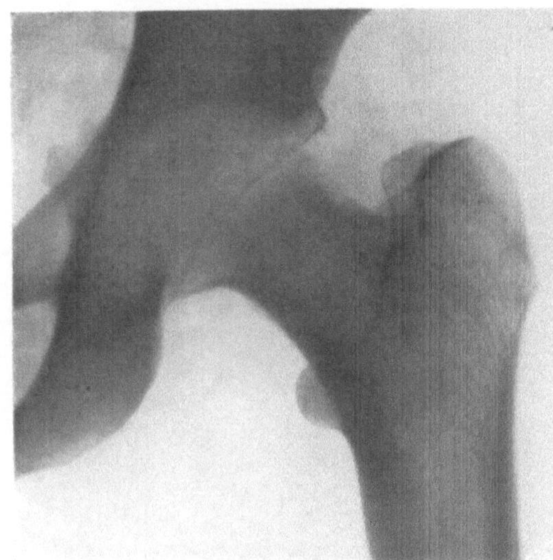

Nach 10 Wochen hat diese Kalkatrophie noch
zugenommen.

After ten weeks this chalk atrophy had increased.

4.

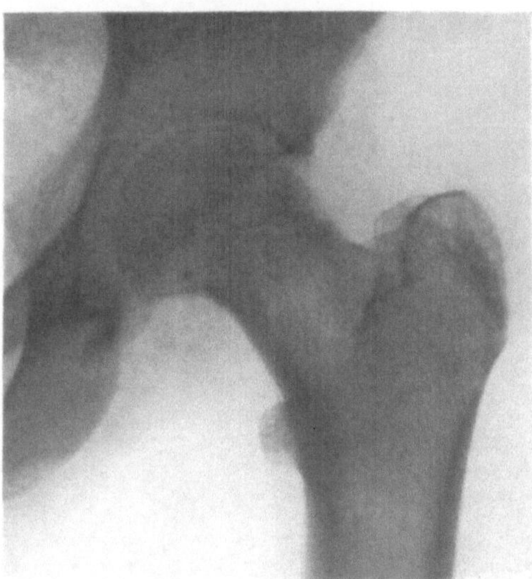

Nach 15 Wochen ist der Knochen wieder kalkreicher
geworden, so daß die Konturen und der Gelenkspalt wieder hervortreten.

After fifteen weeks the bone had become richer in
chalk so that the outlines and the joint cleft are
recognizable.

5.

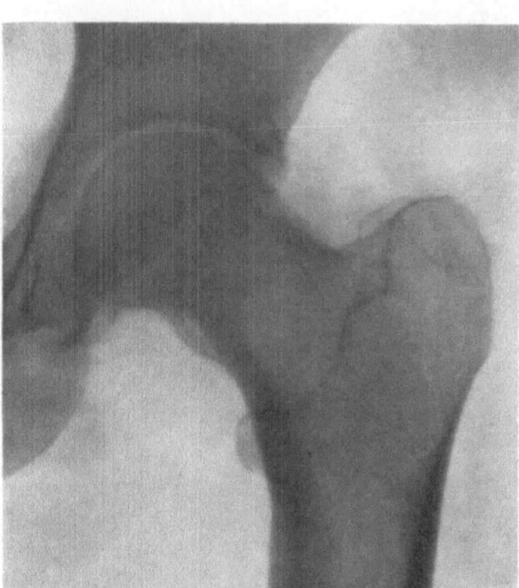

Nach 5 Monaten sind Kopf und Pfanne wieder normal gebildet, die Beweglichkeit ist weitgehend wiederhergestellt.

After five months head and socket are again of normal structure and the mobility is to a very great
extent restored.

Serie 22.

Gonorrhoische Handgelenkentzündung.

Die 33jähr. Frau erkrankte an gonorrhoischer Pelveoperitonitis und wenige Wochen später an der pathognomonisch hochentzündlichen Gelenkmetastase. Die schwere Kapselphlegmone griff auch stellenweise den Knorpel und Knochen an und heilte nach mehreren Monaten mit voller Wiederherstellung aus.

$^1/_5$ n. Gr.   1.

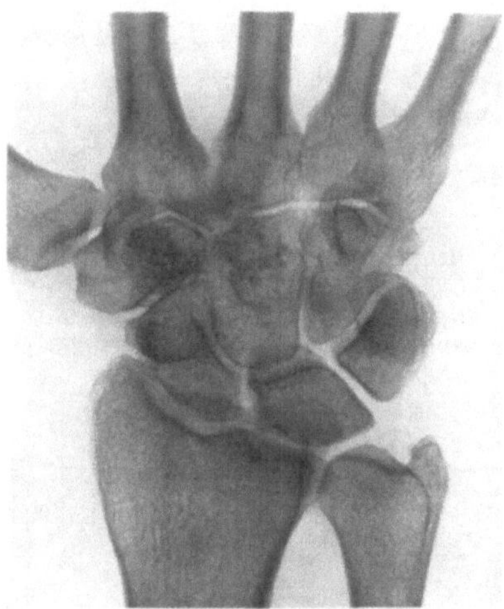

Am 7. Krankheitstag ist der Knochen von der schweren Kapselphlegmone noch nicht angegriffen.

On the seventh day of illness, the bone is not, as yet, attacked by the severe capsular phlegmons.

Series 22.

Gonorrhoeal Inflammation of the Wrist.

A woman of thirty three became ill with gonorrhoeal pelvic peritonitis and a few weeks later with pathognomonic, highly inflamed metastasis of this joint. The severe phlegmons in the capsule attacked the cartilage and bone in places but healed completely after several months.

2.

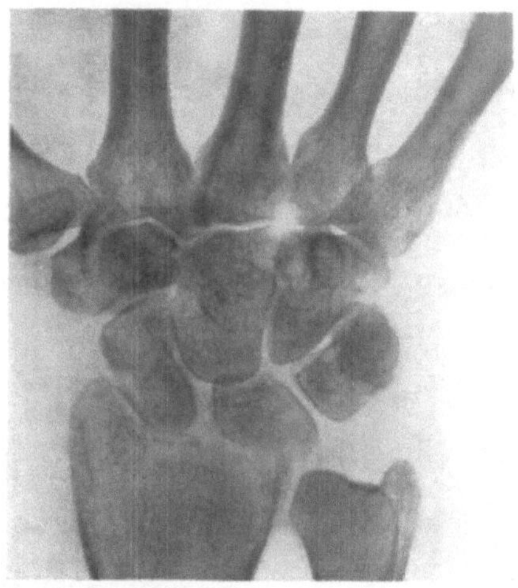

Am Ende der 4. Woche ist die Knochenatrophie und die Usur der Gelenkflächen besonders am Radius deutlich, dabei die Schmerzhaftigkeit noch groß.

At the end of the fourth week the bone atrophy and the destruction of the joint surfaces are particularly clear at the radius. Extremely painful.

Serie 22.

3.

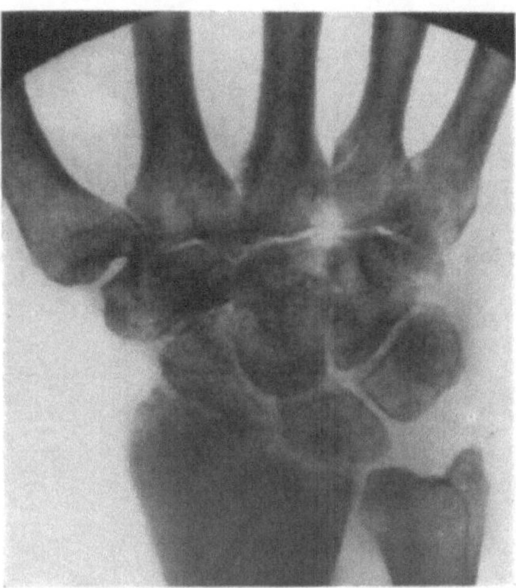

Nach 8 Wochen sind die Gelenkflächen noch stärker aufgelockert bzw. zerstört.

After eight weeks the joint surfaces are further loosened and relatively destroyed.

4.

Nach 10 Wochen ist der Höhepunkt der Entzündung überschritten, so daß mit Bewegungsübungen begonnen werden konnte.

After ten weeks the inflammation climax has been passed, so that movement exercises could be commenced.

5.

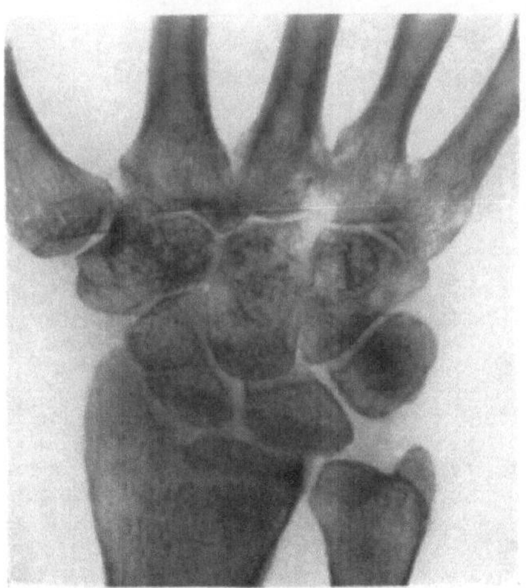

In der 15. Krankheitswoche werden die Gelenkkonturen wieder deutlicher, etwa $^1/_4$ Jahr später ist das Handgelenk wieder frei beweglich.

In the fifteenth week the outlines of the joint are again distinct and about three months later the wrist was movable.

6.

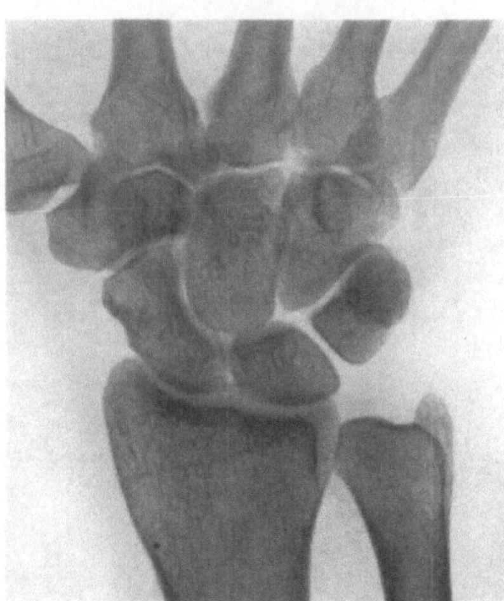

7 Jahre später ist bei vollständiger klinischer Ausheilung die ausgenagte Stelle der Gelenkfläche des Radius noch ein Zeichen der stattgehabten schweren Gelenkentzündung (sekundäre Arthritis def. leichten Grades).

Seven years later, although completely restored, the eroded part of joint-surface of radius shows how severe the inflammation of joint had been (Secondary arthritis def. slight degree).

Serie 23.

Akute Hüftgelenkentzündung.

Der 31 jährige Mann erkrankte plötzlich ohne vorherige Beschwerden mit heftigen Schmerzen in der Hüfte und machte ein wochenlanges hochfieberhaftes Krankenlager durch. Die Hüftgelenkentzündung, für deren Ätiologie die Gonorrhöe auszuschließen war, heilte mit Versteifung. Immerhin war nach Jahren eine unvollständige Wiederherstellung des Gelenkspaltes erkennbar.

$^6/_{10}$ n. Gr.   1.

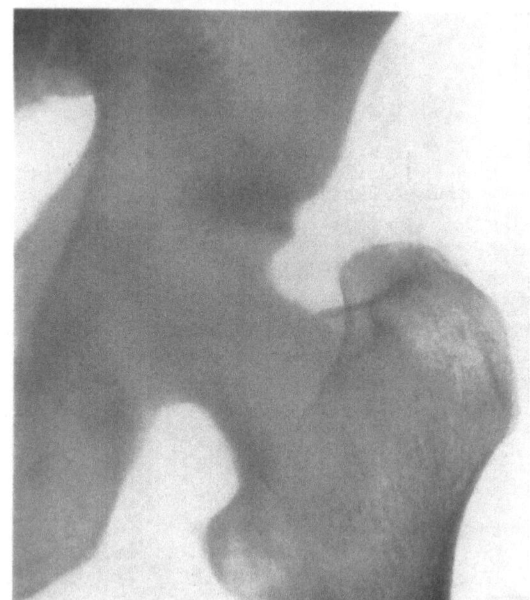

In der 6. Woche der Krankheit ist der Gelenkspalt vollkommen verschwunden.

In the sixth week of the illness, the joint cleft has entirely disappeared.

Series 23.

Acute Coxitis.

A man thirty-one years of age became suddenly ill without any previous complaint and had severe pains in the hip and had high-fever for several weeks. The hip-joint inflammation, which was not due to gonorrhoea, resulted in permanent stiffness. Years afterwards however, an imperfect reconstruction of the joint cleft was recognizable.

2.

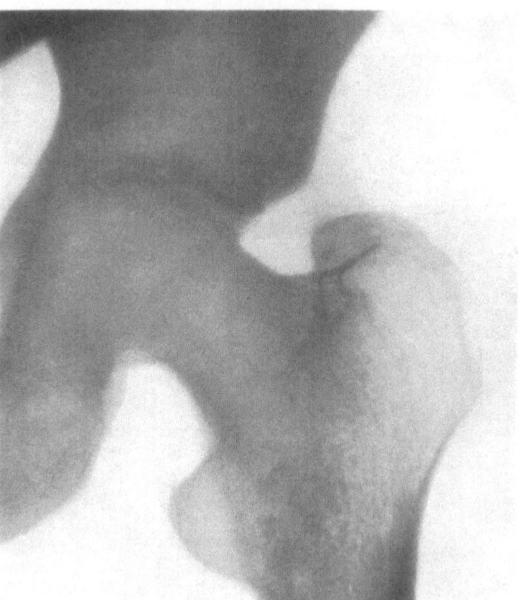

Nach einem Vierteljahr — bei klinischem Rückgang der Beschwerden — beginnt der Gelenkspalt wieder erkennbar zu werden. Der Knochen ist noch atrophisch.

After three months. Upon the clinical recession of the complaints, the joint cleft becomes recognizable again but the bone is still atrophic.

Serie 23.

3.

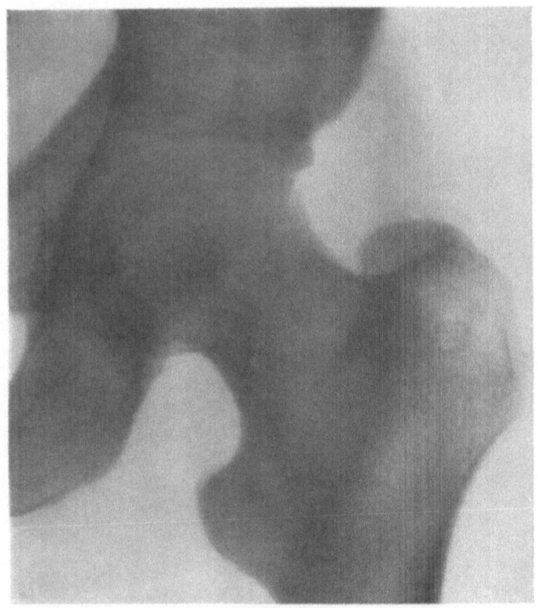

4.

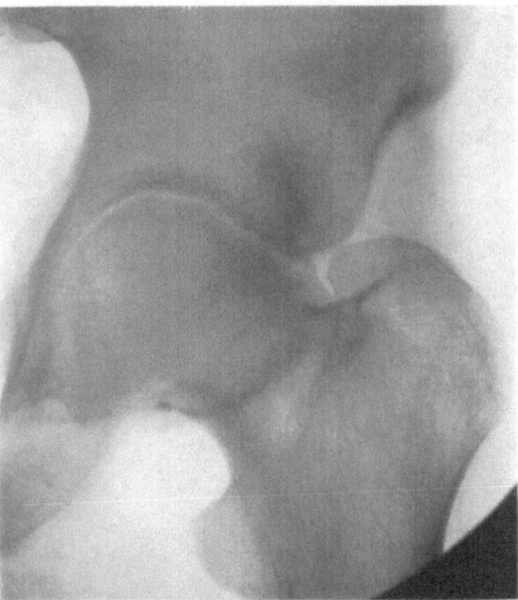

Nach einem halben Jahr, als der Kranke schon arbeitsfähig war, ist der Gelenkspalt noch etwas mehr angedeutet.

After six months. At this time the man was able to work. The joint cleft has become more distinct.

Nach 6 Jahren ist der Schenkelhals verkürzt, das Gelenk deform, aber der Gelenkspalt doch in größerer Ausdehnung wieder entstanden; dabei ist die Hüfte praktisch steif geblieben.

After six years. The femur neck is shortened and the joint deformed, but the joint cleft has become distinct again. The hip remained stiff.

Serie 24.

Akute Hüftgelenkentzündung nach Angina.

Die 40jährige Frau war bereits am 2. Tag einer mit hohem Fieber und Schüttelfrost einsetzenden Angina mit den Erscheinungen einer akuten Hüftgelenksentzündung erkrankt. Das Leiden führte über ein kurzes akutes Stadium in etwa 10 Monaten zu einer Restitutio ad integrum.

$^1/_2$ n. Gr.   1.

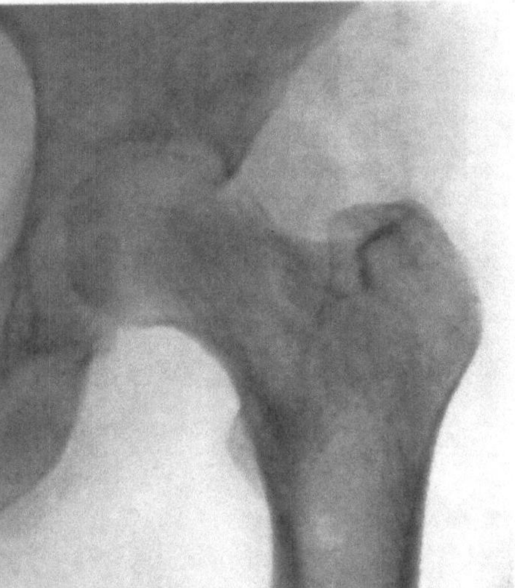

Nach 2 Monaten zeigt das Röntgenbild verwaschene Konturen des Gelenkes bei erheblicher Knochenatrophie.

After 2 months the Röntgen photograph shows indistinct outlines of the joint with considerable atrophy of bone.

Series 24.

Acute Coxitis after Tonsillitis.

A woman of forty had tonsillitis, which commenced with high fever and rigors. On the second day after commencement, an acute hip-joint inflammation set in. After a short acute stage, the malady led to complete recovery in about ten months.

2.

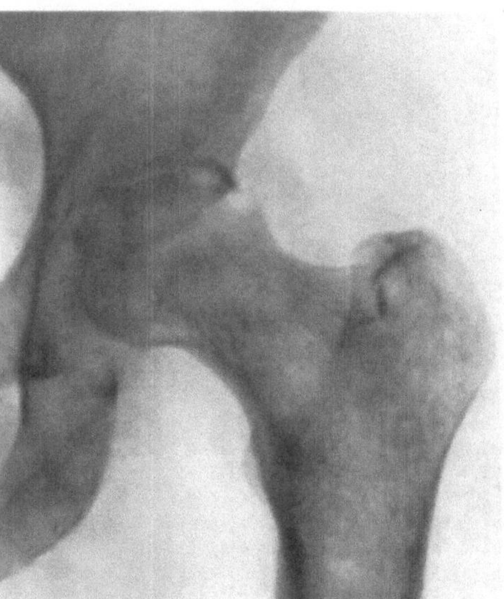

Nach $3^1/_2$ Monaten — als die Kranke bereits mit Gehübungen begonnen hatte — ist der Kopf noch deutlich entrundet und höckerig, der Gelenkspalt noch unterbrochen.

After $3^1/_2$ months when the invalid had commenced walking exercises, the head was still distinctly irregular. The joint cleft is still interrupted.

Serie 24.

3.

4.

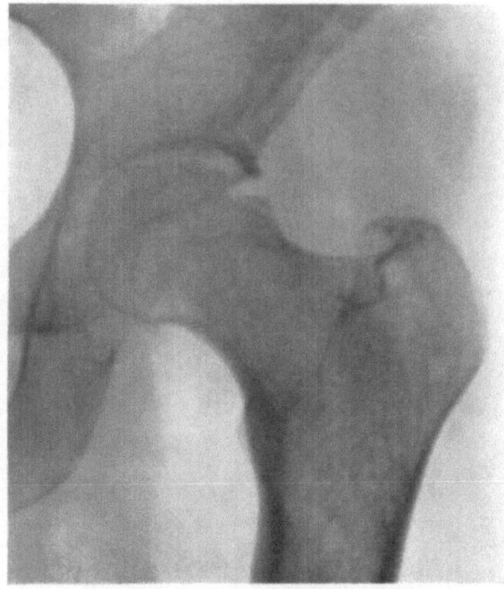

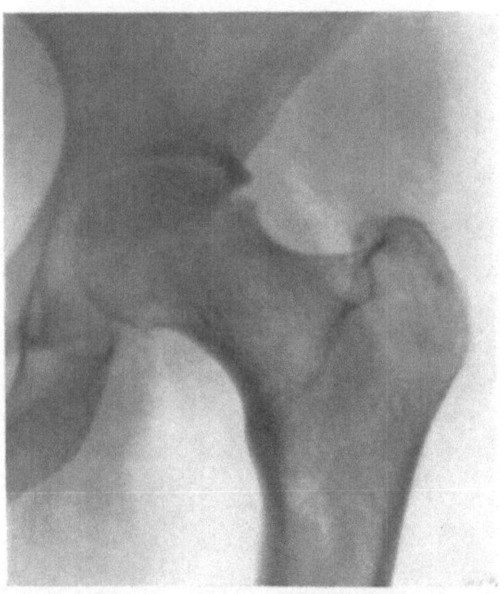

Nach ¹/₂ Jahr ist die günstige Prognose des Leidens aus der Neuformung des Gelenkes ablesbar.

After 6 months the favorable prognosis of the malady is recognisable by the new formation of the joint.

Nach 10 Monaten Ausheilung mit Wiederherstellung der normalen Form und Funktion.

After 10 months. Completely healed and restored to normal form and function.

Serie 25.

Metastatische ossale Hüftgelenkentzündung.

Die 25 jährige Frau erkrankte 6 Wochen nach einem septischen Abort an einer eitrigen Hüftgelenkentzündung, als deren Erreger Streptokokken nachgewiesen wurden. Diese septische Metastase führte zu eitriger Einschmelzung im Gelenk und heilte mit fester knöcherner Ankylose.

$^6/_{10}$ n. Gr.　　　　　1.

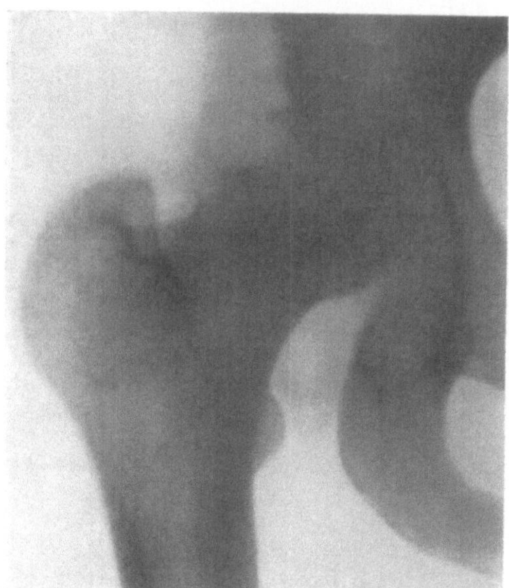

5 Wochen nach Beginn besteht eine ausgedehnte Zerstörung am oberen Teil des Schenkelkopfes und der Gelenkpfanne (Pfannenwanderung).

Five weeks after commencement of illness. Extensive destruction of upper part of femoral head and of the joint socket exists (Wandering of acetabulum).

Series 25.

Metastatic Osteo-Coxitis.

A woman of twenty-five became ill six weeks after a septic abortion with hip-joint inflammation. Streptococci were found in the pus. This septic metastasis led to pyogenic destruction in the joint and permanent osteo-ankylosis.

2.

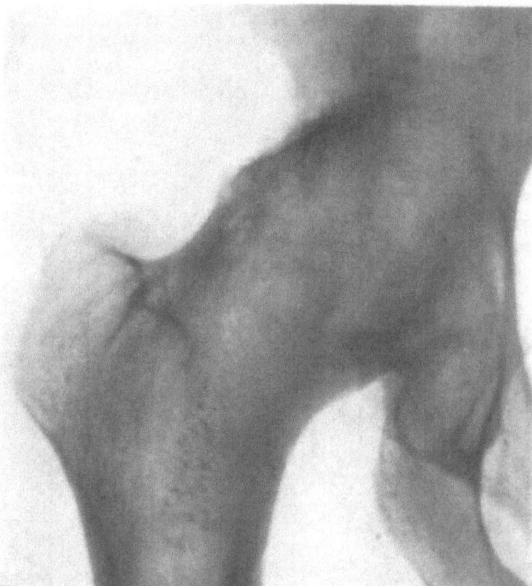

Endzustand nach 6 Jahren: Feste knöcherne Ankylose mit deutlicher Bälkchenzeichnung der Verwachsung.

Final condition after six years. Firm osteo-ankylosis with distinct beam design of the ossified joint.

II. Kapitel.

Chronische spezifische Entzündungen.

A. Tuberkulose der Gelenke.

Die Knochen- und Gelenktuberkulose stellt ihr Wesen und ihre Prognose bezeichnend dar *als eine nagende umschriebene Zerstörung ohne gleichzeitige Reparationsbestrebungen, und läßt auch im Stadium der Heilung immer nur ein Ausflicken mit geringen Mitteln erkennen. Ihre Heilungsaussichten sind abhängig von zwei Faktoren,* von der *Kampfkraft des Körpers* und *von den örtlichen Gewebsverhältnissen.* Im durchseuchten Organismus, wenn ein anderes wesentliches Organsystem, wie die Lungen oder die Nieren schwerer erkrankt sind, fehlt auch der Gelenkerkrankung das Heilbestreben. Das Schultergelenk (Serie 39) oder das Fußgelenk (Serie 30) zeigen den unaufhaltsam fortschreitenden Zerfall unter solchen Bedingungen. Die Heilung geschieht durch die Hebung der immunisatorischen Kräfte des ganzen Körpers. Das beweist u. a. auch die in der Schweiz so großartig durchgeführte Sonnenbehandlung der Knochen- und Gelenktuberkulose. Viel leichter ist sie im kindlichen Organismus herbeizuführen als beim Erwachsenen. Es kann besonders bei unterernährten Kindern lediglich die Herbeiführung geordneter Pflege, ausreichender Ernährung und Hygiene genügen (Serie 26 und 37). Auch die Spondylitis tuberculosa der Frau (Serie 43) kam zur Ausheilung, obwohl lediglich eine kurze Liege- und Stützkorsettbehandlung geschah. — Sind die humoralen Einflüsse eines heilstrebigen Körpers die Voraussetzung der Heilung, so kommt den örtlichen Gewebsverhältnissen die größte Bedeutung dafür zu, ob eine Restitutio ad integrum erreicht wird, oder eine Defektheilung mit fortbestehenden Schlupfwinkeln tuberkulösen Granulationsgewebes. Von diesen kann noch nach Jahren eine Gefahr für den Organismus ausgehen. Wir können erwarten, daß eine rein synoviale Gelenktuberkulose anatomisch und funktionell die besten Heilungsaussichten gibt, müssen aber auch mit der Möglichkeit rechnen, daß der Prozeß auf den Knorpel übergreift, ihn zerstört und dann mit Versteifung des Gelenkes (Serie 27) ausheilt. *Günstig liegen auch reine Knochenherde,* das tuberkulöse Granulationsgewebe wird durch gesunden, wohl strukturierten Knochen vollständig ersetzt. So führte der große, die Wachstumsfuge durchsetzende Herd am Kniegelenk (Serie 26) und ebenso am Oberarm (Serie 37) zu einer idealen Ausheilung mit Wiederherstellung der geschädigten Epiphysenfuge. Nicht immer aber ist die anatomische Heilung der Tuberkulose restlos erfolgt, wenn der Kranke auch klinisch geheilt erscheint. *Die Gewebsverhältnisse prädisponieren bei den ulcerösen Gelenktuberkulosen zum Fortbestehen von Schlupfwinkeln,* welche lebendige Tuberkelbazillen beherbergen. In einem Bezirk von Knorpelresten und Narben kann leicht ein spezifisches Granulationsgewebe abgekapselt werden. So erleben wir es, daß kleine Prozesse noch nach vielen Jahren sogar im Röntgenbild den Zustand einer unvollständigen Ausheilung erkennen lassen. Das gilt z. B. für die Schulter der Serie 38. Auch die klinische Heilung der Kniegelenktuberkulose (Serie 28), welche durch konservative Behandlung erreicht war, erwies sich bei einer späteren Obduktion nicht als anatomisch vollständig geheilt, wie etwa im Falle der Gelenkresektion (Serie 29). *Die Vorgänge der Defektheilung sind verschiedener Art.* Der tuberkulös erkrankte Hüftkopf (Serie 33) wurde nicht nur zerstört, sondern auch restlos resorbiert, als ob er abgesägt und entfernt worden wäre. Oft aber werden so reine anatomische Zustände nicht erreicht. Gewöhnlich erfolgt die Heilung erst dann, wenn das gefäßlose, reaktionsschwache Knorpel- und Synovialisgewebe vernichtet sind, so daß sich breite Knochenflächen berühren, welche einer stärkeren Reaktion fähig sind. Das geschieht gewöhnlich bei der Ausheilung des Hüftgelenkes mit Pfannenwanderung (Serien 31 und 32) und bei der Wirbeltuberkulose mit Gibbusbildung (Serien 43 und 44).

Immer beansprucht die Heilung eines tuberkulösen Knochenprozesses eine lange Zeit, oft auch bei kleinen Herden, wie z. B. am Finger (Serie 42) oder Handgelenk (Serie 41). So wird auch heute noch ein chirurgisches Eingreifen gegebenenfalls sicherer und schneller die Heilung, d. h. die Fortnahme der erkrankten Stelle, herbeiführen. Das geschieht bei gelenknahen Herden (Serie 40), um einen Einbruch in das Gelenk zu verhüten, oder bei fortgeschrittenen Prozessen, wenn eine Defektheilung — Versteifung — unabwendbar ist. Ahmt doch die Natur gewissermaßen chirurgische Maßnahmen nach, wenn sie den Hüftkopf (Serie 33) gradlinig absetzt und restlos entfernt, oder einen Herd im Humerus glättet, als ob er ausgemeißelt wäre (Serie 37).

Chapter II.

Chronic Specific Inflammation.

A. Tuberculosis of Joints.

A circumscribed area of erosion, without coincident attempt to repair the damage, is characteristic of tuberculosis of bones and joints and its prognosis. The cure at the best, is a patching together of inferior material. Healing power depends upon two factors, namely the resistance of the body and the condition of the local tissue. When other organs such as the lungs or kidneys, are seriously diseased, the healing power of joint affections is very seriously impaired. The shoulder-joint (Series 39) or the foot-joints (Series 30) show the unarrestable and progressive degeneration under these circumstances. The power of resistance must be increased throughout the whole body before a cure can be established. We have an example of this in the magnificent results of sun treatment for bone and joint tuberculosis, which is carried out in Switzerland. Children are more easily influenced than adults. Indeed, even ill nourished children can be cured by proper food, correct hygiene and good nursing. (Series 26 and 37.) The woman (Series 43) who suffered from tuberculous spondylitis was also cured, although she had to undergo short recumbent treatment and wear a supporting corset in addition. Presuming that the cure is dependant upon the humoral influences of the body endeavouring to overcome the disease, then it depends upon the condition of the local tissue as to whether complete recovery is obtained or, whether an incomplete result may endanger the patient's life for many years by the formation of nooks and crannies of tuberculous granulation tissue. We may take it for granted that a genuine tubercular condition of the synovial membrane has exceptionally good healing capabilities, both functionally and anatomically, but we must also consider the possibility of the process attacking and destroying cartilage, which would only cause healing with subsequent stiffness of the joint (Series 27). The prognosis for genuine tuberculous bone and joint areas is, as a rule, favourable because the tuberculous granulation tissue is repaired by healthy well constructed bone. The extensive process which involved the epiphysis at the knee-joint (Series 26), healed in an ideal manner with regeneration of the injured epiphyseal area. The anatomical healing however, is not always as complete as this, even when the patient appears to be clinically cured. In ulcerative joint tuberculosis, the tissue condition affords hiding places for the tubercle bacilli, which may exist for many years. Specific granulation tissue may be found as a scar in an area of cartilage remains and other scars. Sometimes after many years, we are able to recognize the incomplete healing of a small process, in a Röntgen picture (e. g. in the shoulder — Series 38). The clinical healing of the tuberculous knee joint (Series 28) which was obtained by conservative treatment, showed during an examination which followed amputation how imperfect the anatomical healing had been. This was also the case in the joint resection seen in series 29.

The changes which occur prior to defective healing are numerous. The tuberculous head of the femur (Series 33) was not only destroyed, but was entirely resorbed, just as if it had been sawn off and removed. It often happens though that such a clean anatomical condition is not obtained. Generally speaking, only after destruction of the bloodless, weakly resisting cartilage and synovial tissue, which thus permits the apposition of the bone surfaces, does the healing commence, because they are then more capable of a sturdy reaction. The healing of the hip-joint accompanied by acetabular ,,wandering" (Series 31—32) usually takes this course and this is also the case with tuberculosis of the vertebrae with gibbus formation (Series 43—44).

The healing of tuberculous conditions in bone always takes a long time, even when such small areas as the finger (Series 42) or the wrist-joint (Series 41) are involved. At the present time, removal of the affected part by operation is the quickest and most effective way of promoting healing. This is done when the infection approaches a joint (Series 40) in order to prevent the joint becoming involved. Resection is also preferred in advanced cases, when defective healing (absolute stiffness) is inevitable. When nature removes the femoral head as cleanly as if it had been sawn off (Series 23) and causes it to be entirely absorbed, or levels an area in the humerus as if it had been chiselled out (Series 37), she is merely imitating surgery.

Serie 26.

Fistelnde fungöse Kniegelenk-tuberkulose.

Bei dem 9jähr. Mädchen bestand seit mehreren Monaten eine schmerzhafte derbe Anschwellung des Kniegelenkes, die 3 Fisteln aufwies und mit Fieber einherging. Auf konservative Behandlung (lediglich Röntgenbestrahlung und Hygiene des Krankenhauses) kam der ausgedehnte Krankheitsprozeß in kurzer Zeit zur Heilung.

$^2/_3$ n. Gr.   1 a.

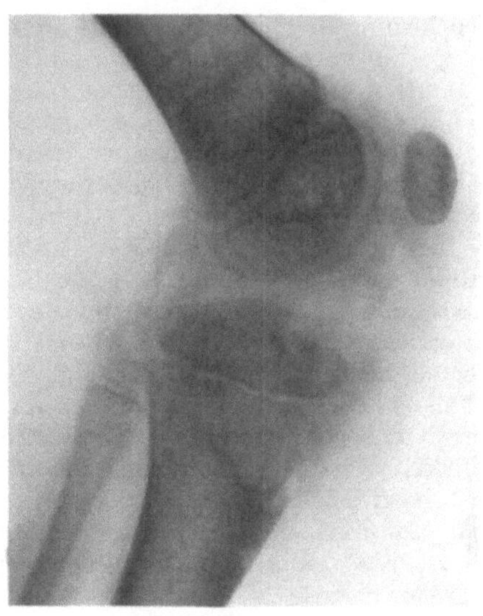

1 b.

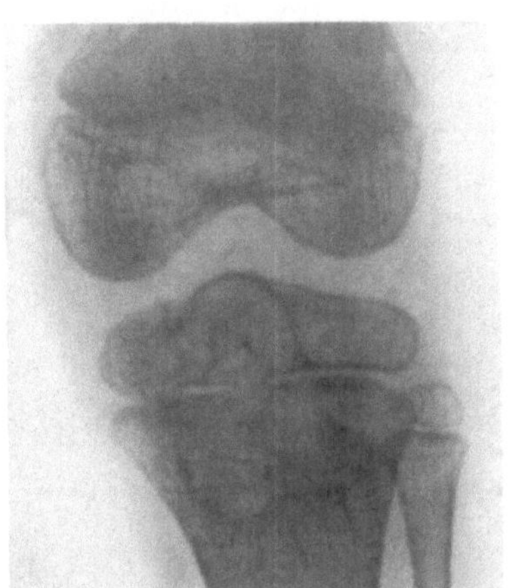

Zustand des Gelenkes etwa $^1/_2$ Jahr nach Beginn der Erkrankung: Außer dem Gelenkfungus der große tuberkulöse Herd der Tibia, welcher die Epiphysenfuge durchsetzt und fast in das Gelenk eingebrochen ist.

Condition of joint about 6 months after commencement of illness. In addition to the joint fungus, the large tuberculous area of the tibia which penetrates into the epiphyseal line, has almost broken into the joint.

Series 26.

Fistulous Fungus of the Knee-Joint.

The nine year old girl suffered for several months with a painful swelling of the knee-joint, which presented 3 fistulae and which was accompanied by fever. The extension of the disease was prevented by conservative treatment (simple Röntgen-rays and hospital hygiene).

2 a.

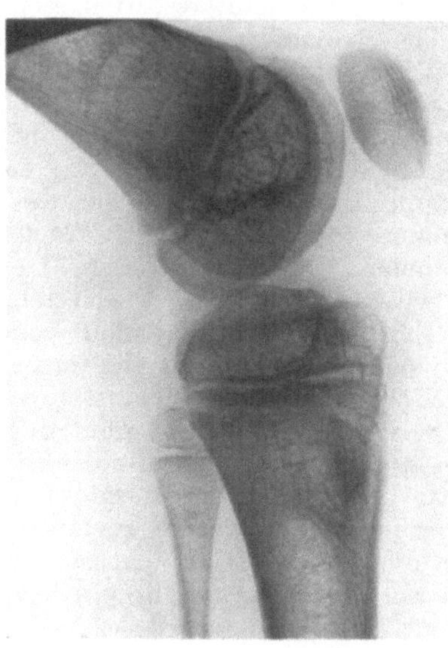

2 b.

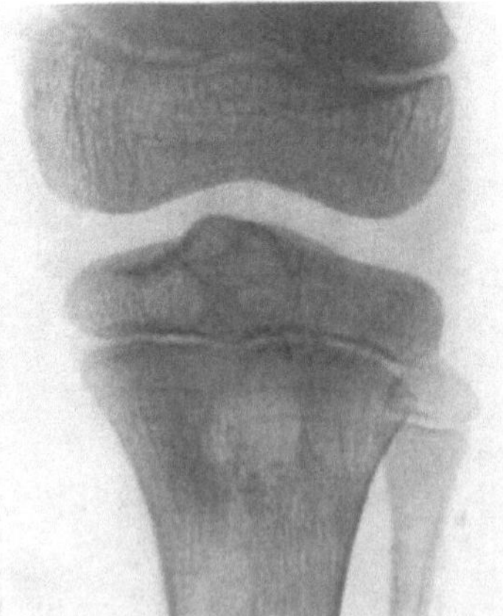

Nach einem weiteren halben Jahr ist der Herd durch Knochen ersetzt, das Wachstum in keiner Weise beeinträchtigt, das Gelenk klinisch geheilt.

6 months later the area is replaced by bone; growth in no way influenced; the joint clinically cured.

Serie 26.

3 a.

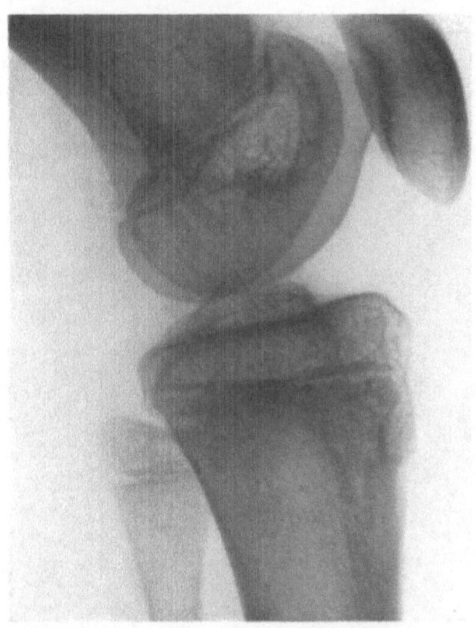

3 b.

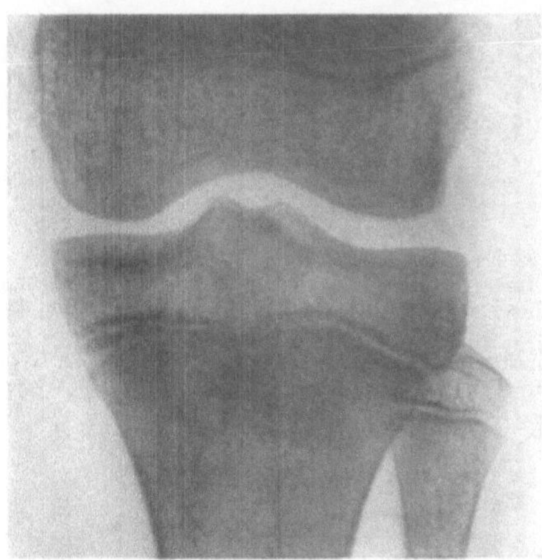

3 Jahre später ist am Knochen nichts mehr von der Erkrankung festzustellen, sein Wachstum trotz einstmaliger Beteiligung der Epiphysenfuge unvermindert fortgeschritten.

3 years later the bone shows no trace of the disease. The growth is undiminished, despite the former involvement of the epiphyseal line.

Series 27.

Serie 27.

Primär-synoviale Kniegelenk-tuberkulose.

Der 13 jähr. Knabe war ganz schleichend mit einer schmerzhaften Schwellung des Kniegelenkes erkrankt. Deswegen wurde er 2 Jahre klinisch mit Sonnen- und Stauungsbehandlung sowie vorübergehend mit Gipsverbänden behandelt, wodurch der Krankheitsprozeß nicht aufgehalten werden konnte, sondern eine deutliche Verschlimmerung zeigte. Dann geschah therapeutisch nichts mehr und es kam zu einer völligen Ausheilung der Tuberkulose, allerdings mit einer knöchernen Versteifung des Gelenkes.

Series 27.

Primary Synovial Tuberculosis of the Knee-Joint.

The 13 year old boy was affected by a very gradual and painful swelling of the knee-joint. For this reason he received for two years, clinical sun and ligature treatment and transiently, plaster of Paris bandages, by which however the process of disease was not arrested. On the contrary the illness became distinctly worse. Then treatment was suspended and the tuberculosis was completely cured, though ossification of the joint remained.

$^6/_{10}$ n. Gr.　　　　1.　　　　　　　　　2.

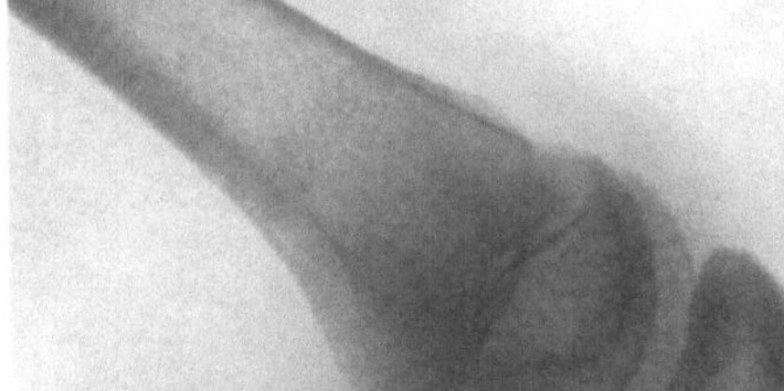

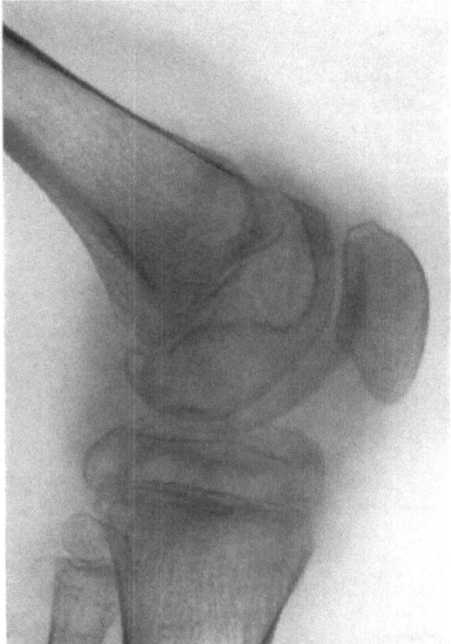

Fungus des Kniegelenkes etwa 5 Wochen nach Beginn der Erkrankung ohne Ergriffensein des Knochens.

Fungus of the knee-joint about 5 weeks after commencement of illness. Bone not affected.

Nach 1 Jahr ist der objektive Befund etwa unverändert, nur die Knochenatrophie stärker.

After one year the actual condition is scarcely altered; only the bone atrophy has increased.

Serie 27.

3.

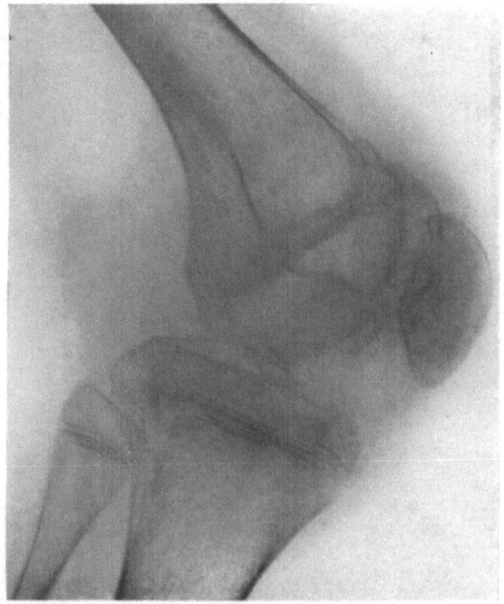

4.

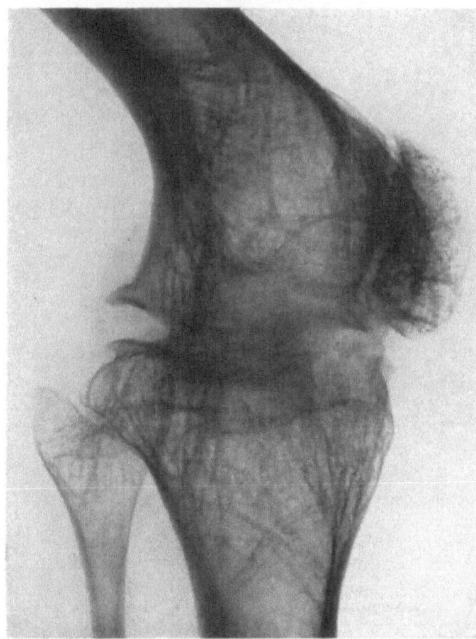

Nach 2 Jahren hat der Zerstörungsprozeß auf die knorpeligen Gelenkflächen übergegriffen und bietet das Bild eines schweren tuberkulösen Fungus.

After two years the process of destruction had spread over the cartilaginous joint surface, showing a serious tuberculous fungus.

Vollständige Ausheilung mit knöcherner Ankylose, die nach den klinischen Daten in etwa einem weiteren Jahr erreicht war und als Endzustand (etwa 11 Jahre später) im Bild festgehalten wurde.

Complete cure with bony ankylosis in about one year according to clinical dates. Final condition in picture (about 11 years later).

Serie 28.

Fungöse Kniegelenktuberkulose.

Trotz frühzeitiger Behandlung kam es bei dem 22jähr. Mädchen schnell zu einer hochgradigen Zerstörung der Gelenkflächen und nach 3jähr. Aufenthalt im Hochgebirge zur klinischen Heilung bei völliger Versteifung des Gelenkes.

$^2/_3$ n. Gr.   1.

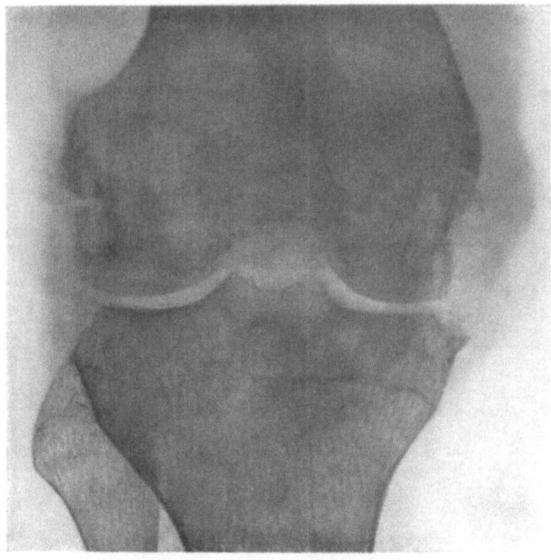

Etwa $^1/_4$ Jahr nach Beginn der Erkrankung: Fungus mit beginnender Usurierung der Gelenkflächen.

About 3 months after commencement of illness: fungus with beginning erosion of the joint surfaces.

Series 28.

Fungoid Tuberculosis of the Knee-Joint.

Girl, 22 years of age. Despite early treatment, intensive destruction of the joint surfaces set in rapidly. After 3 years sojourn in the mountains a cure was effected but the joint remained absolutely stiff.

2.

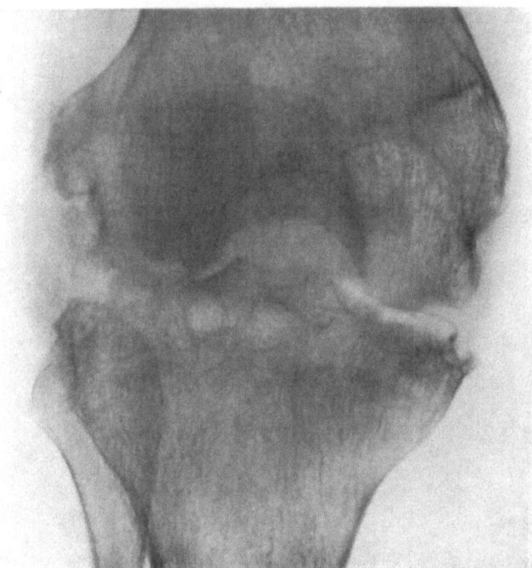

$^1/_2$ Jahr später trotz Gipsverband und Röntgenbestrahlung hochgradige Zerstörung der Gelenkflächen.

Six months later despite plaster of Paris bandages and Röntgen irradiation treatment, intensive destruction of the joint surfaces.

Serie 28.

3.

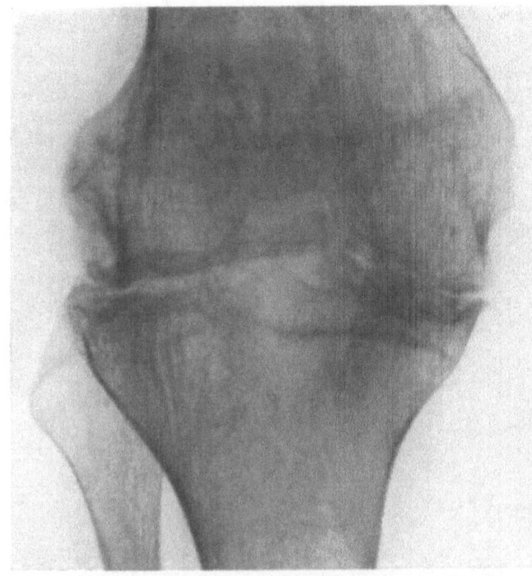

Nach 2 jähr. Sonnenbehandlung im Hochgebirge
Ausheilung im Gang: Die Glättung der Konturen.

After two years sun treatment in the mountains,
cure in progress: Contour becoming smooth.

4.

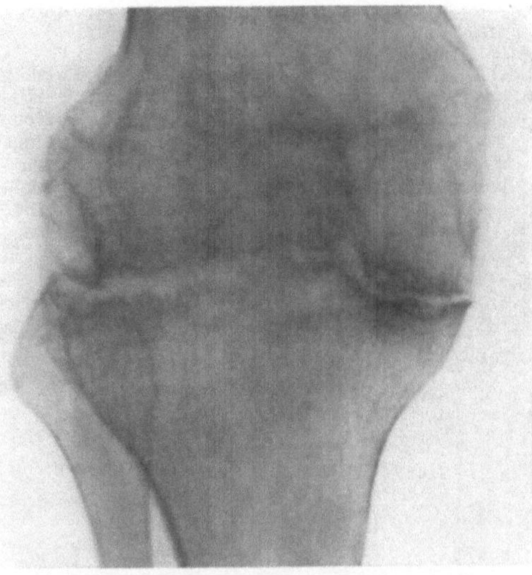

Nach einem weiteren Jahr sind die zerstörten Gelenkflächen noch mehr ausgeflickt und geglättet.

After another year the destroyed joint surfaces are
further restored and smoothed.

5.

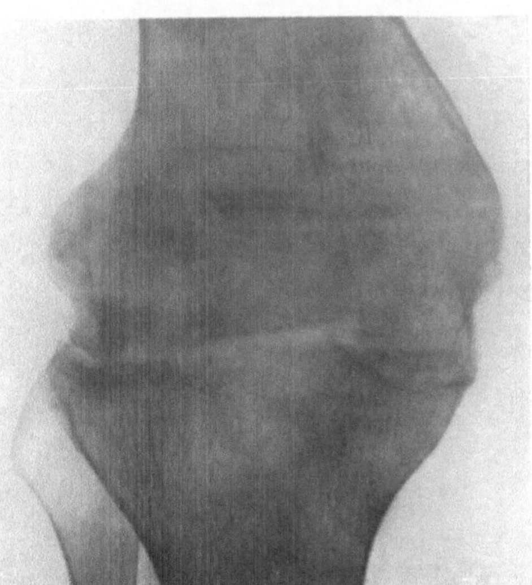

Endzustand nach 6 Jahren (klinisch mit völliger Versteifung geheilt).
Final condition after 6 years (clinically cured with complete stiffness).

Serie 29.

Fistelnde fungöse Kniegelenk-
tuberkulose.

Das Leiden stellte sich bei dem 22 jährigen Mädchen
im 19. Lebensjahr ein und erfuhr trotz der Behandlung im letzten halben Jahre eine erhebliche
Verschlimmerung; es bestand ein Gelenkfungus
mit 4 Fisteln und Absceßdurchbruch in die Knie-
kehle sowie zum Oberschenkel. Die Resektion
beseitigte die Tuberkulose des Knochens, führte
rasch die Ausheilung herbei, das Mädchen
blühte auf.

$^2/_3$ n. Gr.   1.

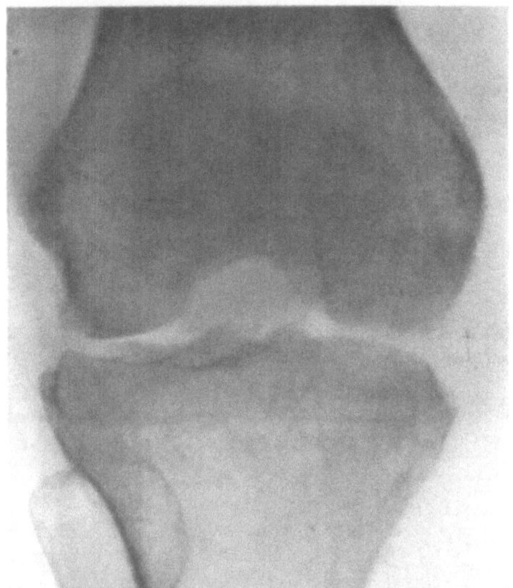

Schwere Zerstörung der Gelenkflächen.

Severe destruction of the joint surfaces.

Series 29.

Fistulous Fungoid Tuberculosis
of the Knee-Joint.

The illness began when the girl was in her nine-
teenth year. In spite of continual treatment for
three years she had become considerably worse
during the last six months. There was a joint
fungus with four fistulae present and abscesses
had broken through in the knee and upper-leg.
Resection removed the bone tuberculosis. The
recovery was rapid and the girl became perfectly
healthy.

2.

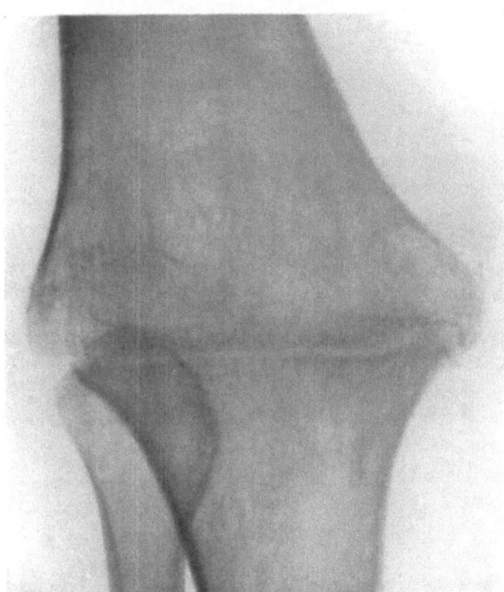

Befund nach der Resektion.

Condition after the resection.

Serie 29.

3.

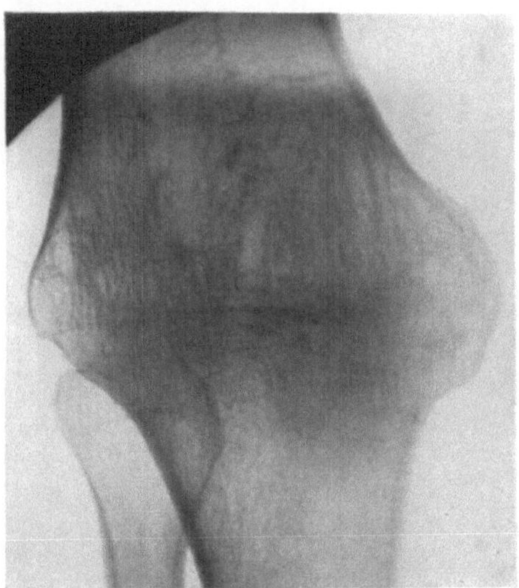

Nach 1¹/₂ Jahren sind die beiden Knochen fest
verwachsen.

After one year and a half. Both bones are
firmly united.

4.

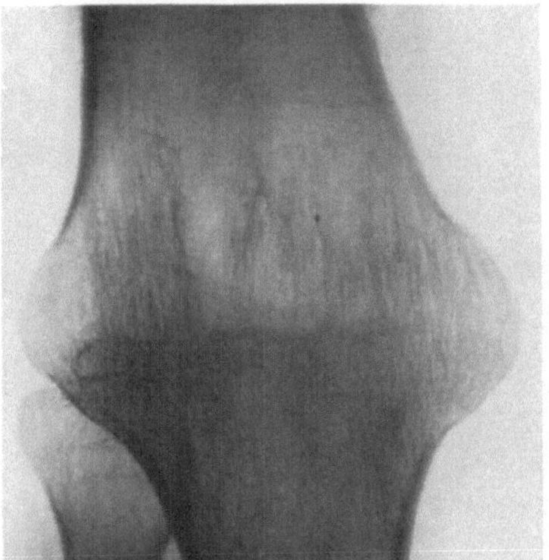

Nach 4 Jahren beweist die feine Bälkchenstruktur
noch deutlicher als schon früher die sichere
Ausheilung des tuberkulösen Prozesses.

After four years. The delicate beam structure
shows still more plainly how complete is the cure.

Serie 30.

Fußgelenktuberkulose.

Der 30jährige Mann litt an Lungen- und Nierentuberkulose. Etwa ³/₄ Jahr vor seinem Tode wurde auch ein Fußgelenk ergriffen: Die primär synoviale Entzündung griff rasch zerstörend auf den Knochen über, nachdem dieser extrem entkalkt und die Widerstandskraft des Organismus gebrochen war.

³/₄ n. Gr.   1.

Series 30.

Foot-Joint Tuberculosis.

A man thirty years of age suffered with tuberculosis of the lungs and kidneys. About nine months previous to his death the foot-joint was attacked. The primary synovial inflammation speedily destroyed the bones as they were almost chalkless and the power of resistance broken down.

2.

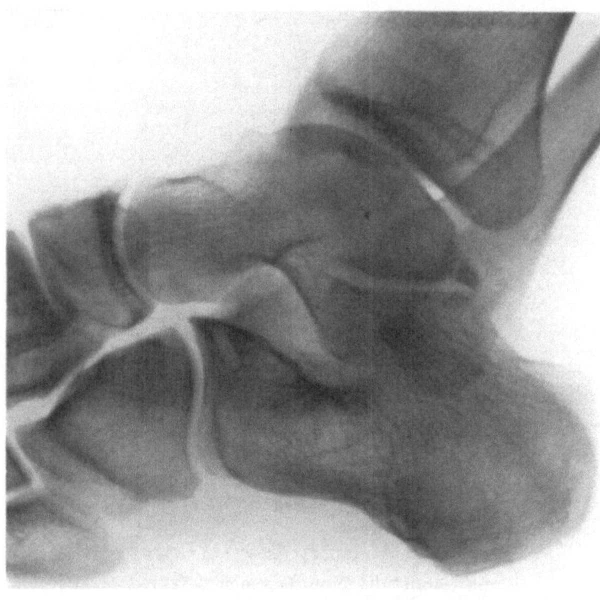

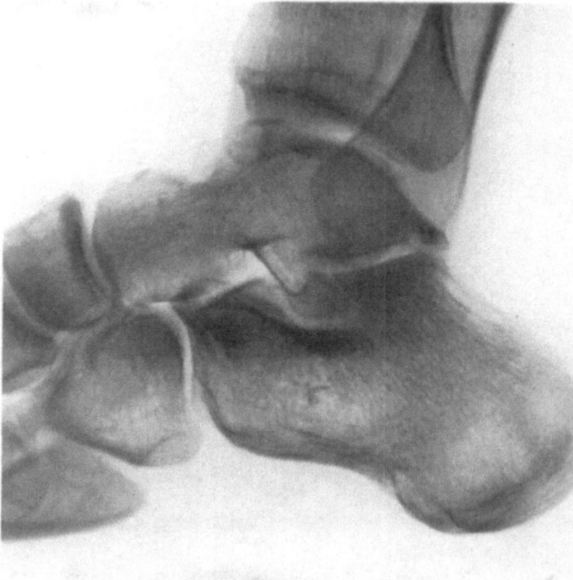

4 Wochen nach Beginn der Weichteilschwellung ist der Knochen noch völlig intakt.

Four weeks after the beginning of swelling of fleshy part, the bone is still quite intact.

2 Monate später ist eine beginnende Knochenatrophie festzustellen.

Two months later, the commencement of bone atrophy is noticeable.

Serie 30.

3.

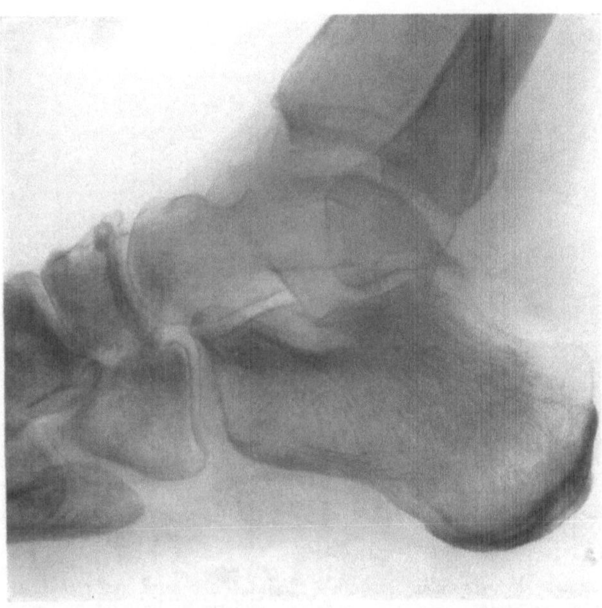

4.

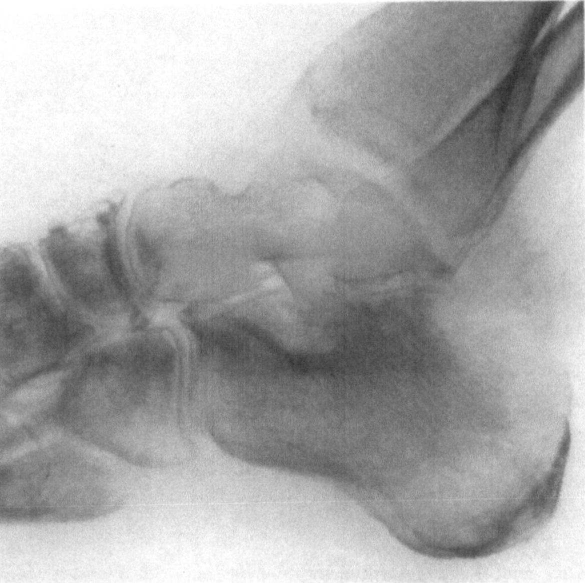

Nach weiteren 2 Monaten hat der *Kalkschwund* insbesondere am Talus erheblich zugenommen.

After another two months, the decalcification particularly at the talus, has considerably increased.

Noch 2 Monate später — kurz vor dem Tode — hat bereits ein Zerfall der Gelenkenden, der Tibia und des Talus, eingesetzt; die Kalkverarmung ist noch weiter fortgeschritten.

Again two months later, just before death. The joint surfaces of the tibia and talus are already destroyed; the decalcification has increased.

Serie 31.

Tuberkulöse Hüftgelenkentzündung.

Die tuberkulöse Entzündung des Hüftgelenkes griff von
einem kleinen Herd der Pfanne rasch auf den Schenkelkopf
über und kam trotz fortgesetzter Behandlung (ruhigstellende
Verbände, Röntgen- und Sonnenbestrahlung) erst zur Ausheilung, als das ganze Gelenk zerstört und verödet war;
der Prozeß machte erst nach 4 Jahren nagender Zerstörung
an „typischer Stelle" Halt, nachdem er den frisch aus-
sehenden Knaben im 5. Lebensjahr befallen hatte.

Series 31.

Tuberculous Inflammation of Hip-Joint.

The tuberculous inflammation of hip-joint spread rapidly
from a small area in the socket to the femur-head and in
spite of constant treatment (bandage, Röntgen-ray and
sun) it was not arrested until the entire joint was destroyed.
The afflicted patient was a healthy looking boy of five
years of age and the eroding destruction at "typical site"
continued for four years.

³/₄ n. Gr.   1.   2.   3.

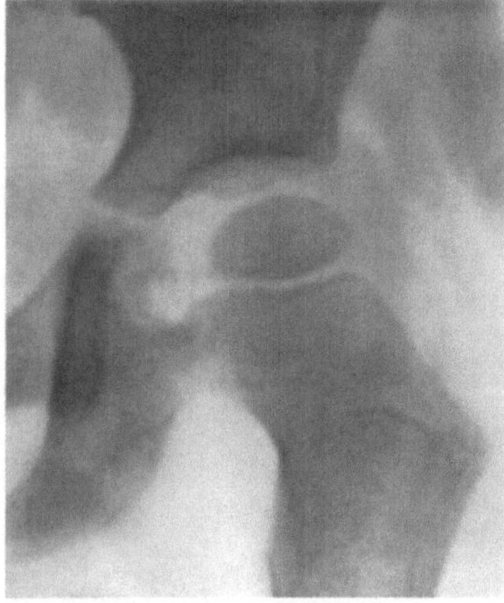 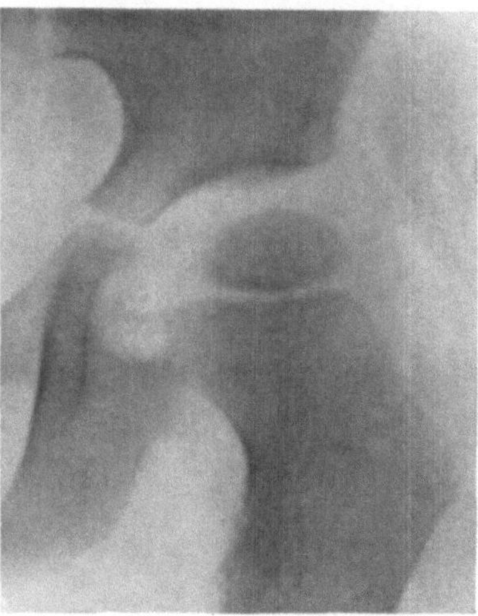 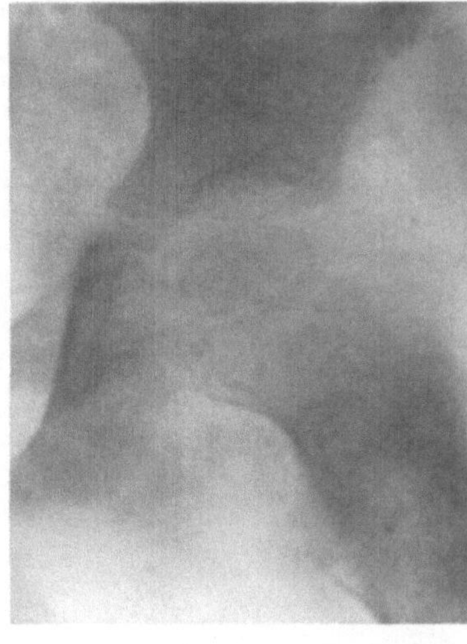

Kurz nach Beginn der Beschwerden ist ein
kleiner Herd der Gelenkpfanne nachweisbar.

Shortly after commencement of complaint
a *small tuberculous area in the acetabulum*
can be seen.

3 Wochen später ist dieser tuberkulöse
Herd bereits größer geworden.

Three weeks later, the area has already
become larger.

Nach 2 Monaten ist auch der *Gelenkko-*
ergriffen: hochgradig kalkverarmt und
angefressen.

After two months, the *joint-head is al.*
attacked; extensively eroded and
decalcified.

Serie 31.

4.

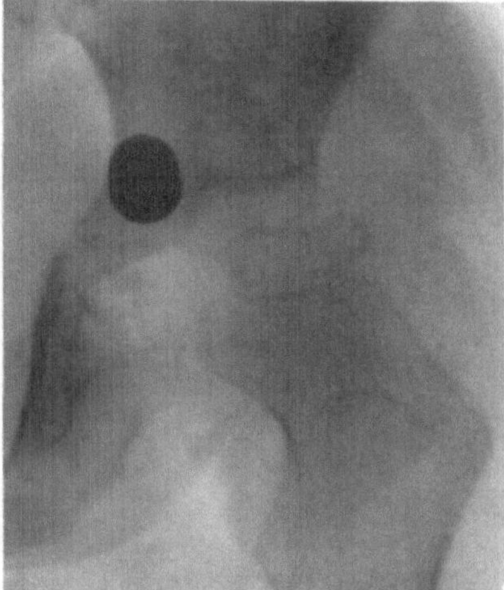

Nach 4 Monaten hat sich die Zerstörung der Pfanne weiter ausgedehnt und die Kopfepiphyse ist zusammengeschrumpft.

After four months, the destruction of the socket has spread and the epiphyseal head has shrunk.

5.

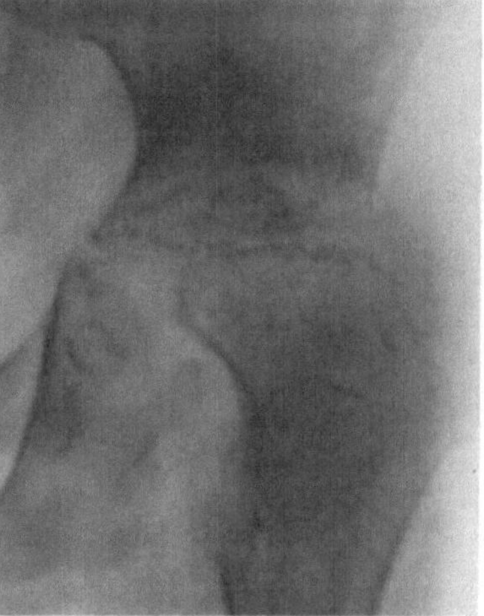

Nach 1 ¼ Jahr ist die *Kopfepiphyse gelöst* und *abgeglitten*, die *Pfanne* noch mehr *gewandert*.

After fifteen months, the *head epiphysis has loosened and slipped off*, the socket has "wandered" further.

6.

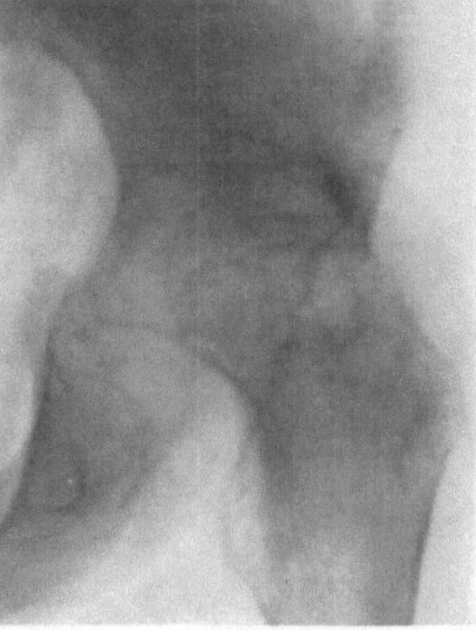

Nach 1 ½ Jahren *scheint die knöcherne Verwachsung* der Wandflächen die Ausheilung des tuberkulösen Prozesses *zu beginnen*.

After a year and a half, the *bony growth* of the wound-surfaces *appears to be the commencement* of the healing process.

7.

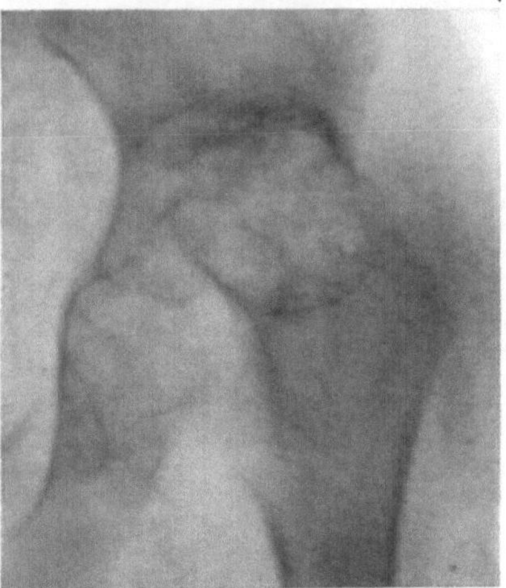

Nach 2 ¾ Jahren aber ist — trotz sachgemäßer Therapie — die *Gelenkpfanne wieder noch mehr darmbeinwärts ausgenagt und von Schenkelkopf und -hals nur noch ein Schatten vorhanden.*

After two years and three quarters, despite correct treatment, the *socket is still more eroded towards the ilium and only a shadow of head and neck of the femur remains.*

8.

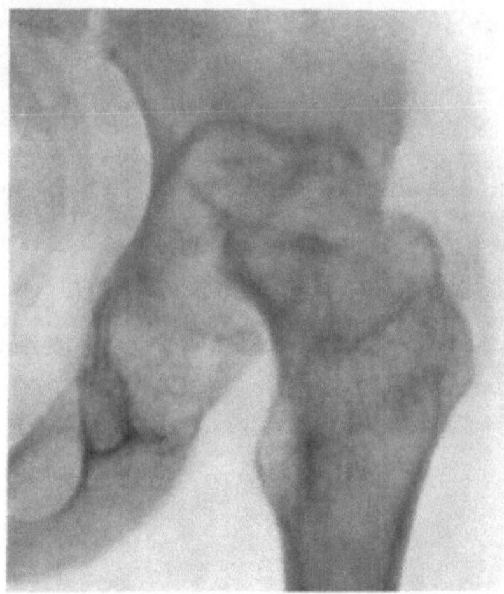

Nach 3 ¾ Jahren zeigt die *gute Knochenstruktur der Ankylose* die endlich eintretende Heilung.

After three years and three quarters, *the good bone structure of the ankylosis* shows that healing has at last begun.

Serie 32.

Tuberkulöse Hüftgelenkentzündung.

Das Leiden begann schon im 2. Lebensjahr und begleitete den Knaben, bis im 10. Jahr der Krankheitsprozeß schließlich ausgeheilt war. Aller Therapie zum Trotz erfolgte die Heilung der Gelenktuberkulose nach anfänglicher Besserung erst, als das ganze Gelenk zerstört war, und zwar mit knöcherner Ankylose. Dabei war die Entwicklung des Kindes gut.

Series 32.

Hip-Joint Tuberculosis.

The illness began at the age of two and lasted until the boy was ten years of age when it was at last cured. Despite all treatment and a slight improvement at first, the disease was only arrested after the entire joint had been destroyed — moreover with ossified ankylosis. The development of the child progressed well.

$^{6}/_{10}$ n. Gr.   1.   2.   3.

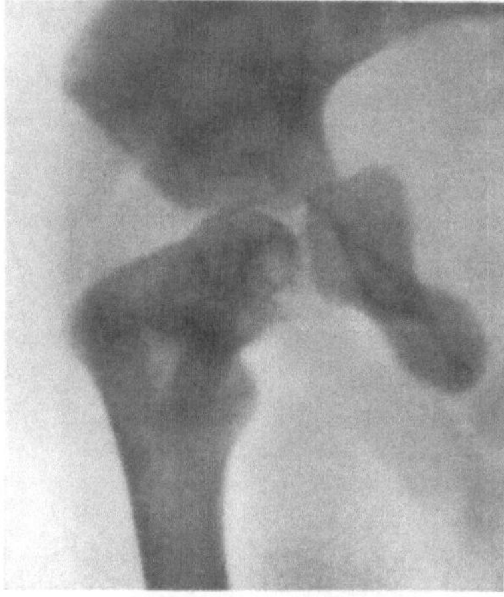 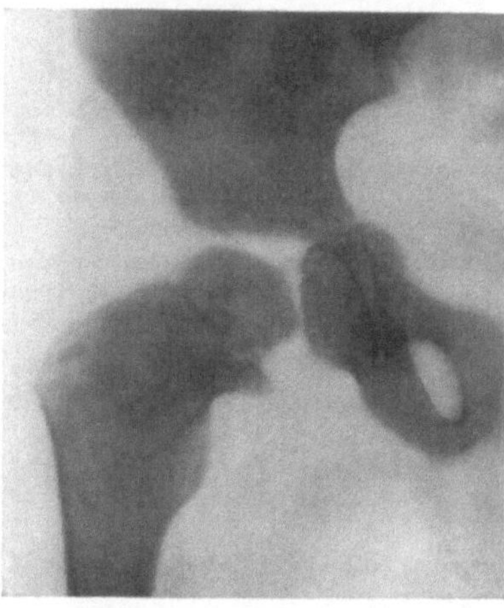 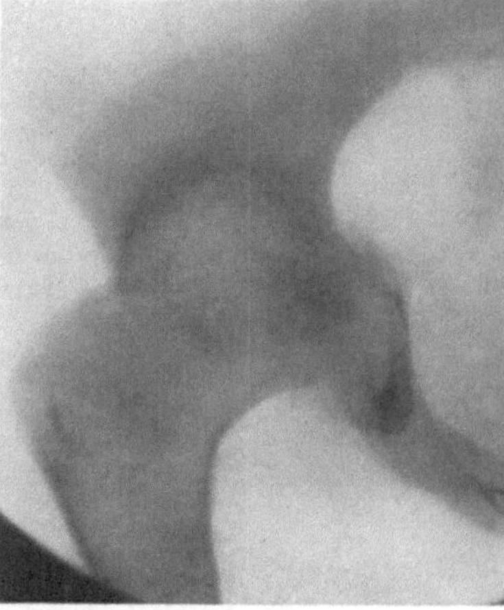

Lebensalter: $2^{1}/_{2}$ Jahre.
Es besteht ein gelenknaher tuberkulöser *Knochenherd* am Oberschenkel (in Höhe der Rollhügel).

Two and a half years of age:
A tuberculous bone process exists near the joint, on a level with the trochanter of the femur.

4 Jahre.
Der Knochenherd scheint ausgeheilt und das Hüftgelenk selbst zeigt keine pathologischen Veränderungen.

Four years of age:
The affected area appears to have healed and the hip-joint shows no pathological alteration.

$5^{1}/_{2}$ Jahre.
Überraschend weit fortgeschrittene Zerstörung des Gelenkes: die Pfanne ist eingebrochen und „gewandert", der Kopf abgeglitten und in Auflösung begriffen.

Five and a half years of age:
Amazingly advanced destruction of the joint: The acetabulum has broken in and „wandered". The head has slipped off in dissolution.

Serie 32.

4.

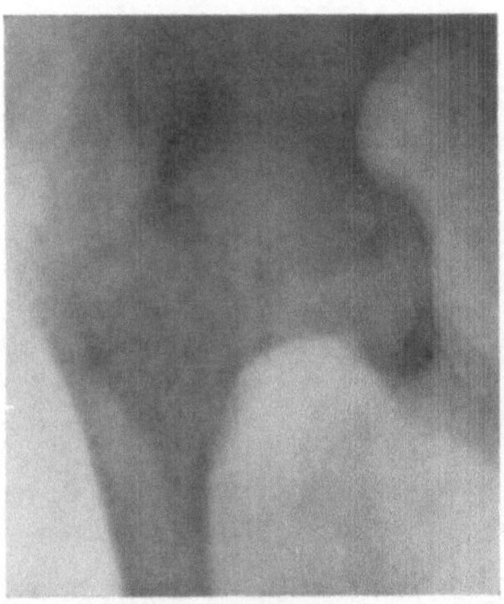

6 Jahre.
Der Zerfall der Gelenkenden hat den
Höhepunkt erreicht.

Six years of age:
The destruction of joint surfaces has
reached its height.

5.

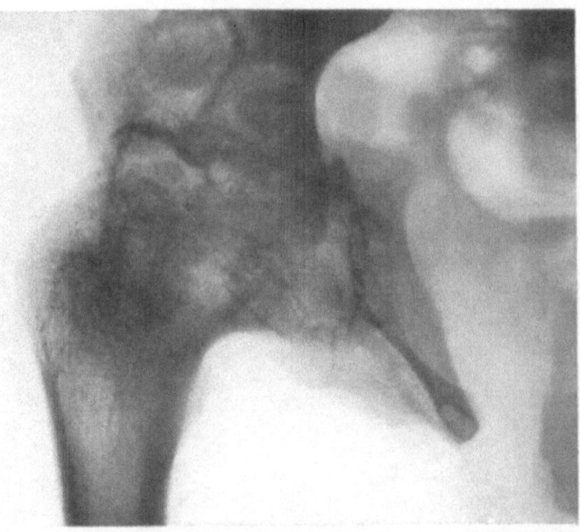

10 Jahre.
Die ausgenagte Gelenkpfanne ist mit dem Schenkelhalsstumpf knöchern verwachsen, die kranke Beckenhälfte
im Wachstum (s. die Symphyse) stark zurückgeblieben.

Ten years of age: The eroded acetabulum has become
joined to the femur-neck stump by ossification, the
affected half of the pelvis (the symphysis) remained very
undeveloped.

Serie 33.

Tuberkulöse Hüftgelenkentzündung.

Der 19jährige Mann trat etwa $^1/_2$ Jahr nach Beginn seines Hüftleidens in klinische Behandlung. Damals war die Hüfte bereits versteift und das Röntgenbild zeigte eine ausgedehnte Zerstörung. Der tuberkulöse Gelenkprozeß heilte unter zeitweisen entlastenden Verbänden langsam in der Weise aus, daß der Schenkelkopf zerstört bzw. aufgelöst und *vollständig resorbiert,* die zerfressene Pfanne solide knöchern geflickt wurde. — Die Hüfte war steif, nicht schmerzhaft. In der Zwischenzeit aber mußte der Kranke wegen verkäsender Nebenhodentuberkulose operiert werden.

$^6/_{10}$ n. Gr.   1.

Series 33.

Tuberculous Hip-Joint Inflammation.

A young man of nineteen had been troubled with his hip for about six months before he sought clinical treatment. By that time the hip had already become stiff and the Röntgen picture showed extensive destruction. The tuberculous joint process was very slow, the femur head was destroyed, dissolved and entirely *resorbed.* Supporting bandages were used, the eroded socket became fairly well patched with bone. The hip was stiff but not painful. In the meantime the patient had to undergo an operation for cheesy tuberculosis of the epididymis.

       2.

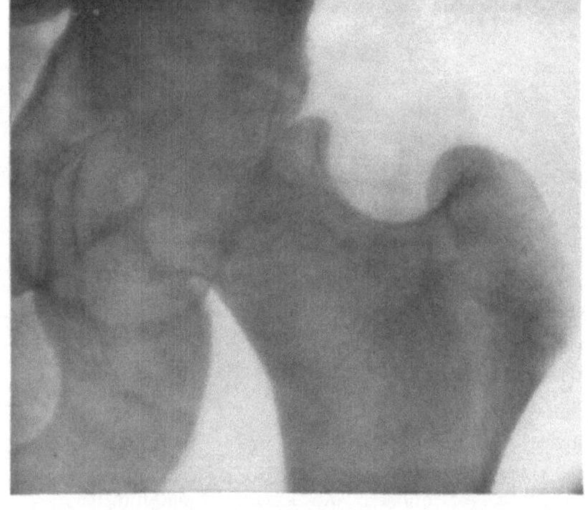

$^1/_2$ Jahr nach Beginn der Beschwerden besteht schon eine fortgeschrittene Caries: der Pfannenrand ist angenagt, *der Kopf kalkarm, geschrumpft und zerlöchert.* — Ein freier Gelenkspalt ist nicht mehr vorhanden.

Six months after commencement of illness. Advanced caries already exists, the acetabular edge eroded and the *head is decalcified, shrunken and perforated.* A free joint cleft no longer exists.

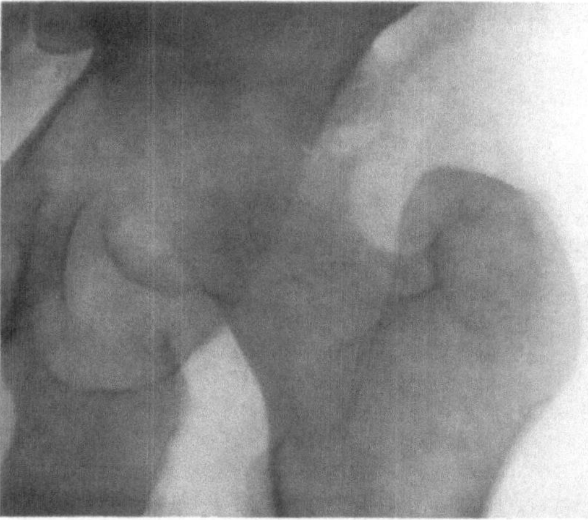

1 Jahr später ist die Pfanne weiter „gewandert", der Kopf gleichmäßig kleiner geworden und noch mehr entkalkt.

One year later. The acetabulum has "wandered" further, the head has become uniformly smaller and the decalcification greater.

Serie 33.

3.

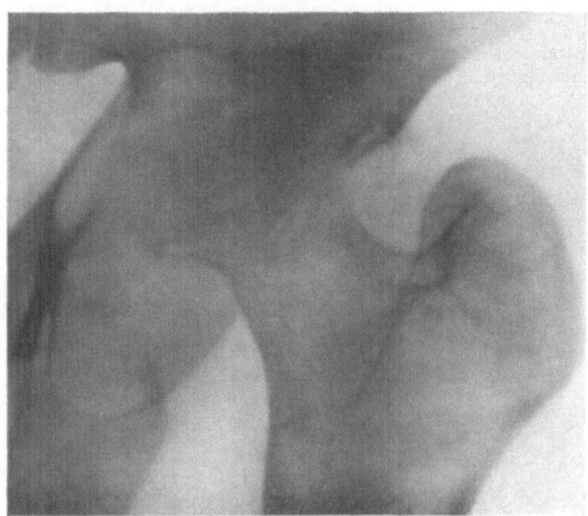

Nach 2 Jahren ist die „Caries sicca“ des
Schenkelkopfes noch fortgeschritten.

After two years. The "caries sicca" of the
femur-head has advanced.

4.

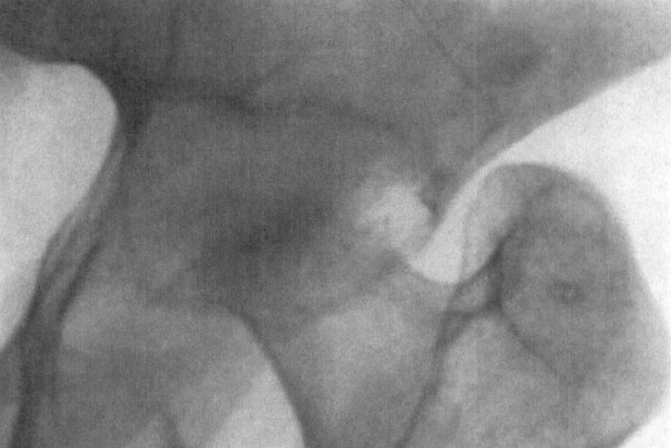

Nach 3 Jahren sind nur noch *schattenhafte
Umrisse des Gelenkkopfes* erkennbar.

After three years. Only *faint shadowy outlines
of the joint-head* are recognizable.

5.

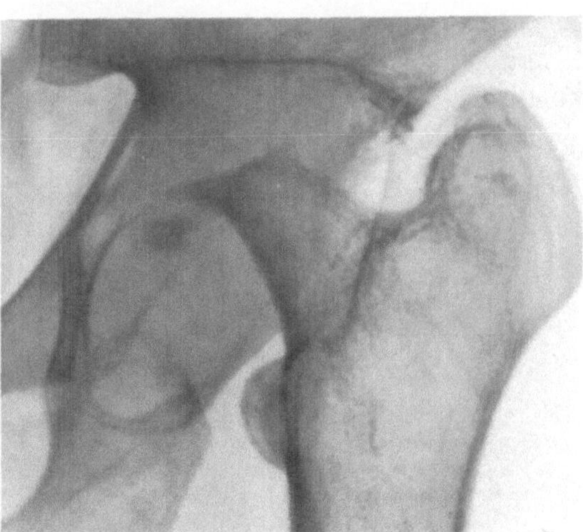

Nach 5 Jahren *fehlt der Schenkelkopf ganz* und der Schenkelhals ist ein glatter Stumpf, als wenn er abgesägt wäre. —
Die ausgenagte Gelenkpfanne zeigt überall feine Knochenstruktur.

After five years. The *femur-head is missing entirely* and the femur-neck is a smooth stump, as smooth as if it had
been sawn off. The eroded socket shows fine bone-structure everywhere.

Serie 34.

Tuberkulöse
Hüftgelenkentzündung.

Das Hüftleiden des 20jährigen Mannes begann schleichend, verlief fieberfrei und heilte mit Versteifung. Wegen bestehender Drüsentuberkulose wurde eine tuberkulöse Hüftgelenkentzündung angenommen. — Ein Kapselprozeß ohne Beteiligung des Knochens, im Röntgenbild ohne charakteristisches Gepräge.

Series 34.

Tuberculous
Hip-Joint Inflammation.

A twenty year old man had hip-disease. It progressed very slowly, ran its course without fever and resulted in stiffness. As the patient had tuberculous glands it was concluded that the hip-joint inflammation was tuberculous also. It was a capsular process without involvement of the bone and there were no characteristic signs in the X-ray picture.

$^6/_{10}$ n. Gr.   1.   2.

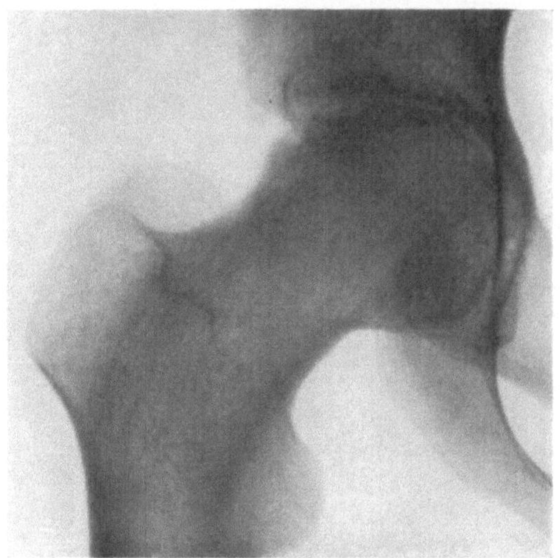

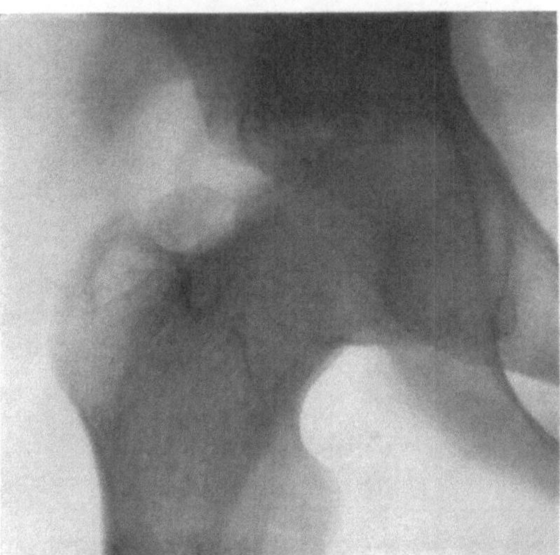

Der Gelenkspalt ist verschmälert und unscharf.
The joint cleft has narrowed and is not distinct.

$^1/_4$ Jahr später sind die Gelenkumrisse ausgelöscht.
Three months later. The joint outlines have disappeared.

3.

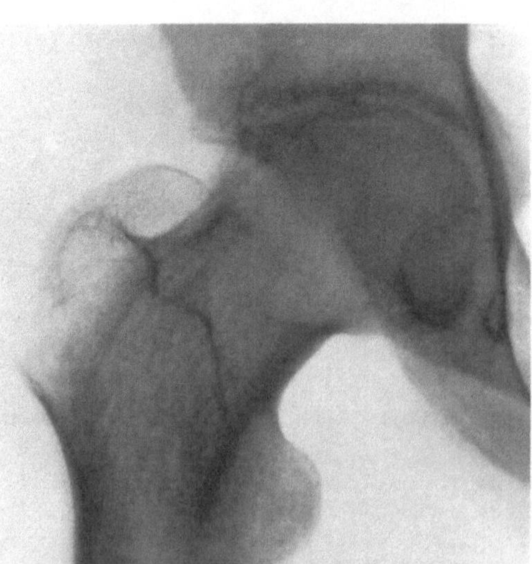

Nach 2 Jahren besteht wieder ein deutlicher Gelenkspalt.
After two years. There is a distinct joint cleft again.

Serie 35.

Ellenbogentuberkulose.

Bei dem zarten 7jährigen Mädchen entwickelte sich in 5 Monaten ein *tuberkulöser Fungus* des Ellenbogengelenkes mit ausgedehnter Zerstörung der knöchernen Gelenkenden. Konservative Behandlung — Röntgenbestrahlung und eine Freiluft-Sonnenkur in einer Heilstätte der Ebene — führte in $2^1/_2$ Jahren eine solide Ausheilung des Krankheitsprozesses herbei; eine Wiederherstellung der Funktion war infolge der ausgedehnten Zerstörung nicht mehr möglich.

Series 35.

Tuberculosis of the Elbow.

A delicate girl of seven developed a *tuberculous fungus* of the elbow-joint with extensive destruction of the bony joint-ends in five months. Conservative treatment — X-Ray, open air and sun cure in a sanatorium in the plains —, led, within two years and a half, to a real healing of the diseased process. The extensive destruction however, made the functional restoration impossible.

$^3/_4$ n. Gr.   1.

2.

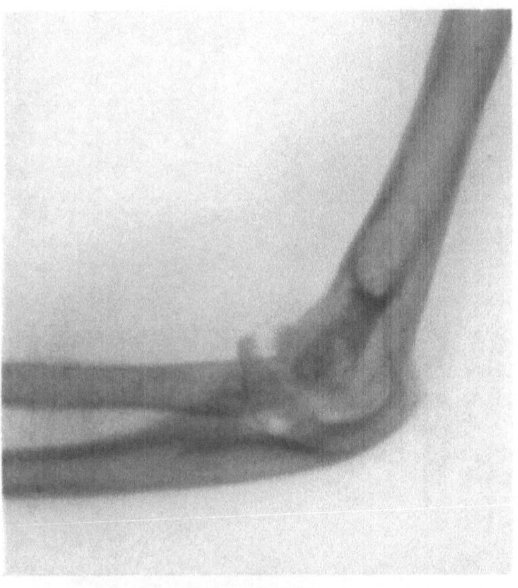

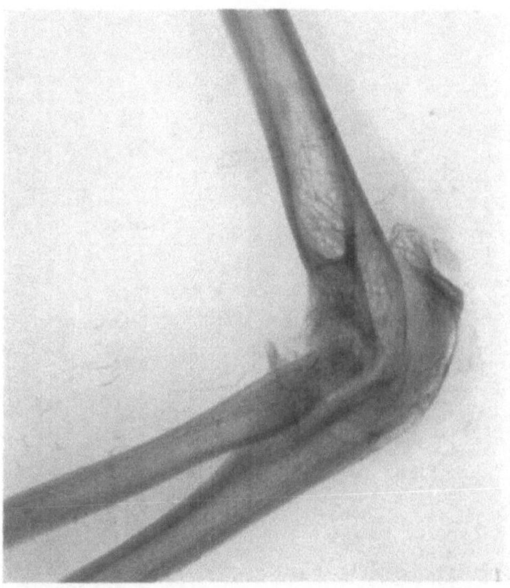

5 Monate nach Beginn der Erkrankung besteht bereits eine hochgradige Zerstörung der Gelenkenden.

Five months after commencement of disease a vast destruction of joint-ends exists.

Nach $2^1/_2$ Jahren läßt die *solide Wiederherstellung der Knochenstruktur* die Ausheilung des tuberkulösen Prozesses erkennen.

After two years and a half the *solid reparation of bone-structure* shows the healing of the Tb. process.

Serie 36.

Fungöse Ellenbogentuberkulose.

Bei der 27 jährigen, sonst gesunden Frau verlief die primär synoviale Gelenktuberkulose unter dem klinischen Bilde eines „Fungus", der trotz frühzeitiger Behandlung (Gipsschiene, Röntgen- und Sonnenbestrahlung usw.) zum Fistelaufbruch und zur Zerstörung der knöchernen Gelenkenden führte. Die Resektion brachte die Tuberkulose zur Ausheilung und im Laufe der Jahre kam es durch Weichteilschrumpfung zu einer Annäherung und gegenseitigen Stützung der Knochenenden, so daß funktionell wieder für leichtere Beanspruchung ein brauchbares Gelenk besteht.

Series 36.

Fungoid Tuberculosis of Elbow-Joint.

A twenty seven year old woman, otherwise healthy, had a primary synovial joint tuberculosis, clinically described as fungous. In spite of timely treatment (plaster-of-Paris splint, X-rays, sun-rays etc.) fistula and destruction of the bony joint ends ensued. Resection cured the tuberculosis and in course of time, by the shrinking of the fleshy parts, the bone-ends were brought nearer together and so supported one another, thus producing a useful joint for slight service.

$^7/_{10}$ n. Gr.   1.   2.   3.

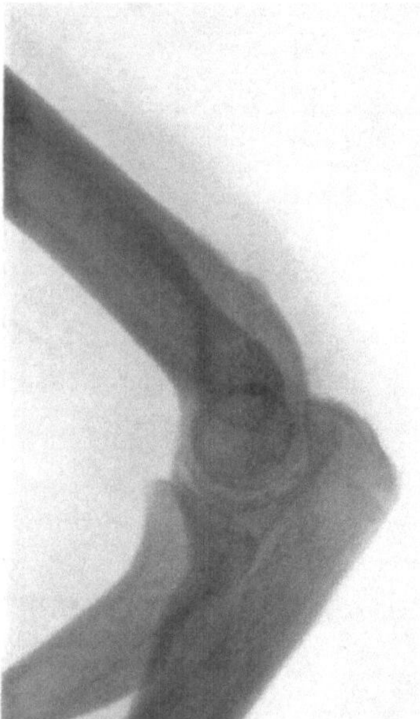 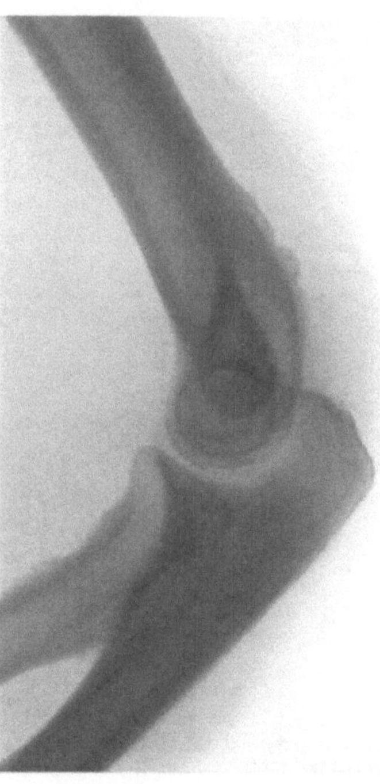 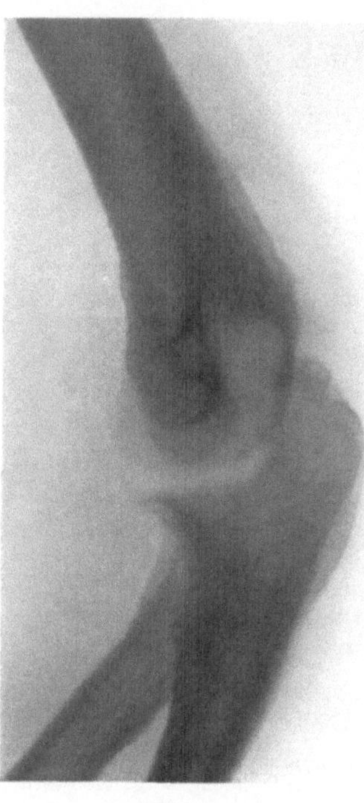

$^1/_4$ Jahr nach Beginn der Erkrankung ist am Knochen lediglich eine geringe Periostitis des Humerus vorhanden.

Three months after commencement of disease there is only a slight periostitis of humerus present.

Nach 5 Monaten ist die Periostwucherung etwas stärker.

After five months, the periosteal growth has increased.

Nach 1 Jahr aber besteht eine *ausgedehnte Zerstörung der knöchernen Gelenkenden*.

After one year *an extensive destruction of the bony joint ends* persists.

Serie 36.

4.

5.

6.

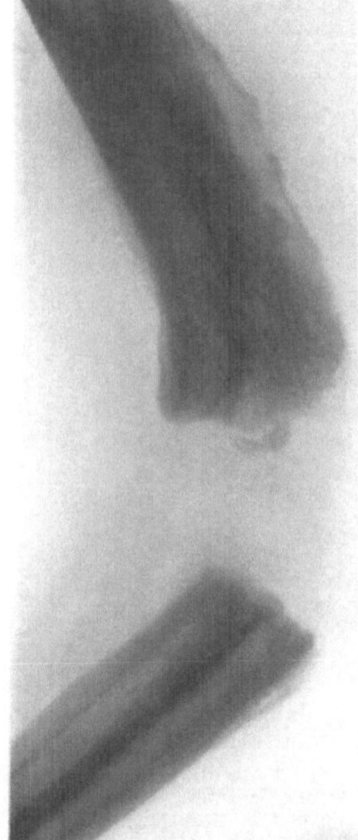

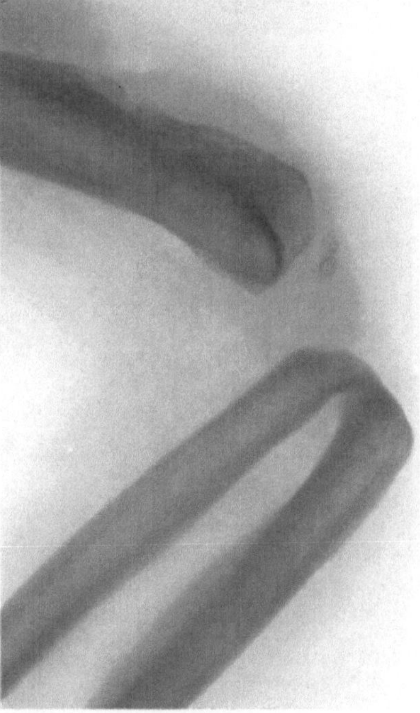

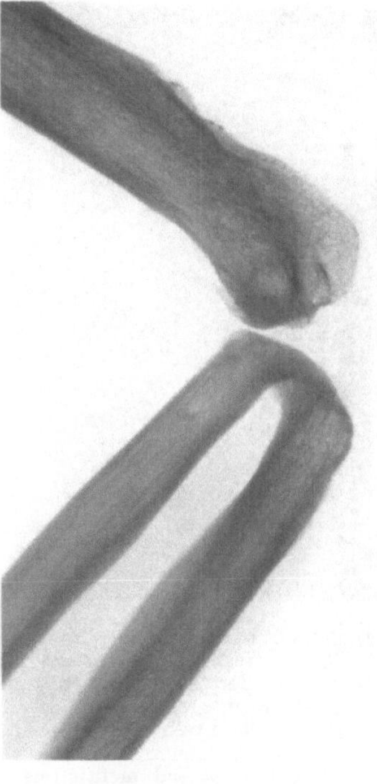

$^{1}/_{4}$ Jahr nach der Gelenkresektion ist noch eine periostale Auflockerung des Humerus und eine weite Diastase
der Knochen vorhanden.

Three months after resection
of joint, a periosteal loosening
of humerus and a wide separa-
tion of the bones exists.

Nach 7 Monaten sind Radius und Ulna
durch eine Brücke verbunden und dem
Humerus genähert; ihre Konturen
sind schärfer geworden.

After seven months radius, and ulna are
connected by a bridge and drawn nearer
to humerus. Their outlines have become
more distinct.

6 Jahre später sind die Knochen geglättet, gut strukturiert und berühren
einander.

Six years later the bones are smooth,
well-built and have come into contact
with one another.

Serie 37.

Schultergelenktuberkulose.

Bei dem 3jährigen unterernährten Knaben kam die
schon fortgeschrittene Schultergelenktuberkulose nach
einmaliger Punktion (8 ccm käsiger Eiter; Tbc-Bac. +)
unter der Hygiene des Krankenhauses und einer Freiluft-
liegekur in der Ebene in $1^1/_4$ Jahr zur Ausheilung: *zuerst*
geschah — an eine operative Ausmeißelung oder Auskratzung erinnernd — *die Ausglättung des Herdes, sodann*
wurde dieser *Defekt regeneriert.*

Series 37.

Shoulder Tuberculosis.

An ill-nourished boy of three had advanced shoulder-
joint tuberculosis, which was brought to a standstill
within one year and a quarter by one single puncture
(8 c c. cheesy matter, Tb. bac. +) and hygienic hospital-
treatment combined with recumbent open-air treatment
in the plains. *First* appeared — what reminded one of a
chiselled or scraped surface — the smoothing or levelling
of the diseased area, and *then* followed the regeneration
of this defect.

$^4/_5$ n. Gr.   1.   2.   3.

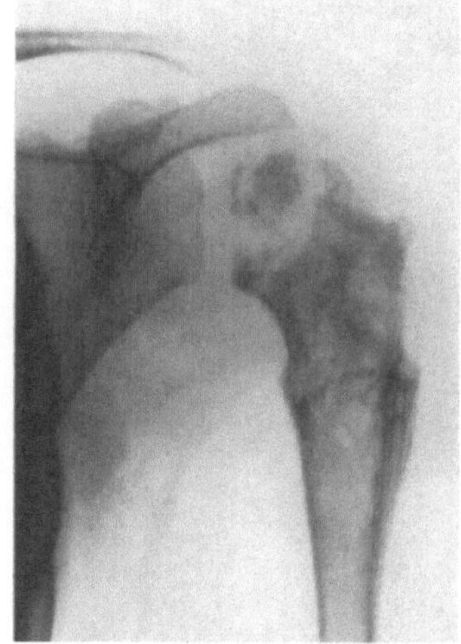

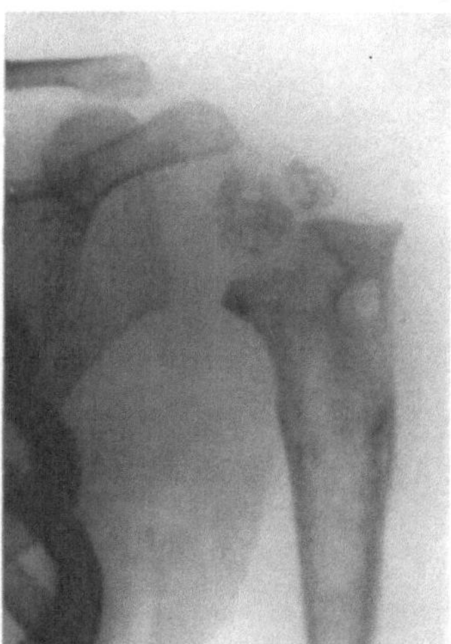

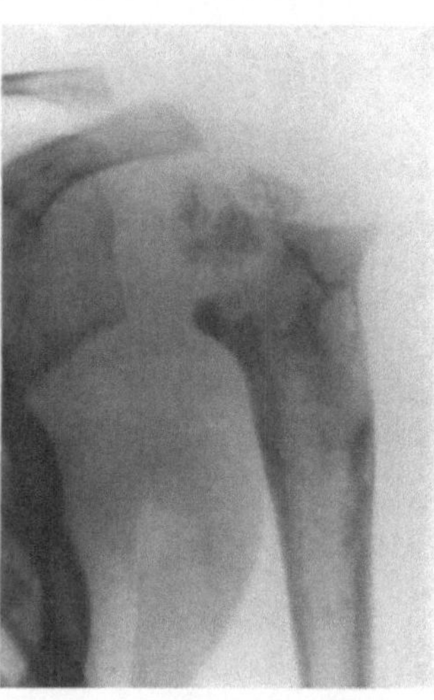

Epi- und Metaphyse des Humerus
sind „zerfressen“; es besteht ein
Herd an der Epiphysenfuge und
ein noch größerer lateral-
diaphysenwärts.

Both epiphysis and metaphysis of
humerus have been eroded. One
diseased area is at the epiphyseal line
and a still larger area lies laterally
towards the diaphysis.

8 Wochen später ist bereits eine
Ausglättung der Herde erkennbar.

Eight weeks later a levelling of the
diseased area is recognizable.

Nach $^1/_4$ Jahr ist der anatomische
Zustand etwa der gleiche.

After three months the anatomical
state is unchanged.

Serie 37.

4.

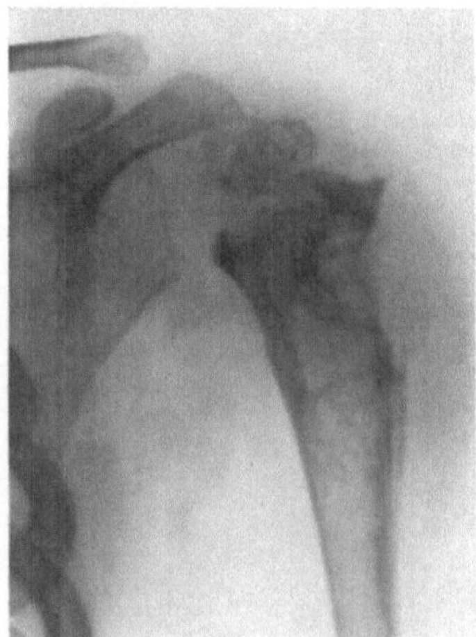

5.

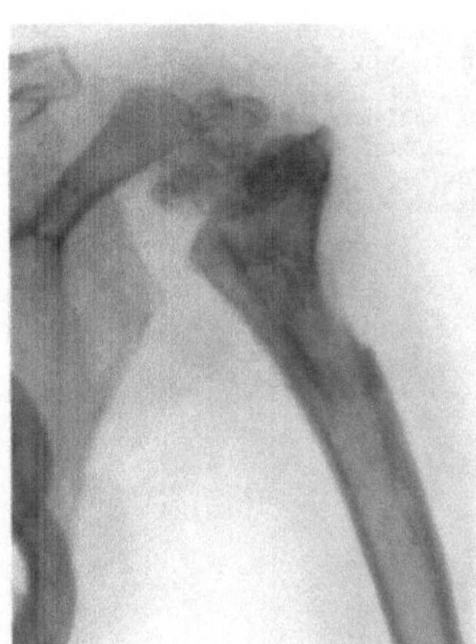

6.

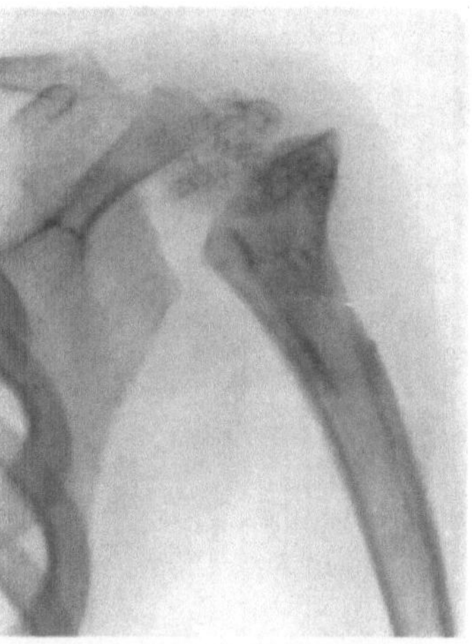

Nach ½ Jahr ist auch noch keine
wesentliche Änderung eingetreten.

After six months the same state
exists.

Nach 8 Monaten ist eine *Caries
nicht mehr vorhanden*. Der große
laterale Herd erscheint
wie ausgemeißelt.

After eight months *caries is no
longer present*. The large lateral
diseased area appears to have been
chiselled out.

Nach 10 Monaten ist der Befund kaum
verändert; immerhin hat die Knochenregeneration den Defekt bereits etwas
abgeflacht.

After ten months no great change has
taken place except that bone-regenera-
tion has already somewhat levelled
the defect.

7.

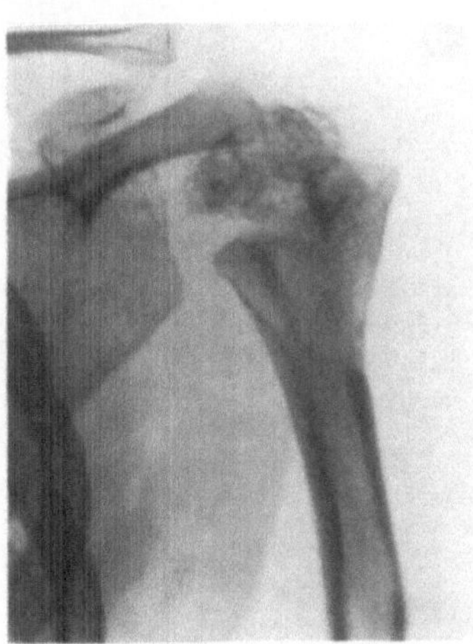

Nach 1¼ Jahr ist die Delle ausgefüllt, der Knochen gewachsen und kalkhaltiger geworden.

After one year and a quarter the cavity has filled out, the bone has grown and has become more calcified.

Serie 38.

Schultergelenktuberkulose.

Bei der 19jährigen früher gesunden Frau stellte
sich eine wenig schmerzhafte Anschwellung der
Schulter ein, die bald zu einer Versteifung führte.
Der tuberkulöse Prozeß führte ganz schleichend
eine Zerstörung des Gelenkes mit Schrumpfung
des Oberarmkopfes (Carries cicca) und war nach
9 Jahren wahrscheinlich noch nicht abgelaufen.

³/₄ n. Gr.   1.

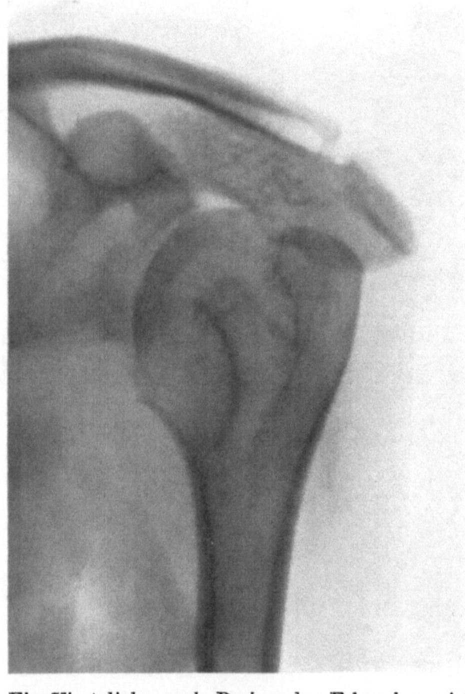

Ein Vierteljahr nach Beginn der Erkrankung ist
ein Zerstörungsherd im Oberarmkopf erkennbar.

Three months after onset of illness, the disease
in the head of the humerus is recognizable.

Serie 38.

Shoulder-joint tuberculosis.

A girl of nineteen who had always been healthy,
was affected with a slightly painful swelling of the
shoulder which became stiff. Very slowly the tuberculous process led to destruction of the joint and
shrinking up of the head of the humerus (caries
sicca) and apparently was still in progress
nine years later.

2.

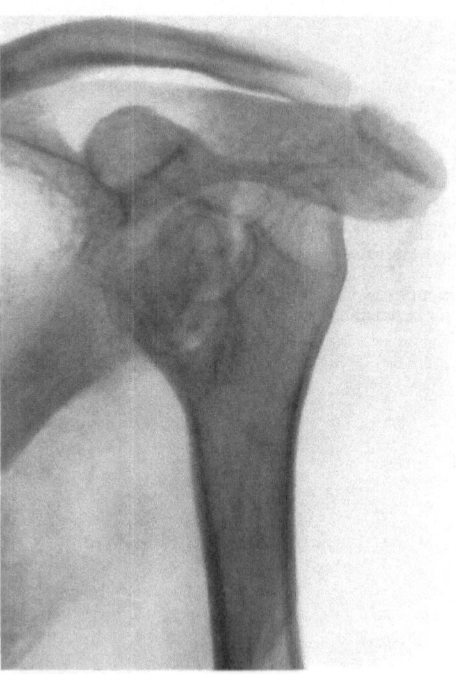

Nach 9 Jahren sind Pfanne und Gelenkkopf weitgehend zerstört und verschmolzen. Die Knochenstruktur ist aber noch stellenweise wolkig.

After nine years. The socket and joint head are
destroyed and dissolved. The bone structure is
still indistinct in some parts.

Serie 39.
Fistelnde Schultergelenk-
tuberkulose.

Bei der seit langem an offener Lungentuberkulose leidenden Frau trat im 68. Lebensjahr eine gleichartige Erkrankung eines Schultergelenkes hinzu. Es kam rasch zum Fisteldurchbruch und — ohne daß ein Heilbestreben erkennbar war — zu einer unaufhaltsam fortschreitenden Zerstörung des Gelenkes.

Series 39.
Fistulous Tuberculosis of the
Shoulder-joint.

A woman who had been suffering for a long time with open lung-tuberculosis, in her sixty eighth year became ill with tuberculosis of the shoulder-joint. A fistula broke through almost immediately. Without any signs of healing being noticeable, the destruction of the joint advanced without cessation.

$^2/_3$ n. Gr. 1. 2.

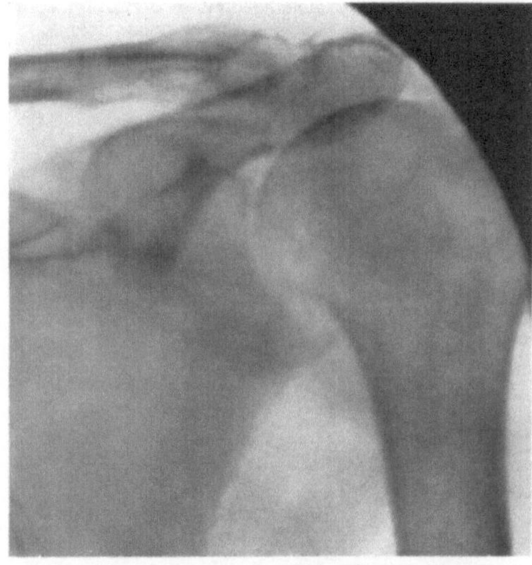

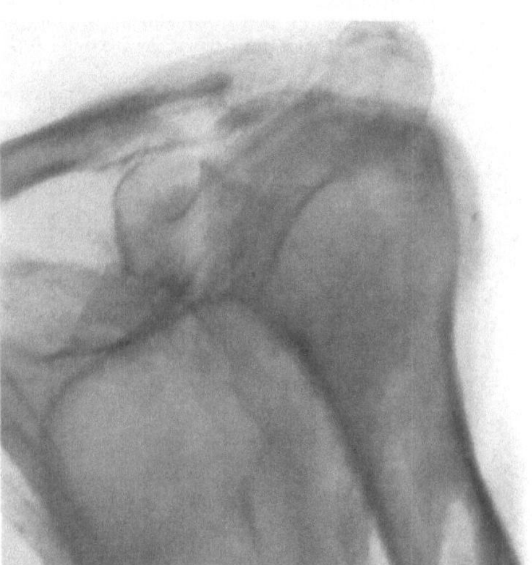

Kurz nach Beginn der Krankheit sind am Gelenkteil des Schulterblattes die Anfänge des Zerstörungsprozesses erkennbar.

Shortly after beginning of illness. The commencement of the process of destruction is noticeable at the joint of the scapula.

Nach 4 Monaten ist die Gelenkoberfläche allenthalben angenagt.

After four months; the joint-surface is entirely eroded.

3.

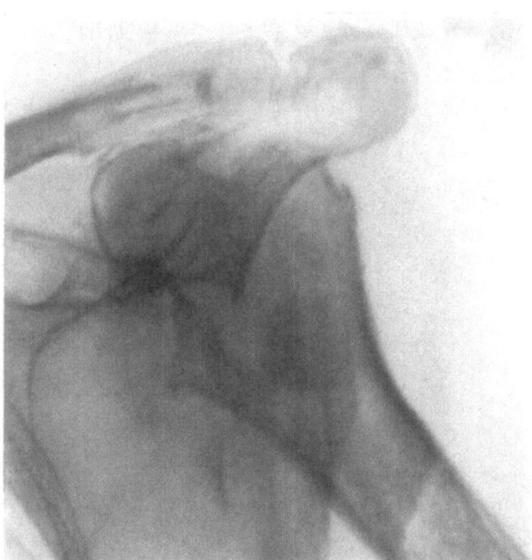

Nach 1 Jahr — kurz vor dem Tode — sind Oberarmkopf und Gelenkpfanne weitgehend zerstört und eine Subluxation ist eingetreten.

After one year, shortly before death, the head of the humerus and the scapular socket are extensively destroyed and subluxation has taken place.

<table>
<tr><td>

Serie 40.

Ulnatuberkulose.

Wegen der Gefahr des Einbruches in das intakte Gelenk wurde der tuberkulöse Herd der Ulna-epiphyse operativ ausgemeißelt und somit die spezifische Knochenerkrankung beseitigt. Die Wundheilung erfolgte ohne Störung; der Defekt wurde langsam bis zur ungefähren Formangleichung regeneriert.

</td><td>

Series 40.

Ulna Tuberculosis.

To prevent the disease penetrating into the still healthy joint, the affected part of ulna epiphysis was removed by operation and chiselled out, thus removing the specific bone malady. The healing of the wound continued without interruption and the part slowly resumed its previous form.

</td></tr>
</table>

$^4/_5$ n. Gr.   1.   2.

<table>
<tr><td>

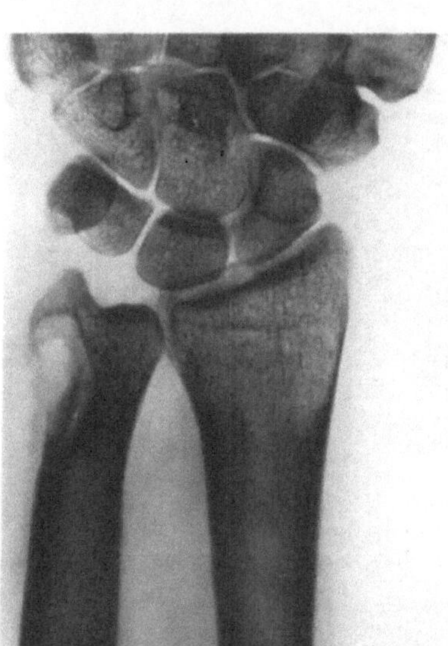

Gelenknaher tuberkulöser Knochenherd der Ulna.

Joint bone tuberculosis. Diseased area of the ulna.

</td><td>

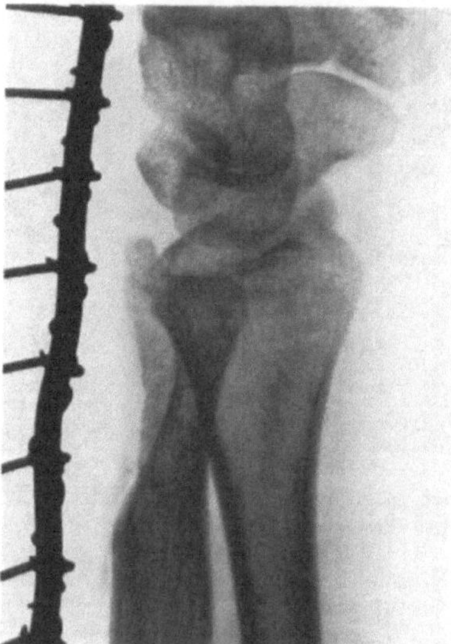

Knochendefekt nach Ausmeißelung des Herdes.

Bone - defect after chiselling out affected part.

</td></tr>
</table>

Serie 40.

3.

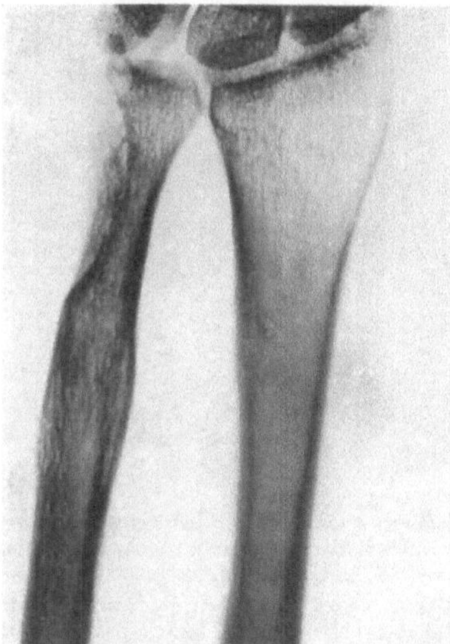

4.

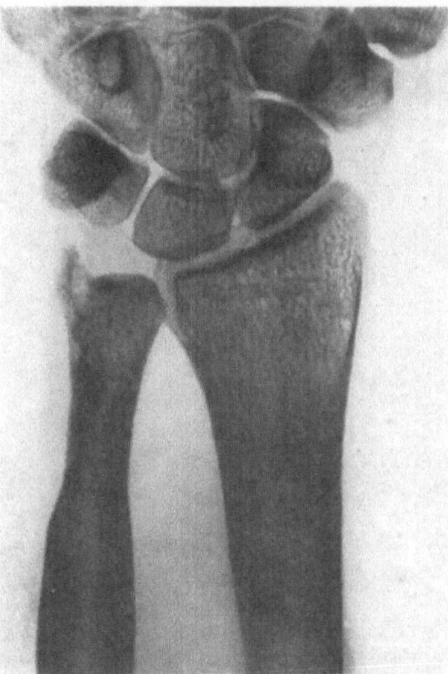

Nach ¹/₂ Jahr ist die Mulde noch deutlich, der
Röhrenknochen aber wieder geschlossen.

After six months the hollow is still distinct but
the tubular bones are again closed.

Nach 1 Jahr ist als Endzustand die Form der
Ulna ungefähr wiederhergestellt.

Finally, after one year, the shape of the ulna has
been restored.

Serie 41.

Handgelenktuberkulose.

Der 18jährige, sonst gesunde Mann erkrankte an einer Handgelenktuberkulose. Die primär synoviale Entzündung griff auf den Knochen über und führte zum Fisteldurchbruch. Trotz entsprechender Behandlung und trotz der Kleinheit des einzigen Herdes zog sich der Krankheitsprozeß über mehr als 4 Jahre hin und kam erst nach operativer Entfernung des cariösen Handwurzelknochens zur Heilung.

Series 41.

Wrist Tuberculosis.

A young man of eighteen, otherwise healthy, was affected with wrist tuberculosis. The primary synovial inflammation penetrated into the bone and led to a fistulous outbreak. Despite suitable treatment and the triviality of the case, a cure was only completed after more than four years and then only by the removal of the carious bone by operation.

$^4/_5$ n. Gr. 1.

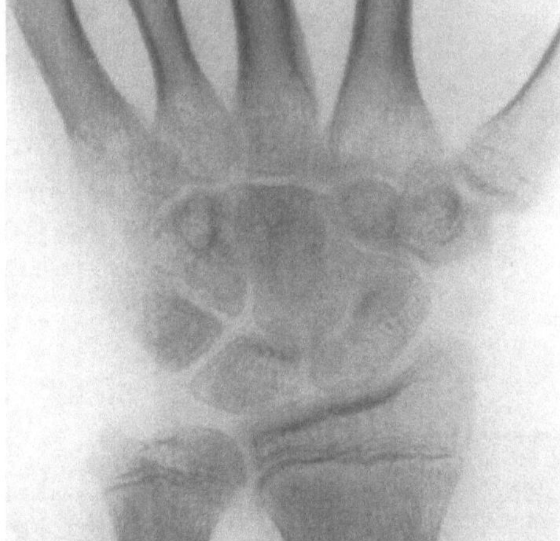

Wenige Wochen nach Beginn der Weichteilschwellung besteht eine starke Atrophie des Knochens.

A few weeks after the commencement of swelling, a marked atrophy of the bone exists.

2.

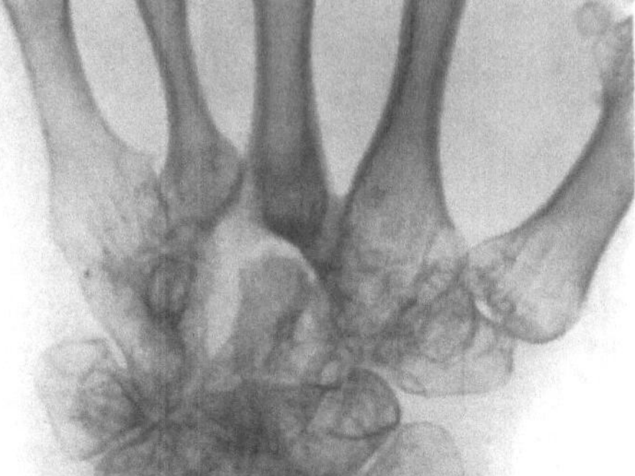

Nach über 4 Jahren ist das Os capitatum zum Teil zerstört, die übrigen Metacarpalien dagegen sind fest strukturiert.

After four years the os capitatum is partly destroyed but the other metacarpals are of firm structure.

3.

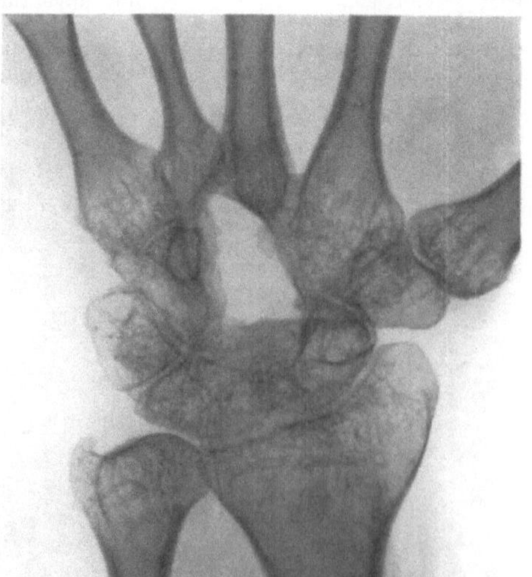

1 Jahr später ist noch die Lücke vorhanden; das Knochengefüge ist in sich abgestützt. Es besteht volle Funktionsfähigkeit.

One year later the gap is still present. The bone-structure supports itself. Entire function restored.

Serie 42.

Spina ventosa.

Bei dem lungenkranken 18 jährigen Mädchen brauchte die Knochentuberkulose eines Fingergliedes trotz der Kleinheit des Herdes mehr als 3 Jahre zur völligen Ausheilung: unter wiederholten Röntgenbestrahlungen stieß sich das käsig zerfallene Gewebe durch eine Fistel aus, aber die Regeneration des ausgeglätteten Defektes ging außerordentlich langsam vor sich.

Series 42.

Spina Ventosa.

An eighteen year old girl had lung-tuberculosis. One of her finger joints was also infected and despite the smallness of the area, it took over three years to heal. After repeated Röntgen irradiation treatment, the cheesy decayed tissue was expelled through a fistula. The regeneration of the flat defect progressed very slowly.

$^9/_{10}$ n. Gr.　　1.

2.

3.

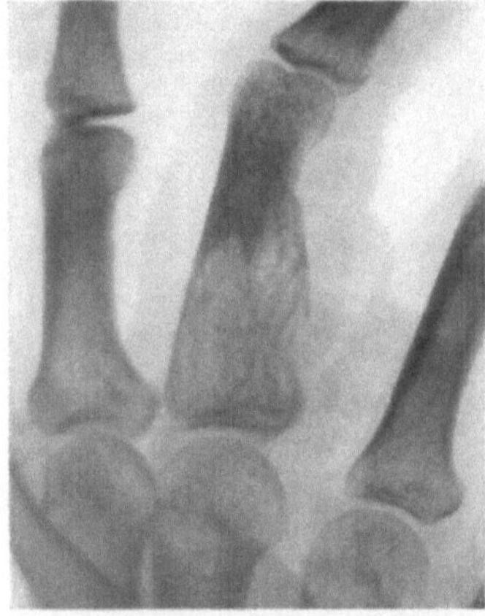

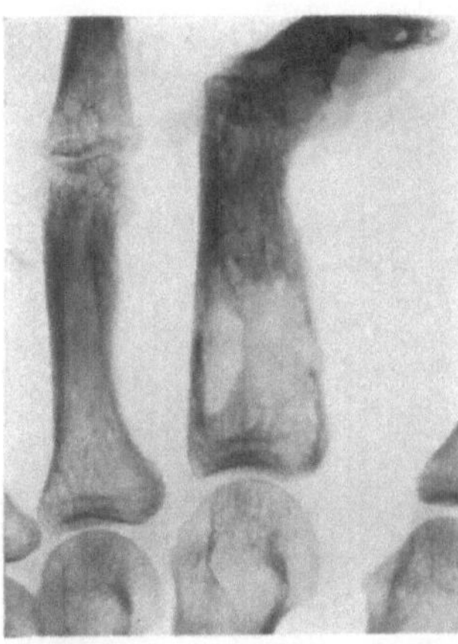

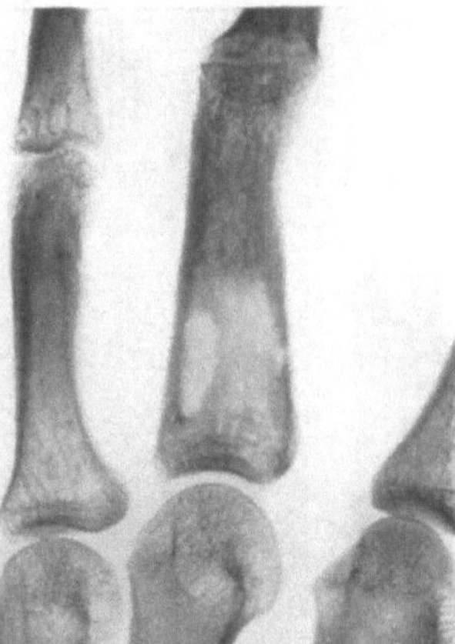

Ausgedehnte Zerstörung der Grundphalanx des Mittelfingers.

Extensive destruction of the basalphalanx of middle finger.

4 Monate später ist die cariöse Partie ausgefallen.

Four months later, the carious portion is expelled.

Nach 1 Jahr ist ein Teil des Defektes regeneriert, die Fistel geschlossen.

After one year, part of the defect is regenerated. The fistula is closed.

4.

5.

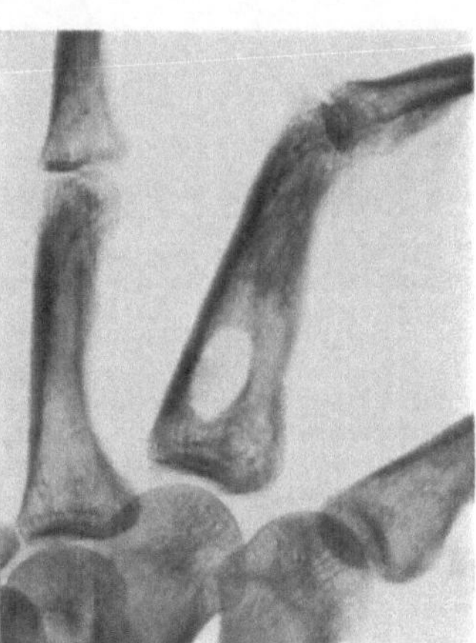

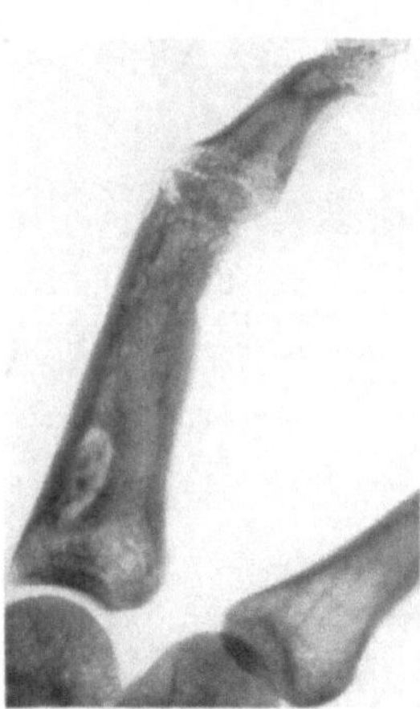

Nach 1½ Jahren besteht noch eine verhältnismäßig große ausgeglättete Knochenhöhle.

After one year and a half, there is still a fairly large flat bone cavity.

Nach 3 Jahren ist dieser Defekt erst zum Teil knöchern ausgefüllt.

Only now, after three years, is this defect partly filled out by ossification.

Serie 43.

Spondylitis tuberculosa.

Bei der 40 Jahre alten Frau bestand 6 Wochen nach
Beginn der Rückenschmerzen bereits eine weitgehende
Zerstörung des 7. und 8. Brustwirbels. Nach einer
etwa 4 Monate durchgeführten Liege-Extensions-
behandlung verließ sie die Klinik und trug noch 1 Jahr
lang ein Stützkorsett. In dieser Zeit besorgte sie bereits
ihren Haushalt und tat nichts mehr gegen das Leiden.
Dennoch war die schwere Knochentuberkulose in etwa
20 Monaten solide und dauernd ausgeheilt.

$^7/_{10}$ n. Gr.   1.

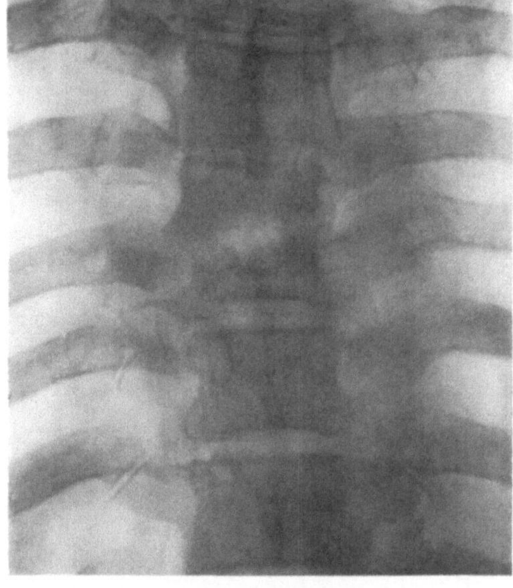

6 Wochen nach Beginn der Beschwerden sind der
7. und 8. Brustwirbel etwa zur Hälfte zerstört und
ineinander gesunken.

Six weeks after commencement of complaint the
seventh and eighth dorsal vertebrae are partially
destroyed and have sunk into one another.

Series 43.

Tuberculous Spondylitis.

A woman of forty complained of pain in the back.
Six weeks after commencement of pain she was found
to be suffering with extensive destruction of the
seventh and eighth dorsal vertebrae. A recumbent
extension treatment was followed for four months, after
which she left the hospital and wore a supporting corset
for one year. During this time, although no other
treatment was administered, she was able to perform
her daily duties in the household and the serious bone
tuberculosis was creditably and permanently cured
within about twenty months.

2.

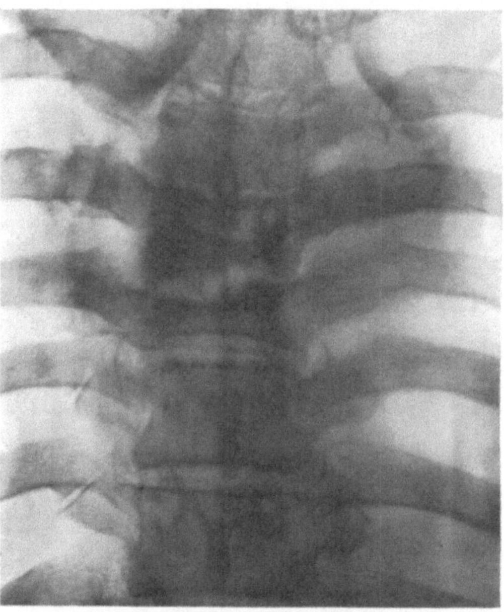

4 Monate später — nach streng durchgeführter Liege-
Extensionsbehandlung — ist der Zerstörungsprozeß
zum Stillstand gekommen, nachdem er zuerst noch
etwas fortgeschritten war.

Four months later, after the strictly carried out
recumbent-extension treatment, the destructive process has come to a standstill, after very slight
further progress.

Serie 43.

3.

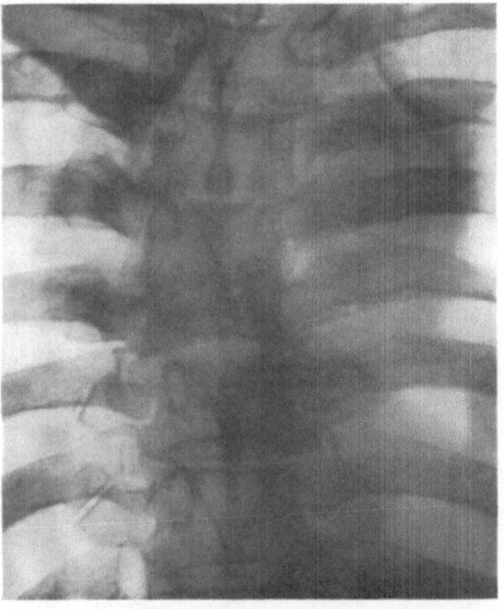

4.

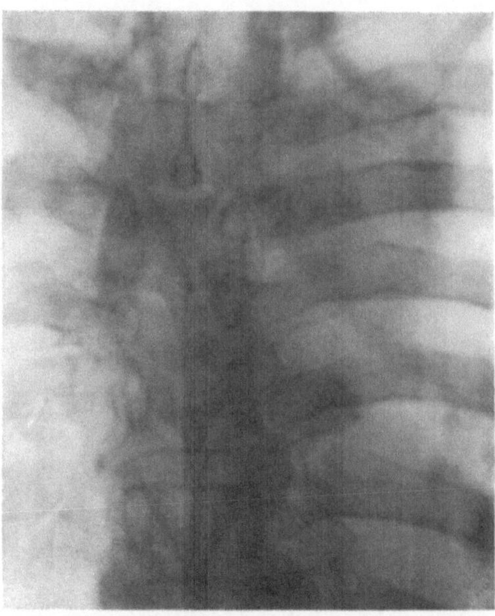

Nach 20 Monaten sind die beiden erkrankten Wirbelkörper knöchern fest verwachsen: der Prozeß ist ausgeheilt.

After twenty months the two affected vertebrae are grown firmly together and the process cured.

Nach weiteren 3 Jahren sind die beiden Wirbelkörper ein fester Knochenblock.

Three years later the two vertebrae are a firm bony mass.

Serie 44.

Spondylitis tuberculosa.

Während des Krankenlagers, das die 22 jährige Frau wegen Tuberkulose der Articulatio sacro-iliaca durchmachte, wurde ein gleichartiger Prozeß am 2. Lendenwirbel festgestellt. Trotz Liegebehandlung im Gipsbett griff die Caries um sich, zerstörte die Zwischenwirbelscheibe, brach in den 3. Lendenwirbel ein und kam erst dann zum Stillstand, als breite Knochenflächen der Wirbelkörper sich berührten. Die Kranke befand sich jetzt in bestem Allgemeinzustand, so daß man die Anbahnung anatomischer Ausheilung annehmen konnte, als kurz danach der Tod an Miliartuberkulose eintrat.

Series 44.

Tuberculous Spondylitis.

A woman of twenty-two was ill with tuberculosis of the sacro-iliac joint. During this time a similar process was established in the second lumbar vertebra. Despite recumbent treatment in plaster of Paris, the caries spread and destroyed the inter vertebral disc and broke into the third lumbar vertebra. Its progress was only arrested when broad bonesu rfaces of the vertebrae touched one another. At this time the patient seemed so very well in general health that it was thought the anatomical healing had commenced, instead of which, she died shortly after of miliary tuberculosis.

²/₃ n. Gr.   1.   2.

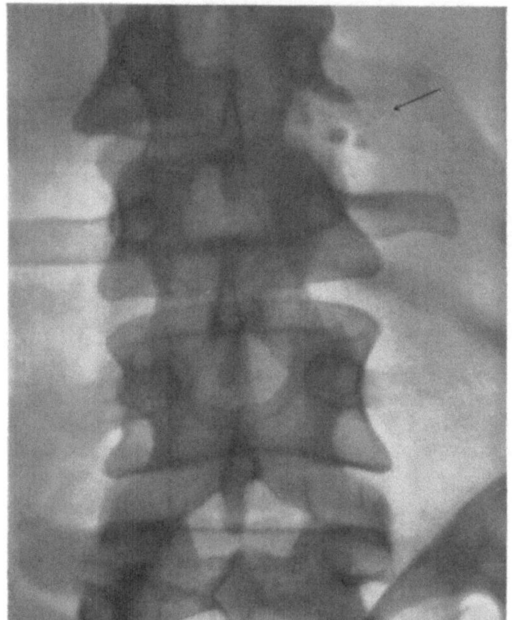

Cariöser Herd in der rechten unteren Ecke
des 2. Lendenwirbels und dem Rand
der Zwischenwirbelscheibe.

Area of caries in the right lower corner of the second
lumbar vertebra and the edge of the intervertebral disc.

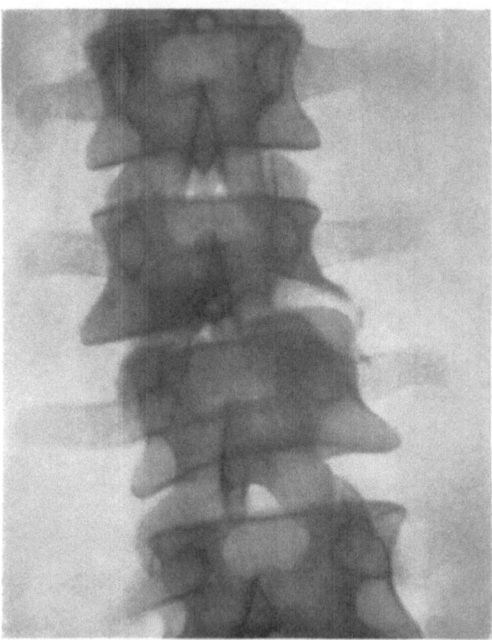

4 Monate später ist der Zerstörungsprozeß nach der
Wirbelmitte zu fortgeschritten.

Four months later, the process of destruction has
advanced towards the centre of the vertebra.

Serie 44.

3.

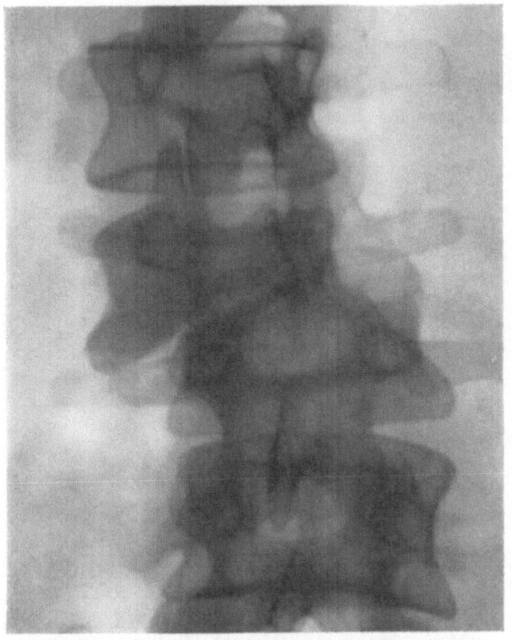

4.

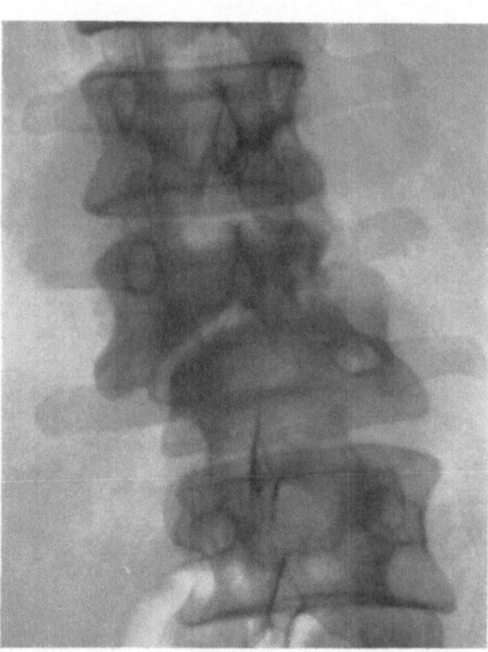

Nach 1 Jahr ist der II. Lendenwirbel zur Hälfte vernichtet, die Zwischenwirbelscheibe zerstört, und auch
ein großer Teil des III. Lendenwirbels fehlt.

After one year, half of the second lumbar vertebra
and the intervertebral disc are destroyed, also a large
part of the third lumbar-vertebra is missing.

Nach 1¹/₂ Jahren ist die Caries nur noch wenig, nach
2 Jahren gar nicht mehr fortgeschritten.

After one year and a half, the caries has advanced
only slightly and after two years, not at all.

Serie 45.

Spondylitis tuberculosa.

Als bei dem 5jährigen Knaben wenige Wochen nach Beginn der Beschwerden die Erkrankung der Wirbelsäule festgestellt wurde, waren bereits zwei Lendenwirbel weitgehend zerstört. Trotz streng durchgeführter Liegebehandlung im Gipsbett griff die Caries im 2. Jahre noch auf den 3. Lendenwirbel über, um dann zunächst wenigstens Halt zu machen. Der nunmehr 8 Jahre alte Knabe sah frisch aus, trug zuletzt ein Stützkorsett und war schmerzfrei; die anatomische Heilung aber ließ noch zu wünschen übrig.

Series 45.

Tuberculous Spondylitis.

The patient was a boy, five years of age. A few weeks after the onset, when the condition was first diagnosed, two lumbar vertebrae had already been partially destroyed. Despite strictly executed treatment (recumbence in plaster of Paris), the destructive process advanced during the second year into the third lumbar vertebra. It then halted. At this time the boy was eight years of age, looked very well, wore a supporting corset and was free from pain. The anatomical healing, however, left much to be desired.

$^4/_5$ n. Gr. 1.   2.   3.

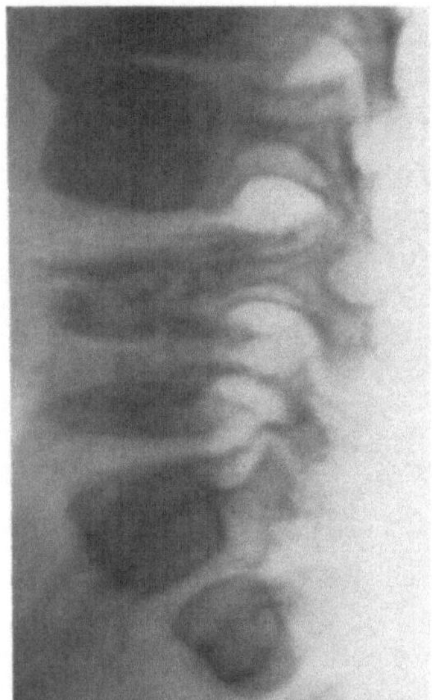
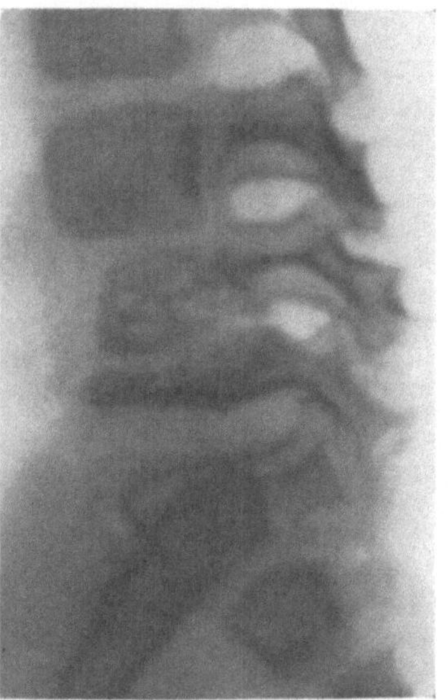
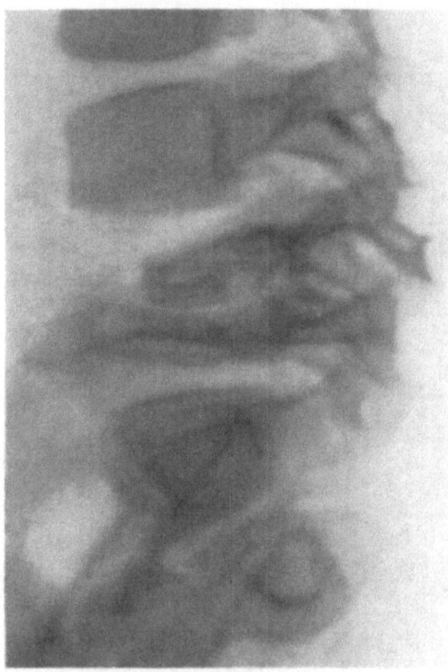

Der 4. und 5. Lendenwirbel sind zerfressen und zusammengesunken.

The fourth and fifth lumbar vertebrae have eroded and sunk into one another.

Nach $^3/_4$ Jahren ist der 5. Lendenwirbel noch mehr zerstört.

After nine months. The destruction of the fifth lumbar vertebra has advanced.

Nach $1^1/_2$ Jahren ist auch der 4. Lendenwirbel weiter zerfallen.

After eigtheen months. The destruction of the fourth lumbar vertebra has also advanced.

Serie 45.

4.

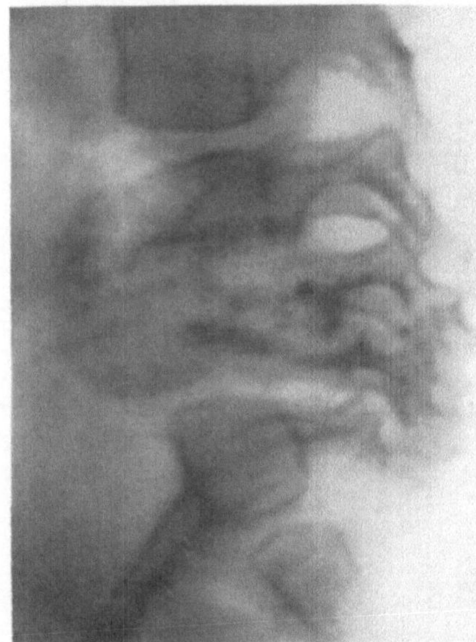

5.

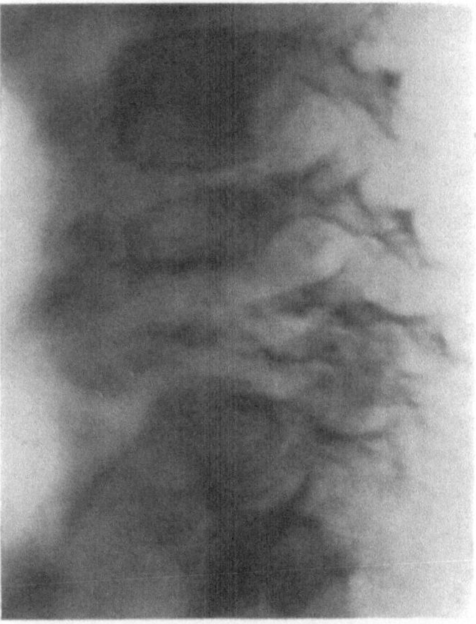

Nach 2 Jahren sind der 4. und 5. Lendenwirbel
fast ganz zerstört und in sich zusammengesunken,
aber auch der 3. ist erkrankt und ein Kongestions-
absceß entstanden.

After two years. The fourth and fifth lumbar-
vertebrae are almost entirely destroyed, the third
is also diseased and a congestion abscess has
developed.

Nach 3 Jahren ist der Befund nicht viel verändert;
es besteht auch noch der kalte Absceß.

After three years. The condition is not much
altered. The cold abscess still exists.

Serie 46.

Schambeintuberkulose.

Die tuberkulöse Caries in der Symphyse führte zur Verkäsung und Absceßbildung mit Fisteldurchbruch. Unter Röntgenbestrahlungen schloß sich schließlich die Fistel, aber der Prozeß in dem Knorpel-Knochenstück schien — nach dem Röntgenbefund — noch nach 7 Jahren nicht solide ausgeheilt.

Series 46.

Tuberculosis of the Pubic Bone.

The tuberculous caries in symphysis led to cheesiness and fistulous abscess formation. After lengthy X-ray treatment, the fistula closed but the process in the cartilage bone area, according to a Röntgenphoto taken seven years later, was apparently not perfectly cured.

³/₄ n. Gr.   1.

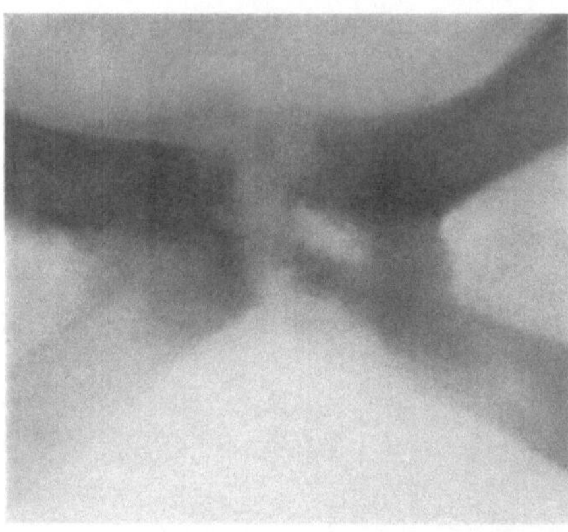

Einige Wochen nach Beginn der Beschwerden besteht eine umschriebene Zerstörung des rechten absteigenden Schambeinastes.

A few weeks after commencement of complaint, a limited destruction of the right upper ramus of the pubis exists.

2.

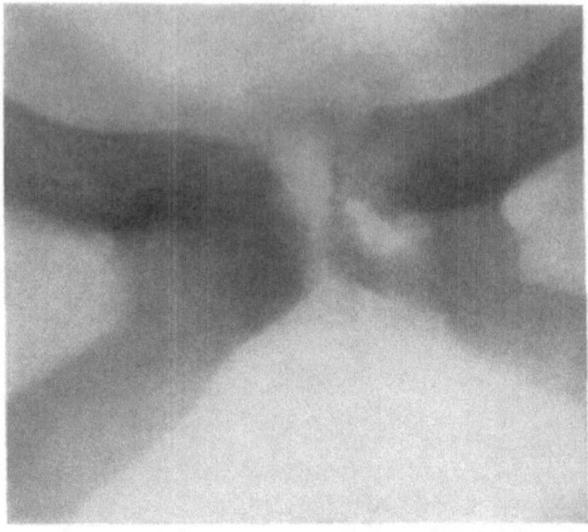

Nach 1 Jahr ist dieser Herd größer geworden und in den Knorpel eingebrochen.

After one year. This area has enlarged and broken into the cartilage.

3.

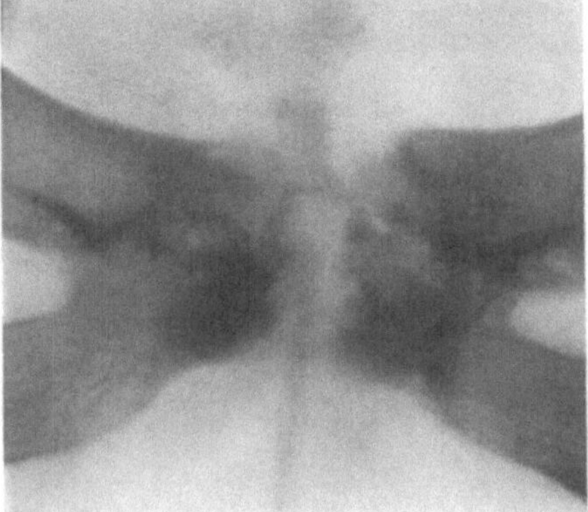

Nach 3 Jahren hat die Caries auch den Knochen der anderen Seite befallen.

After three years. The caries has attacked the bone of the other side.

4.

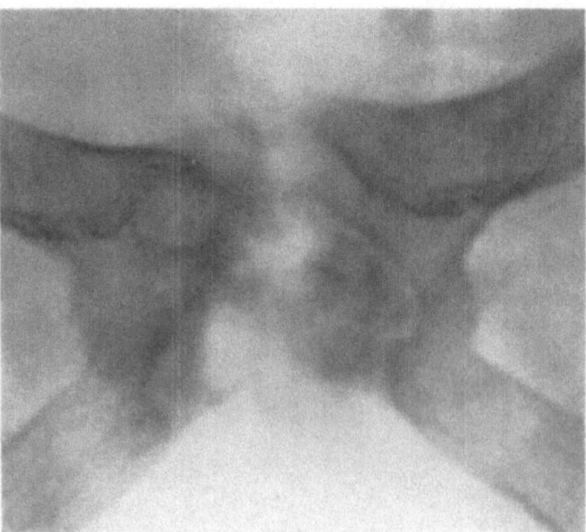

Nach 7 Jahren ist die Synchondrose zerstört, der Schambeinknochen links ziemlich geglättet, rechts aber noch ein Bezirk in Demarkation begriffen.

After seven years. The synchondrosis is destroyed The pubis has become fairly smooth and on the right side there is still an area of demarkation.

Anhang.

Die Serien 47—50 stammen aus der Klinik Prof. Dr. ROLLIER in Leysin (Schweiz), dessen Sonnenheilstätte für die Behandlung der Knochen- und Gelenktuberkulose internationale Bedeutung besitzt.

Sie zeigen den Heilverlauf *fortgeschrittener* tuberkulöser Gelenkerkrankungen unter der Sonnenbehandlung des Hochgebirges.

Supplement.

The Series 47—50 are taken originally from Professor Dr. ROLLIER'S clinic in Leysin (Switzerland), whose sun-sanatorium for the treatment of bone and joint tuberculosis is of international fame. They show the healing process of *advanced* tuberculous joint diseases by the mountain sun treatment.

Serie 47.

Fungöse Ellenbogentuberkulose.
(Knabe von etwa 8 Jahren.)

Series 47.

Fungoid Tuberculosis of the Elbow.
(Boy about 8 years of age).

⁷/₁₀ n. Gr.　　　　1.

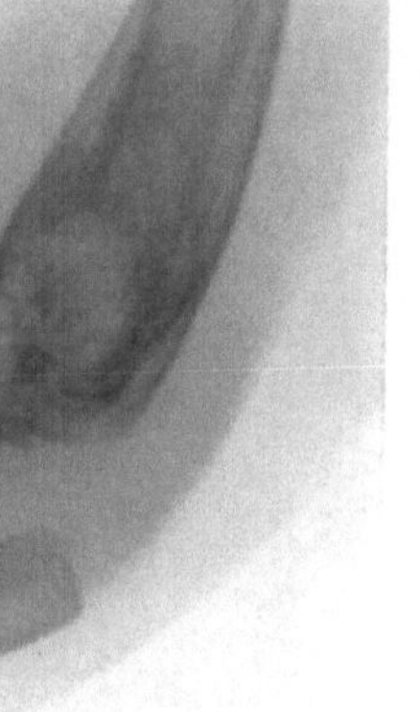

2.

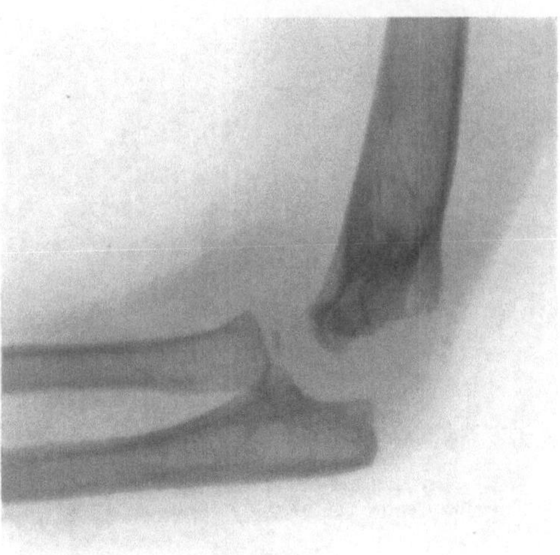

Großer Knochenherd in der aufgetriebenen Humerusepiphyse. Fungus cubiti.

Extensively diseased area in the swollen humerus epiphysis. Fungus cubiti.

Nach 13 Monaten geheilt mit voller Funktion.

Healed after thirteen months with restored function.

6*

Serie 48.

Fungöse Ellenbogentuberkulose.

(Junger Mann.)

²/₃ n. Gr.   1.

Series 48.

Fungoid Tuberculosis of the Elbow.

(Young man.)

2.

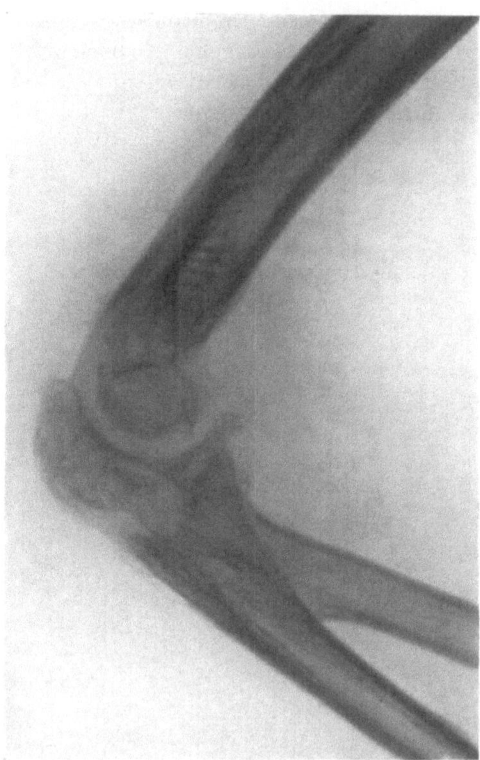

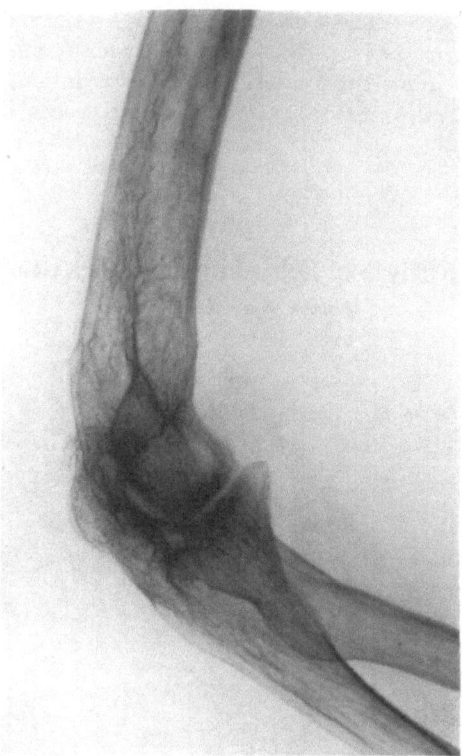

Die Gelenkenden sind atrophisch und teilweise angenagt.

The joint-ends are atrophic and partly eroded.

Nach 15 Monaten Sonnenbehandlung ist der tuberkulöse Prozeß mit solider Strukturbildung ausgeheilt.

After fifteen months sun-treatment, the tuberculous process has healed with solid structure formation.

Serie 49.

Fortgeschrittene Hüftgelenktuberkulose.

(Mädchen von etwa 12 Jahren.)

¹/₂ n. Gr.　　　　1.

Series 49.

Advanced Hip-joint Tuberculosis.

(Girl about 12 years of age.)

2.

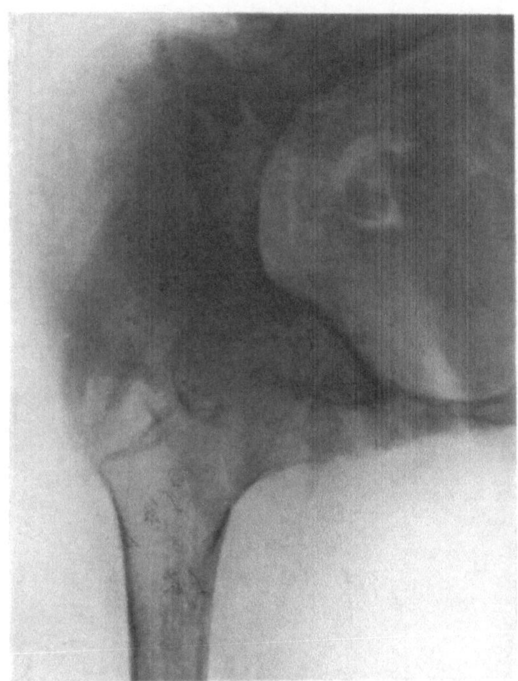

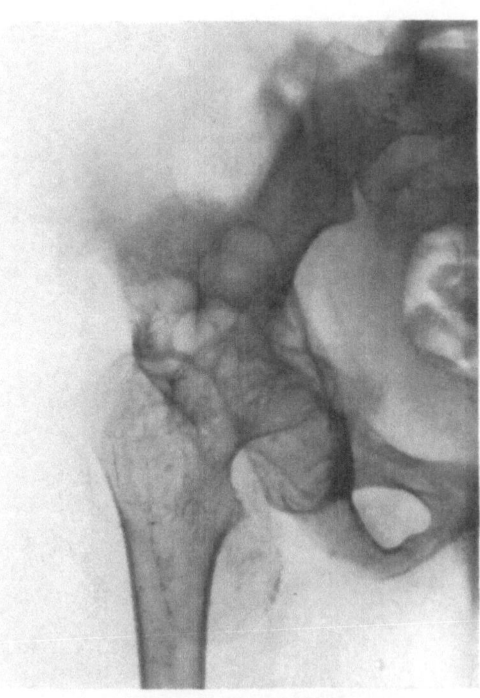

Ausgedehnte Zerstörung von Kopf und Pfanne.

Considerable destruction of head and acetabulum.

„Geheilt unter teilweiser Reorganisation des Gelenkkopfes und guter Strukturbildung in der ganzen Herdgegend."

Healed with partial reorganization of the joint-head and good structural formation in the whole diseased area.

Serie 50.

Fortgeschrittene fungöse Tuber-
kulose beider Kniegelenke.

(Junger Mann von etwa 16 Jahren.)

Series 50.

Advanced Fungoid Tuberculosis
of both Knee-joints.

(Boy of about sixteen years of age.)

$^{6}/_{10}$ n. Gr.   rechts   l.   links

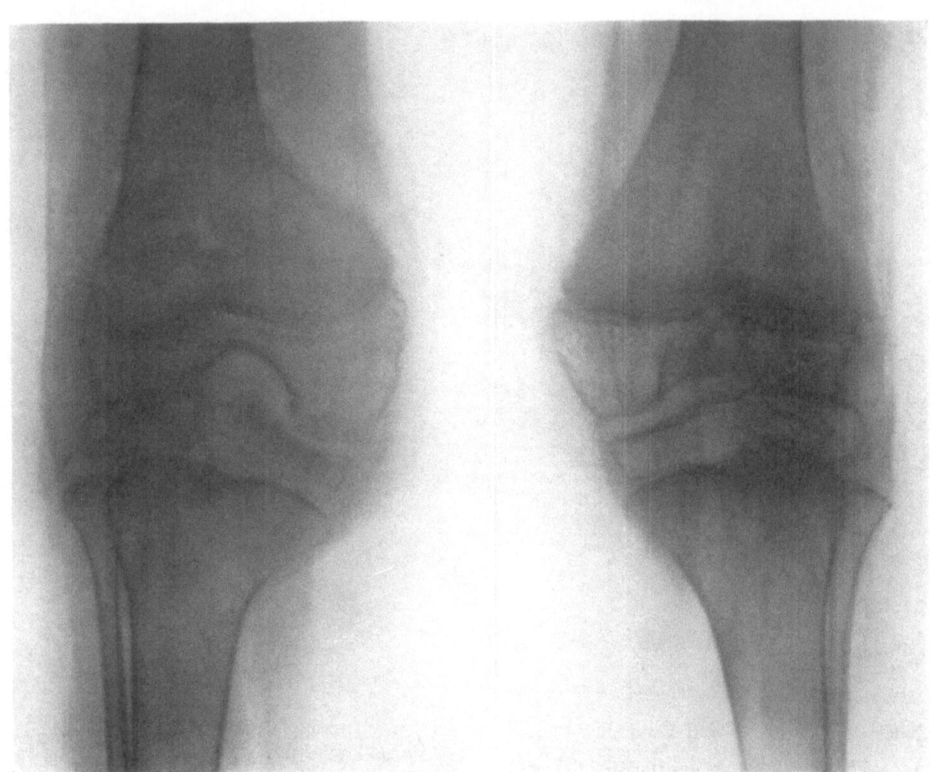

Serie 50.

rechts   2.   links

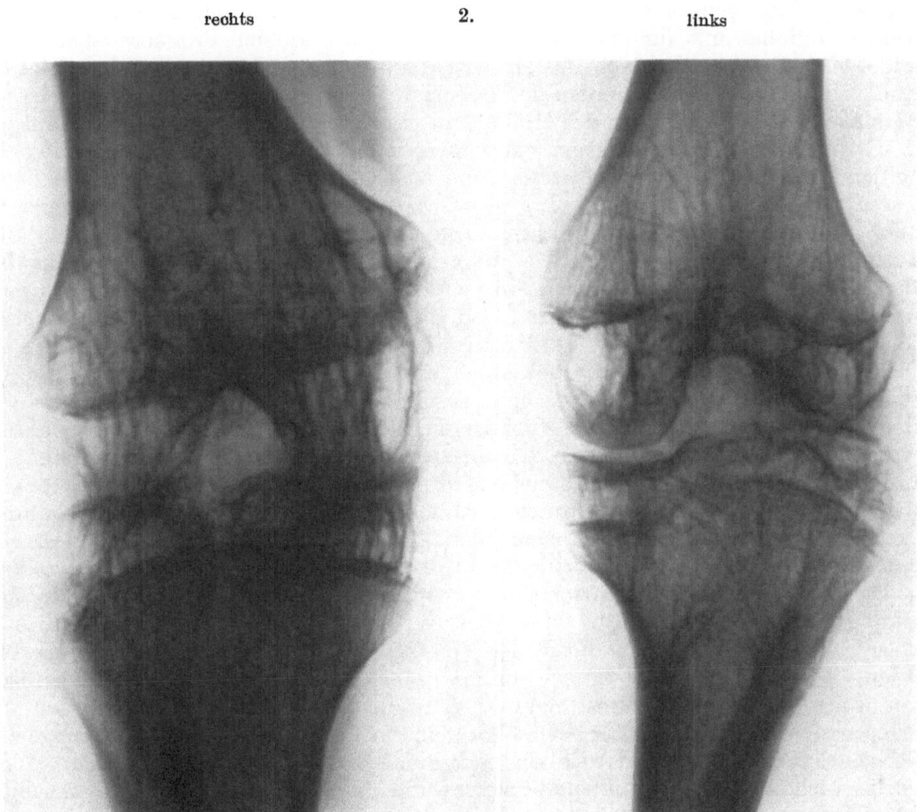

Nach 2 Jahren Sonnenkur: Ankylose des rechten Knies bei starker trabekulärer Struktur, die das alte Herdgebiet durchsetzt und die beiden Gelenkflächen durch solide Brücken verbindet. Links sind die Knochenherde gleichfalls solide knöchern ausgeflickt; der Gelenkspalt ist hier (wenigstens großenteils) erhalten geblieben.

After two years sun-treatment. Ankylosis of right knee with considerable trabecular structure which penetrates the former diseased area, joining both surfaces with solid bridges. On the left side the diseased area is also reconstructed with bone; the joint-cleft however, persists throughout its greatest extent.

B. Angeborene und erworbene Syphilis der Knochen und Gelenke.

Die Syphilis gehört wie die Tuberkulose zu den chronischen spezifischen Infektionen und hat mit ihr auch vielerlei gemeinsam. In der Prognose aber unterscheidet sie sich wesentlich von ihr. Ein Symbol dafür ist das histologische Bild des Granulationsgewebes, das von dem der Tuberkulose vor allem durch das Erhaltensein der Gefäße — den Vermittlern des Heilungsprozesses — abweicht. Auch im Röntgenbild tritt uns die Prognose sichtbar vor Augen, indem eine periostale Knochenwucherung den Zerfallsherd umgibt. *Praktisch unterscheidet sich die Syphilis von der Tuberkulose vor allem dadurch, daß wir auf chemischem Wege die Heilkraft des Körpers mit Sicherheit wecken und fördern können.* Die antiluetische Behandlung ist in allen Stadien der Knochen- und Gelenksyphilis eine vollwertige Therapie. Quecksilber, Jod, am stärksten aber das Salvarsan sind wirksam. In Serie 58 sehen wir die schweren gummösen Veränderungen der Hand lediglich durch eine Quecksilberschmierkur (noch vor der Entdeckung des Salvarsans) heilen. Aber nicht immer sprechen die Knochengummen auf Jod und Quecksilber an. Die Serien 55a und b im Falle der malignen Syphilis zeigen das Versagen dieser beiden Specifica; erst Salvarsan — andere Arsenpräparate nicht — führte die Heilung herbei. Diese Beobachtung beweist zugleich, daß verschiedene, gleichzeitig in demselben Organismus bestehende Manifestationen der Lues auf das gleiche Medikament verschieden ansprechen können: An dem Gumma der Tibia machte sich schließlich die Heilung bemerkbar, während sie zu gleicher Zeit an der Ulna ganz ausblieb. *Heute hängt die Prognose der erworbenen Knochen- und Gelenksyphilis in erster Linie von der rechtzeitigen Salvarsanbehandlung* ab. Das gilt auch für die Spätformen der angeborenen Syphilis, während die *kongenitale Frühsyphilis* — die Osteochondritis — (Serie 51) und die Periostitis (Serie 58) *leichter ansprechen* und auch durch andere Arsenpräparate in Heilung übergeführt werden. Die Heilung eines Knochengummas erfolgt dadurch, daß das spezifische Granulationsgewebe mit seinen charakteristischen knötchenförmigen Herden und Nekrosen sich in ein unspezifisches umwandelt, in welches dann das Knochengewebe der Nachbarschaft einwächst, wie wir es in dem Bild 2 der Serie 55a sehen. Wenn also die Ausheilung des Krankheitsprozesses und die Wiederherstellung des normalen Knochengewebes durch Neosalvarsan durchaus die Regel ist — die Serien 54, 55 und 56 bezeugen dieses — so kann sich eine gummöse Ostitis jeder Therapie, auch dem sonst so wirksamen Salvarsan gegenüber, *refraktär* verhalten, *wenn*, wie in Serie 57, eine schwere *eitrige Mischinfektion* hinzugetreten ist.

B. Hereditary and Acquired Syphilis of Bones and Joints.

Syphilis, like tuberculosis, is a chronic specific infection and they have much in common, though they differ widely as far as their prognosis is concerned. As an example: The histological picture of the granulation tissue, which differs from that of tuberculosis, in that the blood vessels are preserved and are the means by which the healing is effected. In the Röntgen picture also, the prognosis is very clear, because periosteal growth surrounds the area of destruction.

In the first place, syphilis differs practically from tuberculosis, in that drugs assuredly have the power of promoting and establishing healing. For all syphilitic conditions of bones and joints, mercury, iodides and Salvarsan in particular, are invaluable. In series 58, we see how the severe changes in the hand caused by a gummatous tumour, have healed after mercurial inunction treatment. (At that time Salvarsan had not been discovered.) The bone gumma does not always respond to iodides and mercury though. Series 55a. und b. show that both these specific drugs failed in the case of malignant syphilis. Salvarsan alone (no other arsenical preparations) established this cure. This shows that Lues may be manifested in various parts of the same organism at the same time, but in different ways. The gumma of the tibia finally healed, whereas the gumma of the ulna did not. At the present time, the prognosis of acquired bone and joint syphilis primarily depends upon the timely use of Salvarsan. This is also true for cases of late congenital syphilis, whereas the early congenital syphilitic osteochondritis (Series 51) and periostitis (Series 52) are more easily influenced and also cured by the use of other arsenical preparations.

The healing process of a bone gumma is as follows: The specific granulation tissue with its characteristic knot-shaped areas and necrosis, changes into an unspecific area, into which the bone tissue of the neighbouring shaft then grows. (See picture 2 of series 55a). Although healing of the process and reconstruction of the normal bone tissue by the use of Neosalvarsan is far more often the rule rather than the exception (Series 54 and 55), nevertheless a gummatous osteitis may remain obstinate in spite of all treatment. It may even fail to respond to Salvarsan when a serious mixed infection is present, as may be seen in series 57.

Serie 51.

Osteochondritis luetica.

Der 4 Wochen alte Säugling zeigte die kongenital-lueti-
schen Knochenveränderungen der Osteochondritis und
Periostitis in fortgeschrittenem Grade. Unter Arsen-
medikation (Spirocid) heilten die Veränderungen nach
anfänglicher Verschlimmerung in ½ Jahr ab.
Das Wachstum ging in normaler Weise vor sich.

Series 51.

Syphilitic Osteo-Chondritis.

In a baby of four weeks the congenital luetic bone
alterations of osteo-chondritis and periostitis were very
far advanced. Arsenic (Spirocid) was tried and after
appearing somewhat worse at first, the bony changes
healed within six months. In the meantime the growth
of the child was normal.

²/₃ n. Gr.   1.   2.   3.

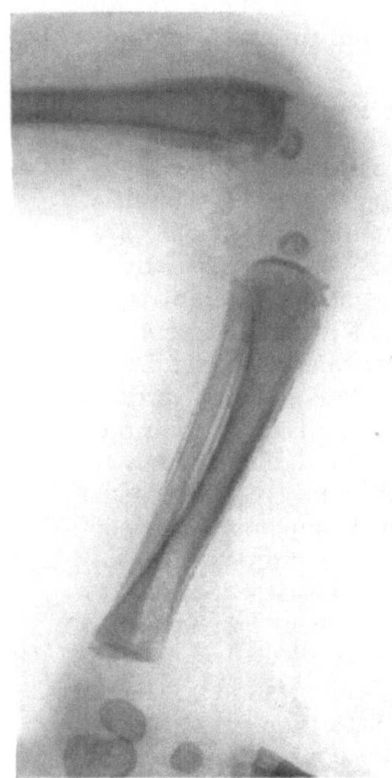
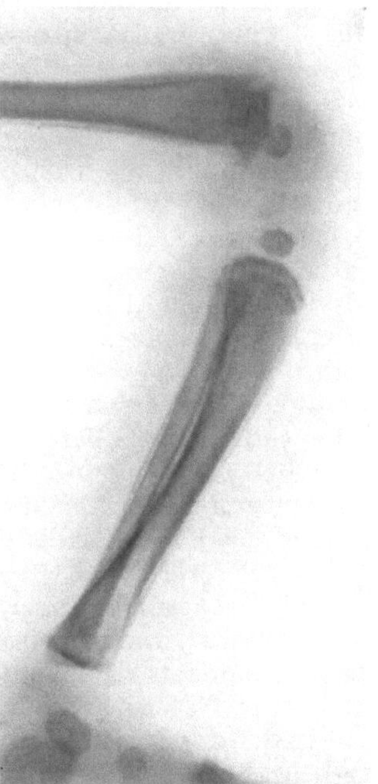
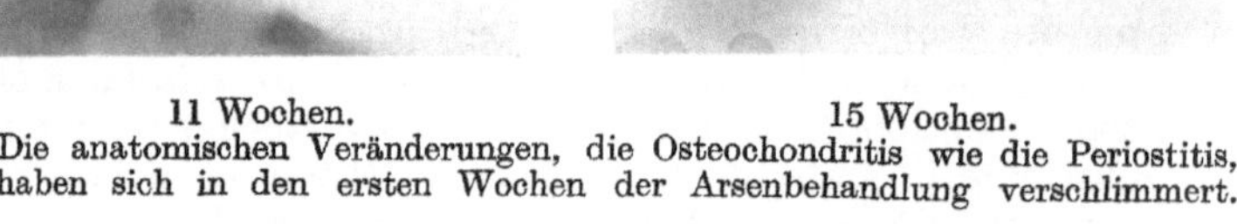

Lebensalter: 4 Wochen.
An dem proximalen *Tibia*ende ist die
provisorische Verkalkungszone verbreitert und verdichtet, durch einen
hellen Streifen (Granulationsgewebe)
diaphysenwärts abgesetzt (sog. doppelte Epiphysenlinie). — Am distalen
Femur ist die Metaphyse unscharf.
— An allen 3 Röhrenknochen besteht
eine starke, streifige *Periostitis.*

11 Wochen.   15 Wochen.
Die anatomischen Veränderungen, die Osteochondritis wie die Periostitis,
haben sich in den ersten Wochen der Arsenbehandlung verschlimmert.

Four weeks old. At the proximal end
of tibia, the provisional calcification
zone is widened and compact, divided
towards the diaphysis — so-called
double epiphysis-line — by a light
stripe (granulation - texture). The
metaphysis of the distal end of the
femur is indistinct. In all three tubular bones there is a severe streaky
periostitis.

Eleven weeks.   Fifteen weeks.
The anatomical alterations, the osteo-chondritis as well as the periostitis,
have become worse during the first few weeks of arsenic treatment.

Serie 51.

4. 5. 6.

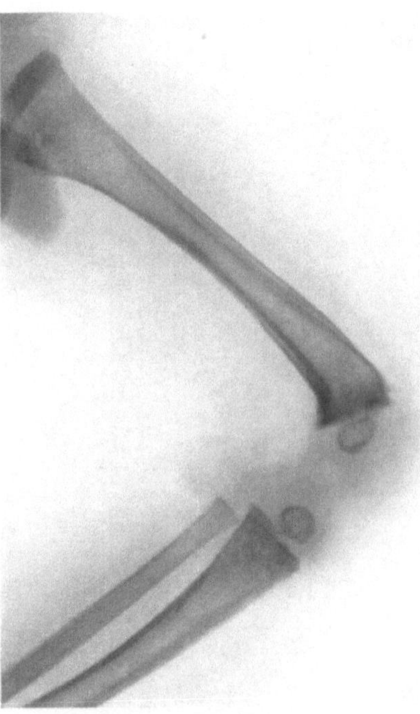

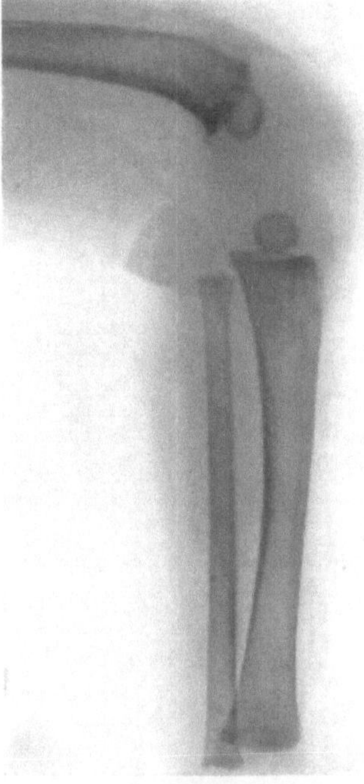

19 Wochen.
In dieser Zeit ist ein deutlicher Rückgang der Symptome im Gang.

Nineteen weeks.
At this time there is a distinct diminution of symptoms.

6 Monate.

Six months old.

7 Monate.
Epi- und Metaphyse der Tibia sind jetzt ganz *normal gebildet,* die des Femur fast geheilt, die ausgedehnte *Periostitis verschwunden.*

Seven months old.
Epiphysis and metaphysis of the tibia are now quite *normal,* the femur nearly healed and the extensive *periostitis has disappeared.*

Serie 52.

Periostitis luetica.

Als Frühsymptom der kongenitalen Syphilis wurde bei
dem 3¹/₂ Monate alten Kind eine ausgebreitete Periostitis
ossificans festgestellt; außerdem bestand eine frische
Humerusfraktur. Unter Arsenbehandlung entstand in
erstaunlich kurzer Zeit ein mächtiger Callus, der sich
ebenso schnell zurückbildete. Die Periostitis verstärkte
sich zuerst noch, ging dann aber an dem wachsenden
Knochen vollständig zurück.

Series 52.

Syphilitic Periostitis.

Periostitis ossificans was an early symptom of congenital
syphilis in a child of three and a half months, besides
which there was a recent humerus fracture. During the
arsenic treatment, an immense callus formed in an
astonishingly short time, and as quickly disappeared.
At first the periostitis increased, but disappeared
entirely with the growth of the bones.

⁶/₁₀ n. Gr.   1.   2.   3.

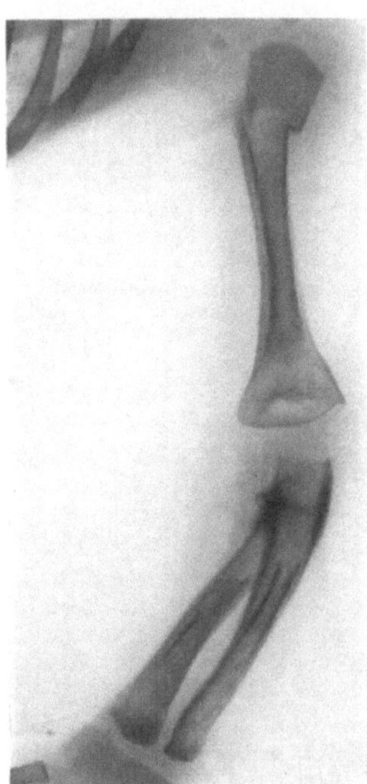

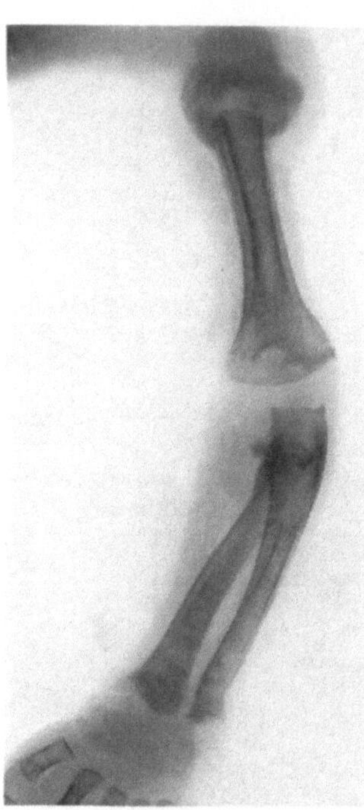

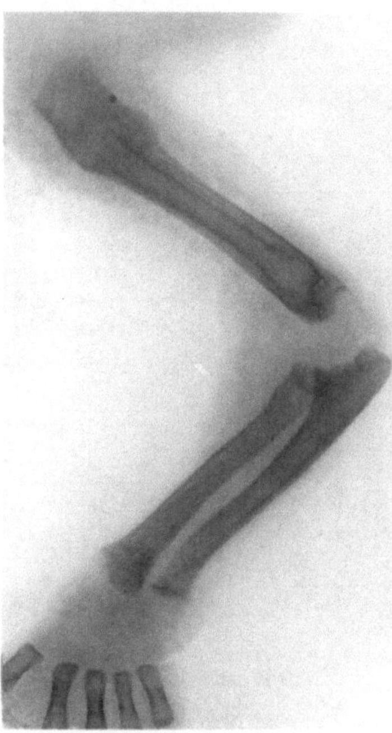

Lebensalter: 3¹/₂ Monate.
Der Humerus zeigt einen gleich-
mäßigen Periost-Knochensaum
und eine frische Fraktur im oberen
Drittel.

3¹/₂ months.
The humerus shows a regular periosteal bone-seam and a recent
fracture in the upper third.

4 Monate.
Die Periostitis hat noch etwas zugenommen, der Bruch ist in den
14 Tagen von einem mächtigen
Callus umwuchert.

Four months.
The periostitis has somewhat increased and in fourteen days an
immense callus has grown around
the fracture.

4¹/₂ Monate.
In weiteren 14 Tagen ist der Callus
fast ganz zurückgebildet, die Periostitis
noch deutlich.

4¹/₂ months.
Within the next fourteen days the
callus has almost entirely disappeared.
The periostitis is still obvious.

Serie 52.

4.

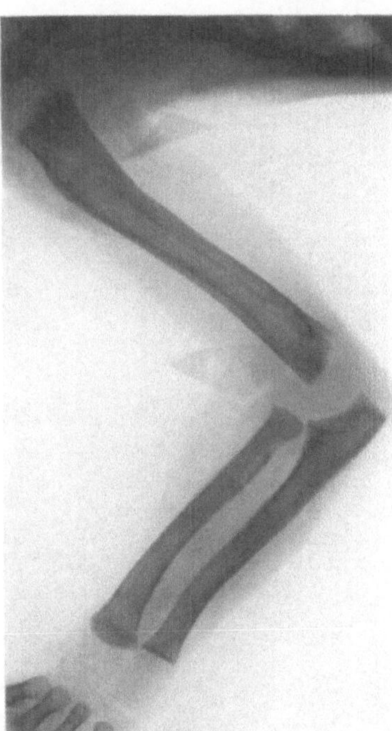

5.

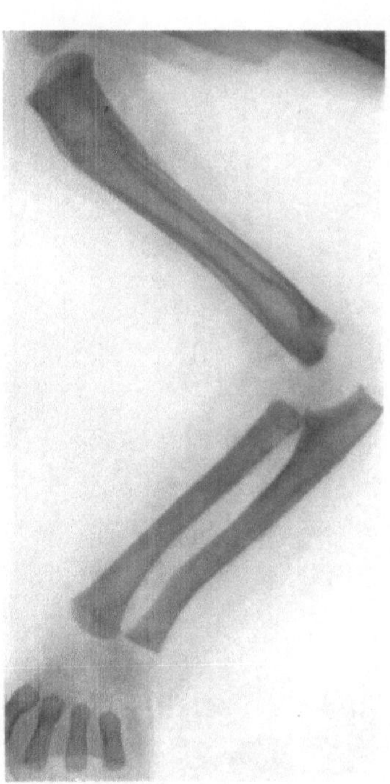

6.

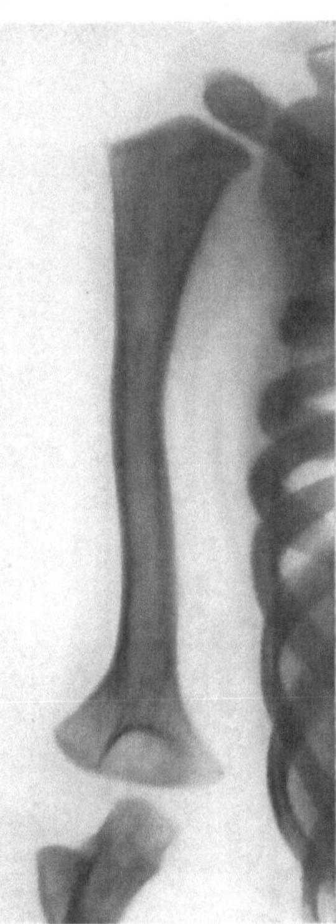

5 Monate.
Der streifige periostale Knochensaum ist besonders am Oberarm noch vorhanden.

Five months.
The streaky periosteal bone-seam is still prominent, especially in the humerus.

6 Monate.

Six months.

1¹/₂ Jahr.
Der Humerus ist gewachsen,
die Periostitis vollständig
verschwunden.

Eighteen months.
The humerus has grown and
the periostitis has completely
disappeared.

Serie 53.
Kongenitale Syphilis.

Bei dem 8 jährigen Mädchen trat die Lues hereditaria tarda unter dem charakteristischen Bilde der Periostitis gummosa an beiden Schienbeinen in Erscheinung. Die Veränderungen heilten auf eine einzige Hg-Salvarsankur restlos ab; die Wa.R. aber blieb stark positiv.

Series 53.
Congenital Syphilis.

A girl eight years of age developed hereditary Lues with the usual characteristic symptoms; periostitis gummosa on both tibiae. The condition in the bone healed after one single Hg-Salvarsan course. W.R. remained strongly positive.

$^6/_{10}$ n. Gr.

1.

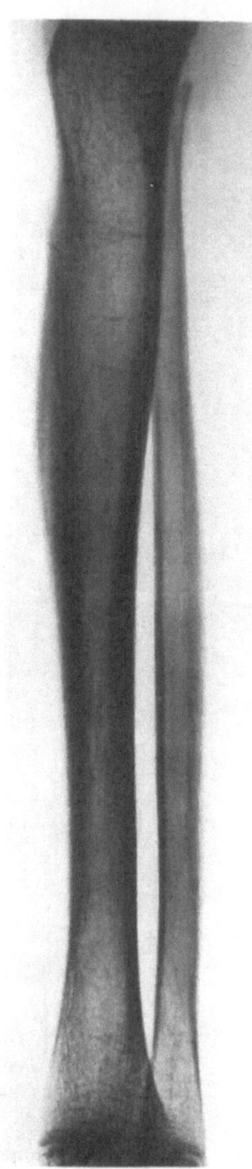

2.

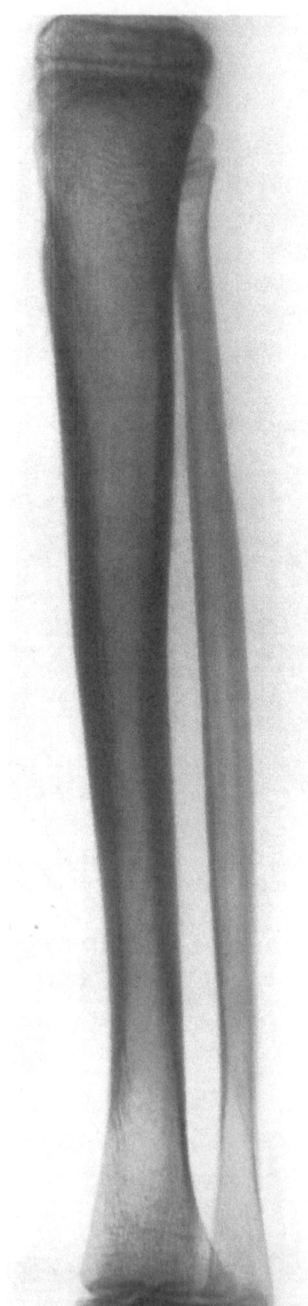

8. Lebensjahr: Periostitis ossificans der Tibiakante.
Eighth year. Periostitis ossificans of the Tibia edge.

11. Lebensjahr: Völlig normaler und entsprechend gewachsener Knochen. — Wa.R. +++.
Eleventh year. Quite normal and corresponding bone-growth. W.R. +++.

Serie 54.

Knochen- und Gelenksyphilis.

Die spezifische Knochen- und Gelenkentzündung (blande Gelenkschwellung) der erworbenen Syphilis heilte auf eine einzige antiluetische Kur bis zur Restitutio ad integrum.

$^2/_3$ n. Gr.   1.

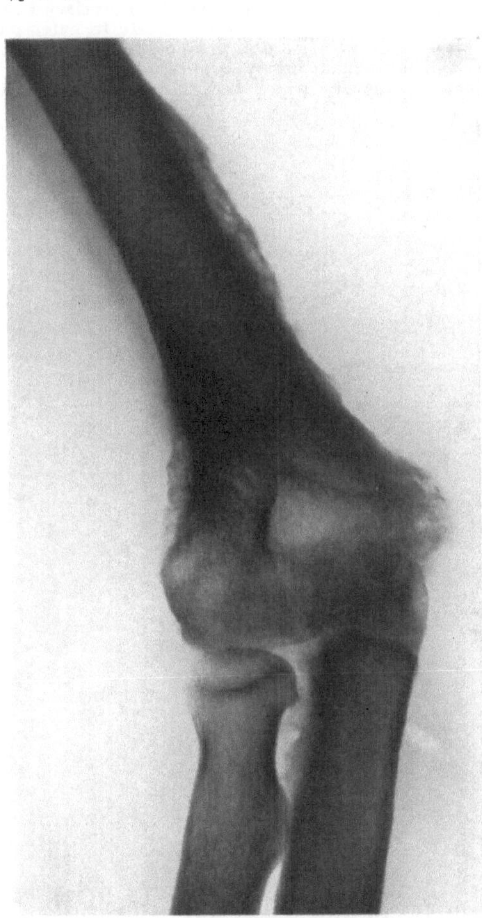

Ausgedehnte gummöse Periostitis am Knochenschaft bis zur Periost-Knorpelgrenze des Ellenbogengelenkes.

Extensive gummatous periostitis of the bone shaft as far as the periosteal cartilage of the elbow-joint.

Series 54.

Syphilis of Bones and Joints.

The specific bone and joint inflammation (mild joint swelling) of acquired syphilis healed absolutely, after one antiluetic course of treatment.

2.

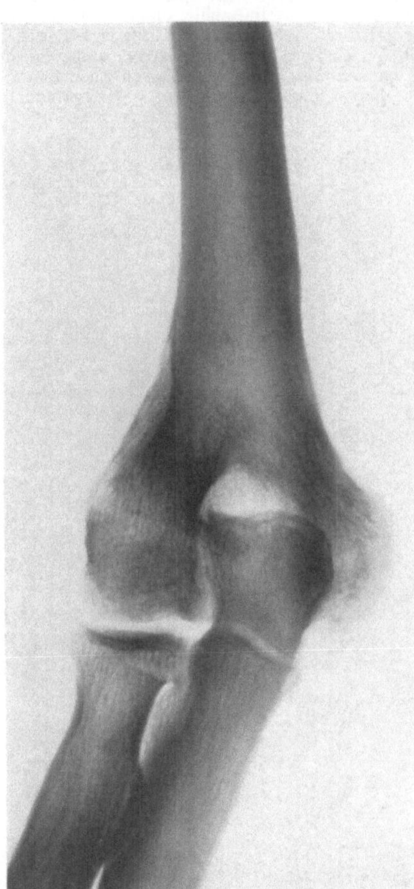

1 Jahr später – nach einer einzigen Hg-Salvarsankur – ist keine Spur der fortgeschrittenen Erkrankung vorhanden.

One year later after a single course of Hg-Salvarsan, not a trace of the advanced disease is to be found.

Serie 55 a.

Gumma der Tibia.

Bei dem 19 jährigen Mann trat die durch die Spirochaeta pallida gesetzte Infektion mehrere Monate nach dem Primäraffekt unter dem Bilde der Syphilis maligna auf und übersäte geradezu den Körper mit spezifischen Veränderungen. Am Knochen entstand ein großes Gumma der Tibia und gleichzeitig ein solches im distalen Ulnaende, welches in das Handgelenk einbrach. Später entwickelte sich noch eine spezifische Arthritis des Ellenbogens. — Die zahlreichen Manifestationen der tertiären Lues sprachen auf ausgiebige Kuren mit Quecksilber, Jod und Arsen *unterschiedlich,* im ganzen *nur wenig* an, heilten aber rasch auf das — damals entdeckte — Salvarsan.

Series 55 a.

Gumma of the Tibia.

A young man of nineteen became infected with spirochaeta pallida. Some months afterwards, syphilis maligna became manifest and practically covered his body with the specific manifestations. A large gumma of the tibia appeared and at the same time one at the distal end of ulna which broke through into the wrist-joint. Specific arthritis of the elbow also developed somewhat later. The numerous manifestations of the tertiary Lues reacted *but little,* and that *diversely* to extensive treatment with iodides, mercury and arsenic but responded immediately to treatment with Salvarsan, a remedy which had just been discovered.

$^7/_{10}$ n. Gr.   1.   2.

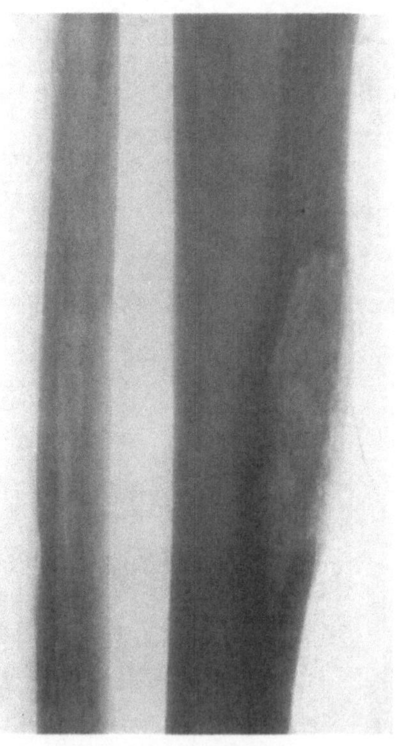

Großes *Gumma der Tibia:* ovaler, von sklerosiertem Knochen und periostitischer Wucherung begrenzter Zerstörungsbezirk.

Large *gumma of the tibia.* Oval area of destruction which is surrounded by sclerosed bone and abundant periosteal growth.

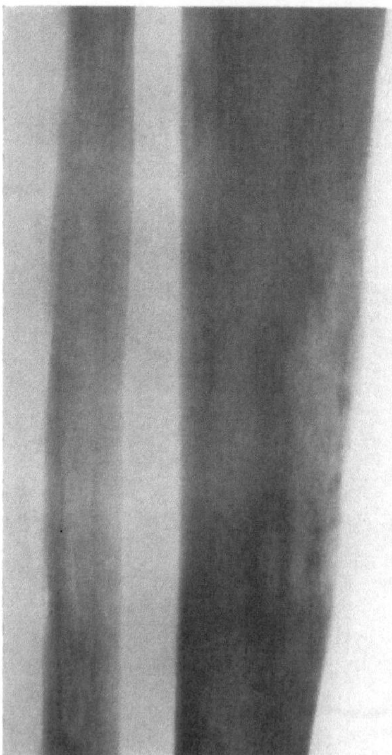

5 Monate später — nach einer Hg-Schmierkur — ist die scharfe Begrenzung des Herdes durch einwachsendes Knochengewebe gesprengt. (Beginnende Heilung.)

Five months later, after treatment with Hg-ointment, the exact margin of the area has been disturbed by the ingrowing bone tissue (Commencement of healing).

Serie 55a.

3.

4.

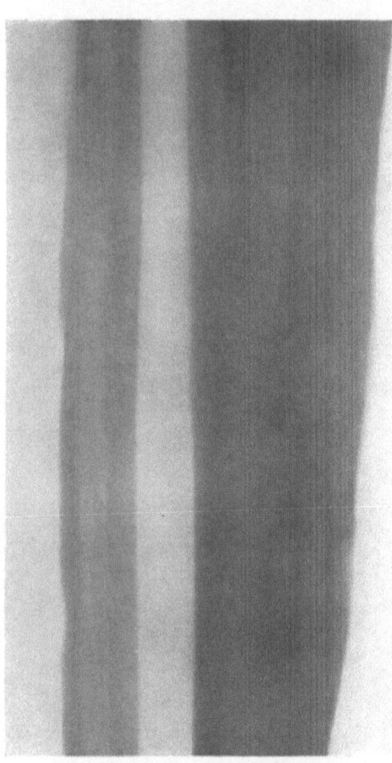

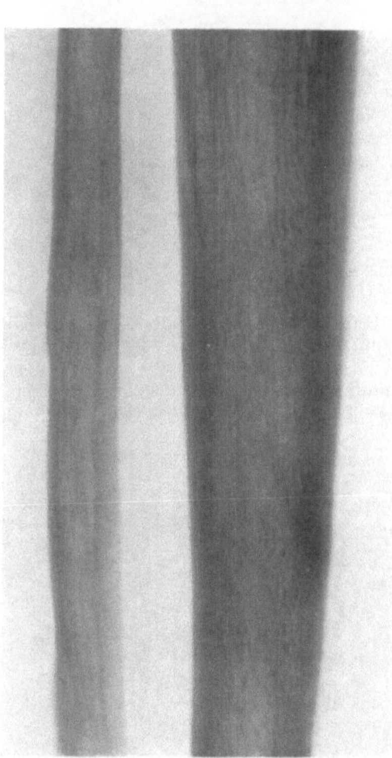

Nach 1 Jahr — unter der inzwischen begonnenen Salvarsantherapie — ist die Stelle vollständig knöchern ersetzt.

After one year. In the meantime the Salvarsan treatment had been commenced and the area has undergone complete regeneration.

Nach 20 Jahren ist auch die feine Bälkchenstruktur wiederhergestellt.

After twenty years, the delicate beam-structure has been renewed.

Serie 55 b.
Ossale luetische Handgelenkentzündung.

Von den spezifischen Knochenprozessen war das Gumma der Ulna auf Quecksilber, Jod und andere Arsenpräparate am meisten refraktär, heilte aber prompt auf Salvarsan.

$^3/_4$ n. Gr.   1.

Series 55 b.
Syphilitic Inflammation of the Bones of the Wrist-Joint.

Of all the specific bone-processes, the gumma of the ulna was most refractory to mercury, iodides and arsenic but healed promptly with Salvarsan treatment.

2.

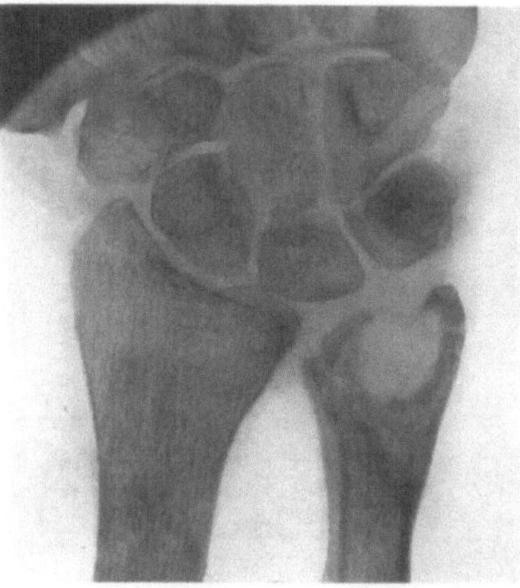

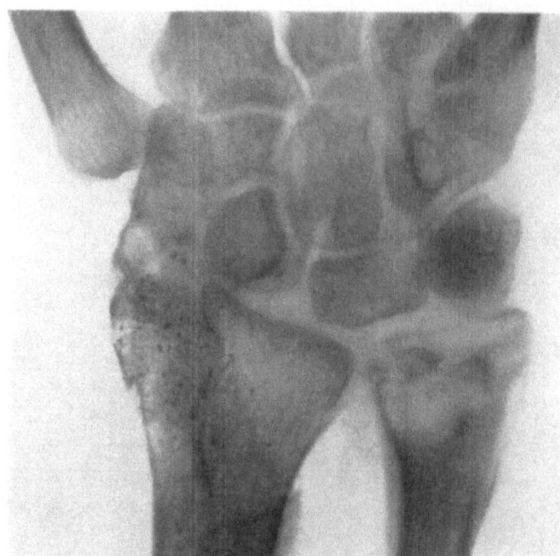

Ein Gumma hat das distale Ulnaende weitgehend zerstört und ist in das Handgelenk eingebrochen.

A gumma has extensively destroyed the distal end of ulna and broken into the wrist-joint.

5 Monate später ist die gummöse *Knochenzerstörung trotz ausgiebiger Hg-Schmierkur fortgeschritten.*

Five months later, the *bone destruction caused by the gumma, has advanced, despite abundant use of Hg-ointment.*

3.   4.

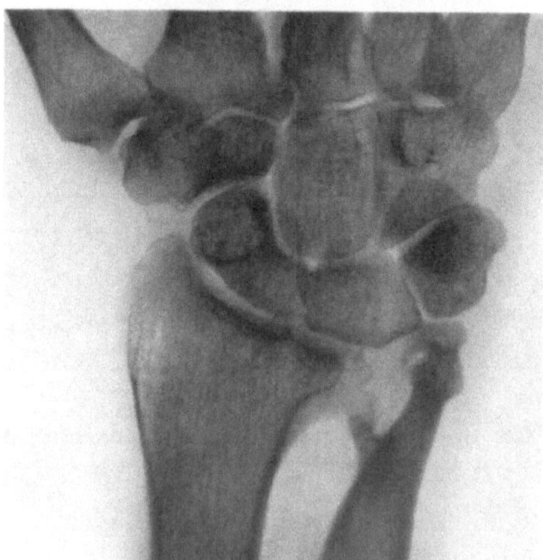

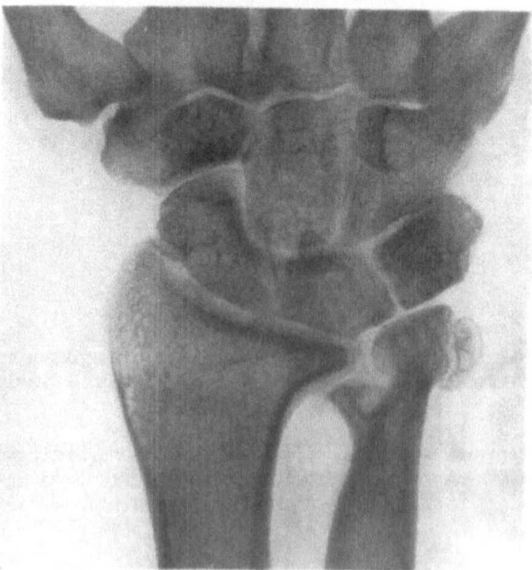

Nach 1 Jahr ist unter der inzwischen erfolgten *Salvarsan*behandlung der tertiär luetische Prozeß *geheilt:* der Knochendefekt gereinigt und geglättet.

After one year. In the meantime, Salvarsan treatment had been carried out and the tertiary luetic process has healed; the bone-defect cleansed and smoothened.

Nach 20 Jahren ist der ulnare Gelenkteil beträchtlich regeneriert, so daß die radio-ulnare Gelenkfläche wieder geschlossen ist.

After twenty years the ulna part of joint has regenerated considerably so that the radio-ulna articulation is again closed.

Serie 55 c.

Ossale Ellenbogenlues.

Ein späterer Rückfall — eine gleichfalls ossale Gelenkentzündung — heilte auf Salvarsan (außerdem Hg-Schmierkur) in kurzer Zeit. — Von da ab blieb der Mann dauernd symptomfrei und war gesund.

$^7/_{10}$ n. Gr.   1.

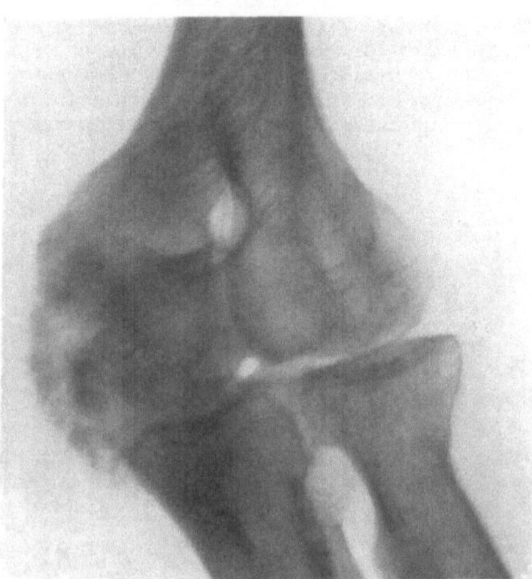

Destruierender, mit periostaler Knochenwucherung einhergehender Prozeß am Condylus medialis humeri.

Process of destruction with abundance of periosteal bone growth at the medial condyle of the humerus.

3.

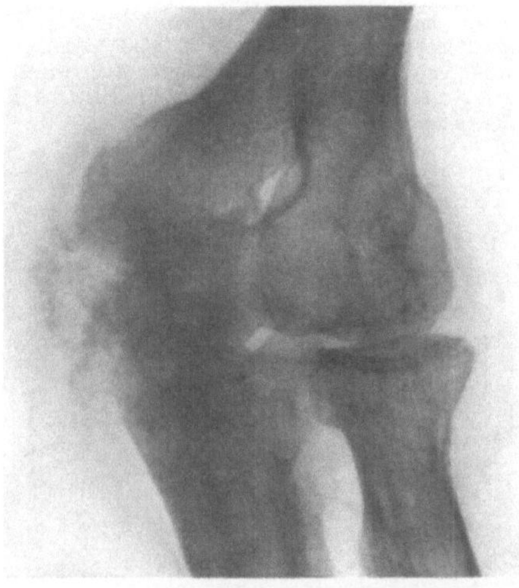

Nach $^1/_2$ Jahr ist die gummöse Entzündung abgeheilt; der mediale Condylus knöchern geflickt, noch etwas uneben umrandet.

After six months, the gummatous inflammation has healed and the medial condyle repaired by bone, but the edges are still somewhat uneven.

Series 55 c.

Syphilitic Osteitis of the Elbow.

A later relapse — also an osteal joint inflammation — healed in a short time by the use of Salvarsan (as well as Hg-ointment). From that time the man had no further symptoms and was quite healthy.

2.

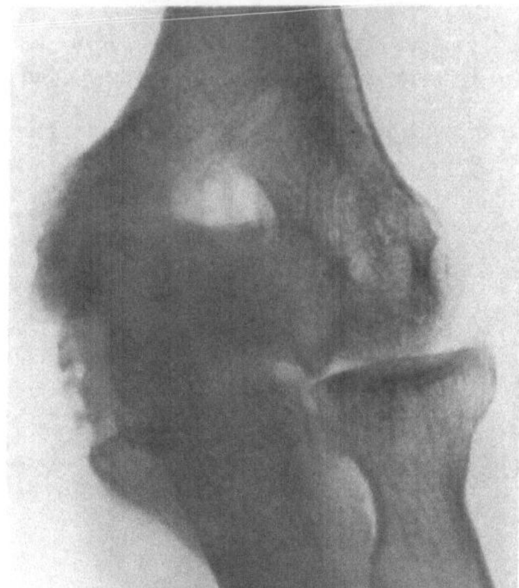

2 Monate später — nach zwei Salvarsaninjektionen — ist die gummöse Osteoperiostitis deutlich in *Rückbildung*, so daß die Knochenkonturen wieder mehr hervortreten.

Two months later. After two Salvarsan injections, the gummatous osteo-periostitis is plainly *diminishing* so that the outlines of the bones are again distinct.

4.

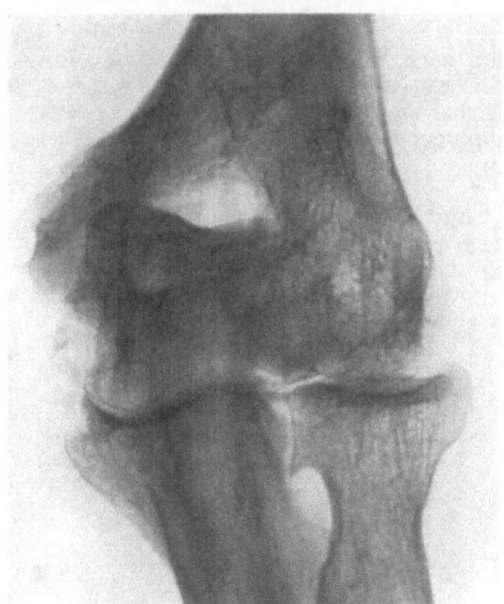

Nach 20 Jahren zeigt der Knochen gute Struktur und glatte Umrisse.

After twenty years, the bone shows good structure and smooth outlines.

7*

Serie 56.

Spondylitis luetica.

Die Krankheit des 45 Jahre alten Mannes wurde erst 1½ Jahre nach Beginn der Beschwerden erkannt. Um diese Zeit hatte der gummöse Prozeß bereits zu einer ausgedehnten Zerstörung des 4. und 5. Halswirbels geführt; dennoch wurde in kurzer Zeit durch Neosalvarsan und Jodkali Beschwerdefreiheit und anatomische Ausheilung erreicht.

⁷/₁₀ n. Gr.   1.

Series 56.

Syphilitic Spondylitis.

The malady of a forty-five year old man was only recognized a year and a half after the commencement of complaint. At this time the gummatous process had already led to an extensive destruction of the fourth and fifth cervical vertebrae, nevertheless, by the use of Neosalvarsan and potassium iodide freedom of disorder and anatomical healing was achieved within a short time.

2.

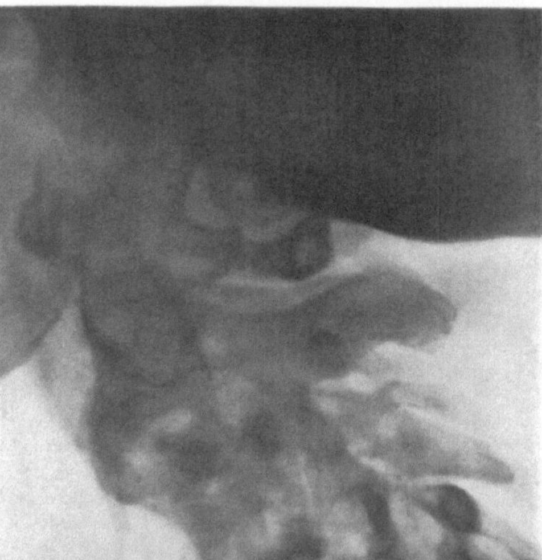

1½ Jahre nach Einsetzen der Schmerzen vor Einleitung der antiluetischen Therapie zeigt der 4. und 5. Halswirbel ausgedehnte Zerstörung, aber auch eine reaktive Knochenwucherung, welche die Wirbelsäule abzustützen sucht. — Wa.R. ++++.

One year and a half after the pain was first felt and before the antiluetic therapy, the fourth and fifth vertebrae showed extensive destruction and also reactive bone-growth which attempts to support the spine.
W.R. ++++.

4 Monate später ist unter dem Einfluß der spezifischen Kur der zerstörte Knochen weitgehend ersetzt.

Four months later, under the influence of the specific treatment, the destroyed bone has been, to a great extent replaced.

Serie 56.

3.

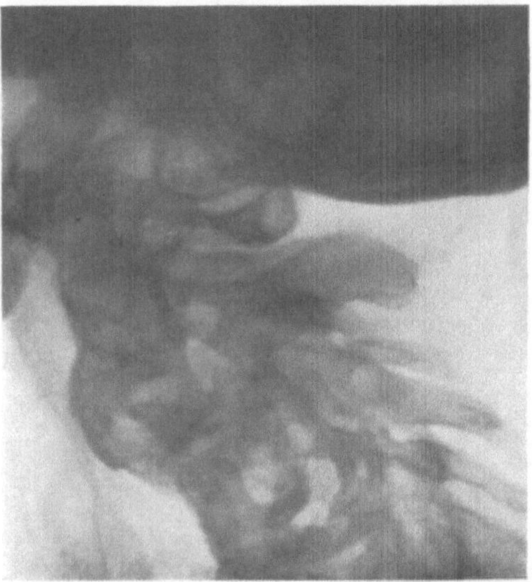

4.

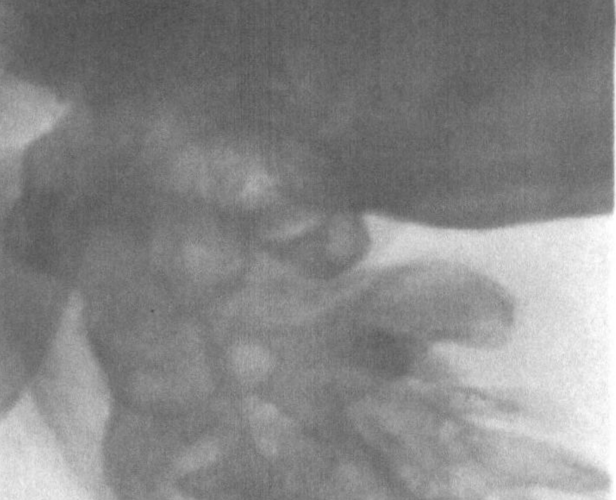

5 Monate nach Beginn der Behandlung ist der zerstörte Bezirk noch mehr wiederhergestellt.

Five months after commencement of treatment, the destroyed area has been further replaced.

Nach 8 Monaten ist der Endzustand erreicht: der Wirbelkörper (C. 5) ist knöchern wiederaufgebaut, eine solide Abstützung ist vorhanden und das Knochengefüge tritt wieder klarer hervor. (Der gleiche Röntgenbefund wurde auch 2 Jahre später nach weiter durchgeführter Therapie erhoben.)

After eight months the final aim has been achieved. The vertebra (C. 5) has been rebuilt with bone, a solid support gained and the bone structure shows again distinctly. Two years later, during which the same treatment was followed, an X-Ray photograph showed the same condition.

Serie 57.	Series 57.

Ostitis gummosa des Schädels.   Gummatous Osteitis of the Skull.

Die fortgeschrittene fistelnde Schädellues der 60jährigen Frau konnte durch wiederholte und ausgiebige spezifische Kuren (Hg, Salvarsan, Jodkali) nicht geheilt werden; vielmehr kam es — bei der Mischinfektion — zu Sequesterbildung und schleichend fortschreitender Zerstörung des Knochens, freilich ohne daß die Kranke in ihrem Allgemeinzustand nennenswert beeinträchtigt wurde. Wa.R. +++.

A woman of sixty suffered with advanced fistulous Lues of the skull. Although copious specific treatment was repeatedly tried (Hg, Salvarsan, pot. iodide) it remained incurable; indeed, the mixed infection led to sequestrum formation and a slowly advancing destruction of the bone. The patient was not greatly inconvenienced by the malady. W.R. +++.

1/2 n. Gr.

1 a.

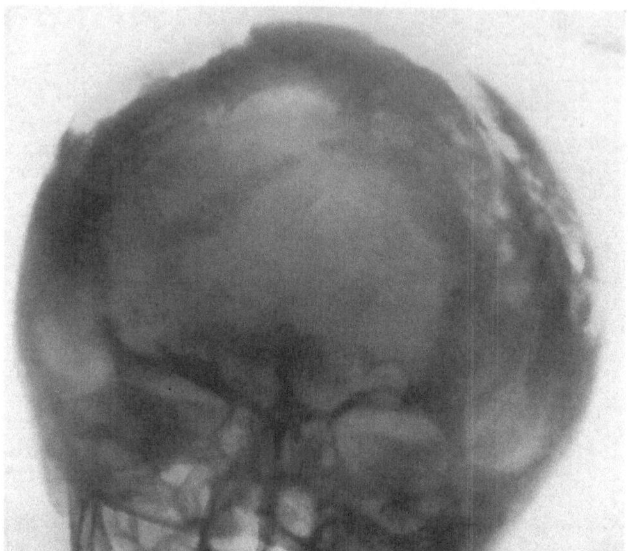

1 b.

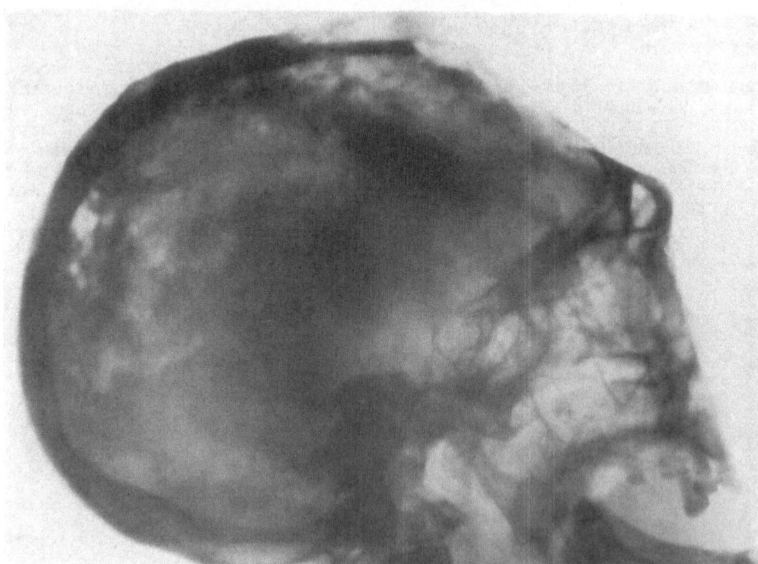

Etwa 10 Jahre nach Beginn besteht eine ausgedehnte Zerstörung des Schädeldaches; ein größerer Sequester ist gelöst.

About ten years after onset of disease there is an extensive destruction of the skull and a large sequestrum is loosened.

Serie 57.

2 a.

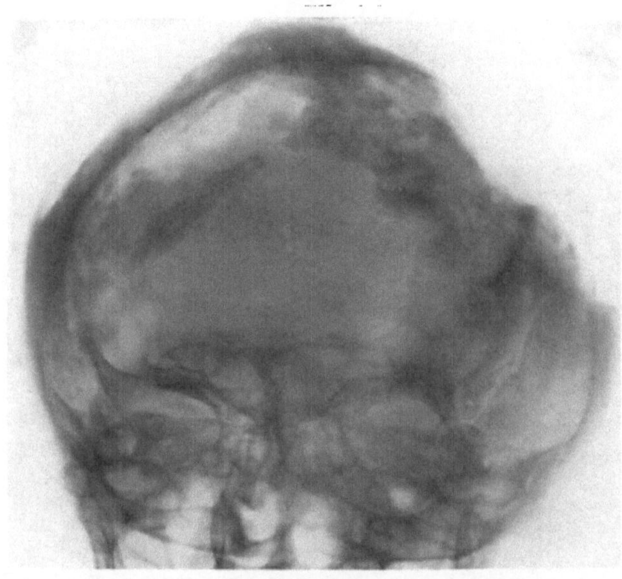

2 b.

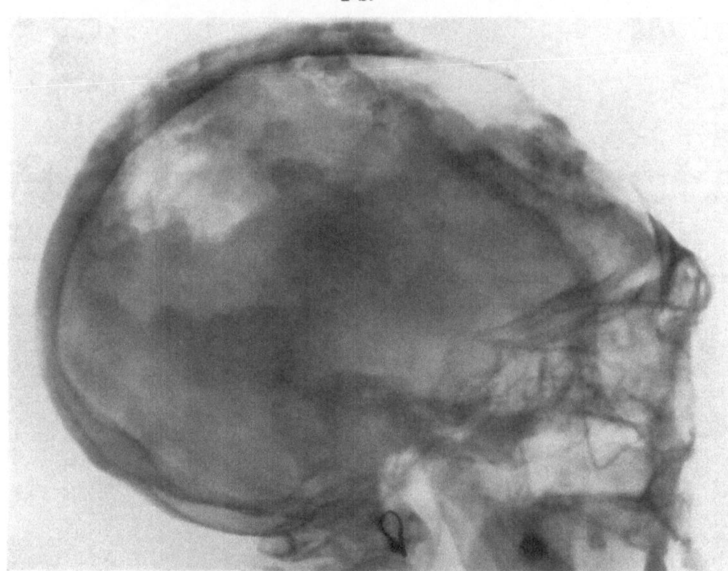

5 Jahre später (nach der Entfernung des Sequesters) ist trotz antiluetischer Kur eine Regeneration des Schädeldaches nicht erfolgt, vielmehr sind die Knochendefekte viel größer.

Five years later (after the removal of sequestrum) in spite of anti-luetic treatment, no regeneration of skull-bone has taken place, but the bony defects have become much larger.

Serie 58.

Ostitis gummosa.

Diese Beobachtung stammt aus der „Vor-Salvarsan-
zeit" und zeigt den die Heilung bestimmenden Einfluß des Quecksilbers bei tertiärer Knochensyphilis.

$^7/_{10}$ n. Gr.   1.

Series 58.

Gummatous Osteitis.

This case was observed before Salvarsan was used
and shows the healing influence that mercury
has over tertiary bone syphilis.

2.

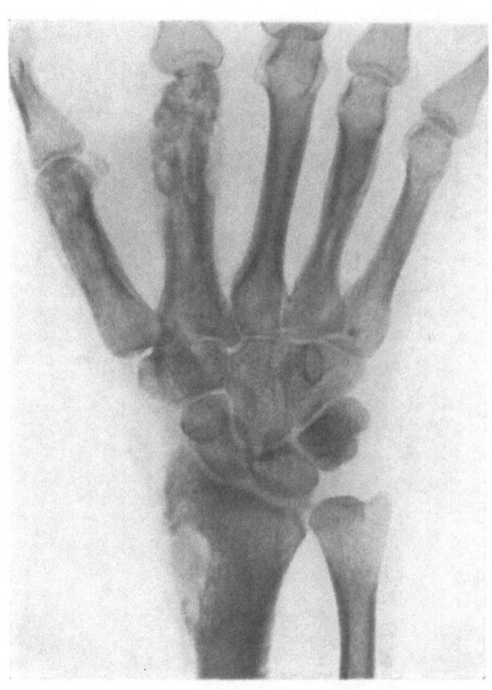

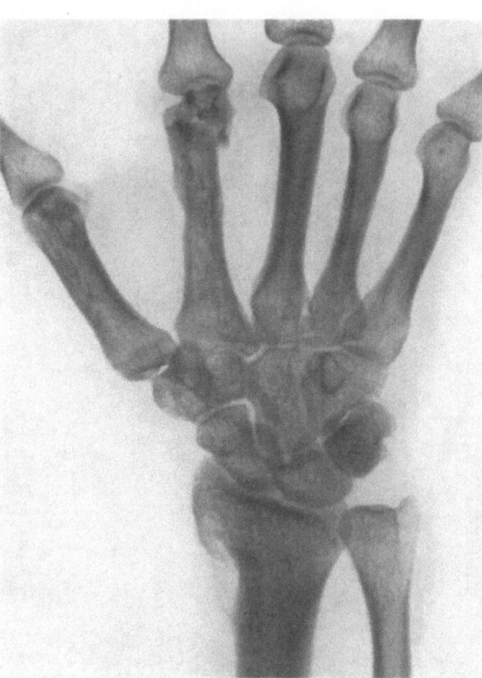

Ausgedehnte Knochenzerstörung besonders des Radius und Metacarpus IV durch die spezifische
Entzündung.

Extensive bone destruction, particularly of radius
and metacarpus IV by the specific process
of inflammation.

4 Monate später nach einer ausgiebigen Quecksilber-
Schmierkur ist der Knochenprozeß nahezu abgeheilt.

Four months later. Almost healed after liberal
mercurial inunction treatment.

III. Kapitel.

Geschwülste.

Primäre und sekundäre Knochengeschwülste.

Die Prognose der bösartigen Geschwülste ist infaust, sofern sie sich nicht im Gesunden operativ entfernen lassen. Dieser Satz der Vor-Röntgenzeit hat für die bösartigen Geschwülste der Knochen auch heute noch seine Gültigkeit behalten. Hat doch noch keine Zentrale der Röntgentherapie trotz der ungeheueren auf dieses Ziel gerichteten Anstrengungen eine *Reihe* dauernd geheilter Knochensarkome bekanntgeben können. Unter den im Schrifttum mitgeteilten Heilungen mögen sich wenige Beobachtungen finden, welche eine Dauerheilung echter Sarkome darstellen. Diese Fälle sind aber seltene Ausnahmen, gewissermaßen Zufallsereignisse, mit denen wir nicht rechnen können. Bei der Mehrzahl ist die Diagnose entweder überhaupt nicht gesichert — die Serie 72 und 73 beweisen die Möglichkeit der Täuschung — oder es handelt sich um sog. Riesenzelltumoren, in deren Reihe die Epulis und die Ostitis fibrosa gehören, die aber heute als Granulationsgewebe erkannt sind und nicht mehr als echte Neubildung aufgefaßt werden. Was die echten bösartigen Knochengeschwülste betrifft, so können in ihrem Verlauf *Veränderungen* auftreten, *welche in die Richtung einer Heilung deuten.* Solche Veränderungen sind Verkalkungen, Verknöcherungen (Serie 64 und 65) oder Abkapselungen. Aber diese sind als regressive oder als Ausreifungsvorgänge ein natürlicher Ablauf und kein Bestrahlungserfolg, ganz abgesehen davon, daß sie stets unvollkommen bleiben. Wissen wir doch, daß eine vorher osteoklastische Metastase nach erfolgter Fraktur des Knochens osteoplastische Fähigkeit annimmt und den Bruch heilt (Serie 67). Auch „Abkapselungen" (Serie 62) sind eine natürliche, von außen unbeeinflußte Reaktion zwischen gesunder Umgebung und der Neubildung. Eine zuverlässige Heilung durch Einwachsen des gesunden Knochens in den untergehenden Geschwulstbezirk, wie wir sie etwa bei den Granulationswucherungen der Serie 26 oder Serie 55a sehen, ist bisher nicht belegt. — Wir haben uns umgesehen, aber außer der Operation noch nichts gefunden.

Chapter III.

Tumours.

Primary and Secondary Bone Tumours.

When the removal of genuine malignant tumours is not possible, the prognosis is of course hopeless. This was so in pre-Röntgen days and as far as bone tumours are concerned, it is still true. Despite tremendous efforts in this direction, no X-ray institute has, as yet, been able to prove a series of permanent cures of bone sarcomata. Among the published cases of permanent cures of genuine bone sarcomata, few are deserving of much consideration. These cases are exceptions — one might say, accidental events, upon which we cannot rely. In the majority of cases, either the diagnosis has not been confirmed (Series 72 and 73 illustrate the possibility of error) or it is a case of so-called giant cell tumour, to which species, epulis and osteitis fibrosa belong. These are now recognised as consisting of granulation tissue and are not genuine new growths. Sometimes changes occur in the course of a genuine malignant bone tumour that seem to indicate healing. Such changes are calcification, deposition of bone (Series 64—65) and scar formation. They are regressive or maturing changes — a natural course which should not be ascribed to the success of Röntgen therapy — apart from the fact that they always remain imperfect. We know that after sustaining a fracture of the bone, an osteoclastic metastasis adopts osteoplastic ability and the fracture heals (Series 67). „Scarring" also (Series 62) is a natural reaction between healthy surroundings and new construction, and is uninfluenced by outside factors. A reliable cure by the penetration of healthy bone into the breaking down tumour area, such as we see in granulation tumours (Series 26 or 55a.) is not yet proved. As far as we know, there is no cure except by operation.

Serie 59.

Spindelzellensarkom des Schienbeins.

Der 54 jähr. Mann erkrankte mit einer zunehmenden Schwellung am Knie, die ihm wenig Beschwerden machte, bis nach 1½ jährigem Bestehen und langsam fortschreitendem Wachstum die Spontanfraktur eintrat. Amputation.

Series 59.

Spindle Cell Sarcoma of the Tibia.

A fifty year old man had slowly increasing swelling under the knee which caused him slight inconvenience. A spontaneous fracture occured after the increasing swelling had existed for eighteen months. Amputation.

$^{7}/_{10}$ n. Gr.   1.

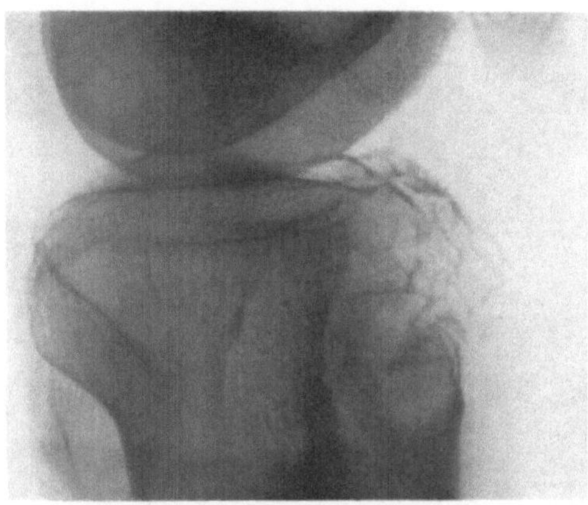

2.

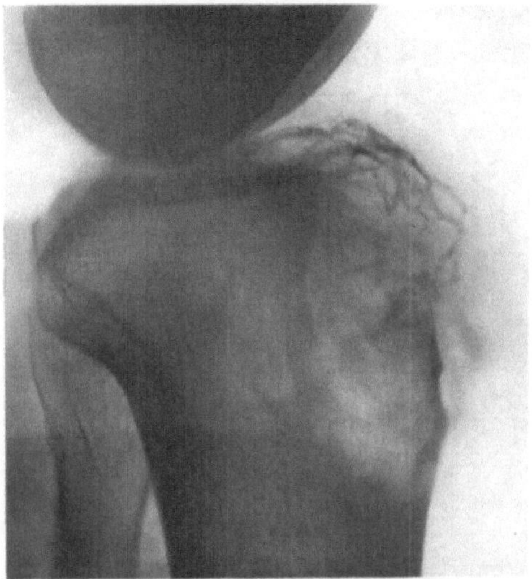

Kurz nachdem die Schwellung bemerkt wurde, bestand bereits ein größerer zentraler Tumor von teilweise wabigem Bau und destruierendem Wachstum.

Soon after the swelling was noticed, a large central tumour was present. It had a honeycomb structure and was very destructive.

Nach 5 Monaten ist das zentrale Sarkom in der vorderen Tibiakante erheblich gewachsen und in die Weichteile eingebrochen.

After five months. The sarcoma has grown considerably into the anterior tibia-edge and extended into the fleshy parts.

3.

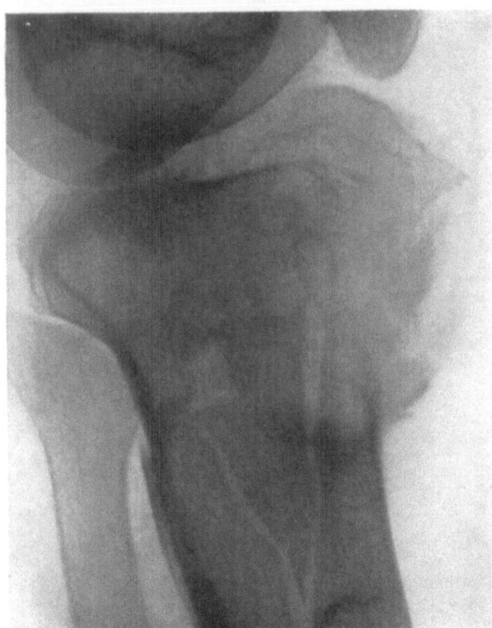

Nach 1½ Jahren ist die Geschwulst knochen- und weichteilwärts noch mehr vorgedrungen und hat zur Spontanfraktur der Tibia geführt.
(Histologisch Spindelzellsarkom.)

After eighteen months. The tumour has penetrated further into bone and fleshy parts and caused a spontaneous fracture of the tibia.
(Histological examination showed spindle cell sarcoma.)

Serie 60.

Spindelzellsarkom des Schenkelhalses.

Das 16 jährige Mädchen erkrankte plötzlich mit einer Spontanfraktur des Schenkelhalses. Wenige Wochen später stellte sich wiederholt Hämoptoe ein, als deren Ursache ausgedehnte Lungenmetastasen festgestellt wurden. Die Kranke verfiel und starb schon nach einem Vierteljahr in extremer Kachexie. In dieser Zeit hatte das Spindelzellsarkom den Schenkelhals vollständig zerstört und war in die Weichteile eingebrochen.

$^6/_{10}$ n. Gr.   1.

Series 60.

Spindle Cell Sarcoma of the Femoral Neck.

A sixteen year old girl suddenly had a spontaneous fracture of the femoral neck. A few weeks later she had repeated attacks of haemoptysis caused by lung-metastasis The patient wasted and three months later died of extreme cachexia. During this time the spindle cell sarcoma had completely destroyed the femoral neck and extended into the fleshy parts.

2.

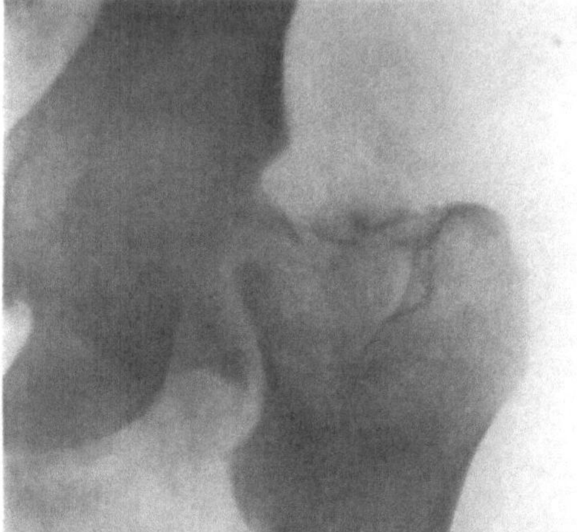

Der Schenkelhals ist eingebrochen, zeigt aber außer der frischen Fraktur deutlich eine Knochenauflösung.

The femoral neck has broken in and a dissolving of bone, as well as the fresh fracture, can be plainly seen.

3.

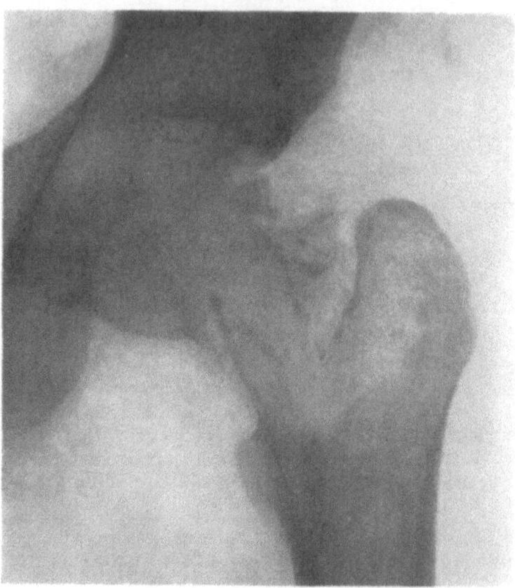

Nach 4 Wochen ist der Knochenuntergang noch deutlicher und ausgedehnter — Frakturcallus fehlt völlig.

After four weeks. The bone decay is plainer and more extensive. There is no fracture callus.

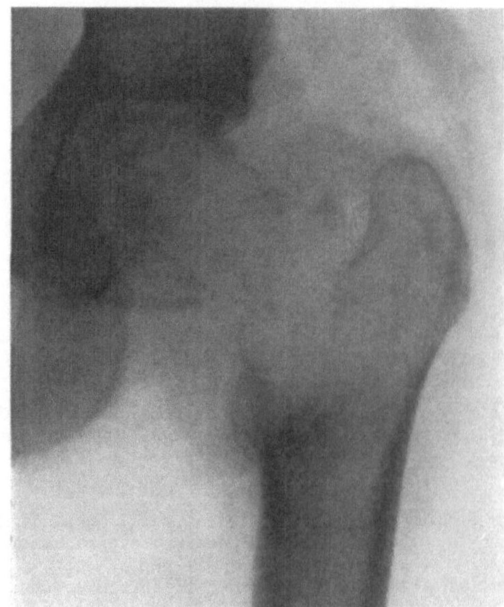

Nach einem Vierteljahr ist der Schenkelhals völlig ausgelöscht.

After three months. The femoral neck is completely destroyed.

Serie 61.

Spindelzellsarkom des Wadenbeinköpfchens.

Die 50jährige Frau erkrankt mit Schmerzen unter dem Knie, die zunächst als Neuralgien gedeutet wurden. Bereits der 1. Röntgenbefund wies ein myelogenes Sarkom nach, wurde aber nicht gewertet. Die Geschwulst wuchs rasch, den Knochen destruierend, und brach in die Weichteile ein. Dann erst erfolgte die Amputation.

$^6/_{10}$ n. Gr.   1.

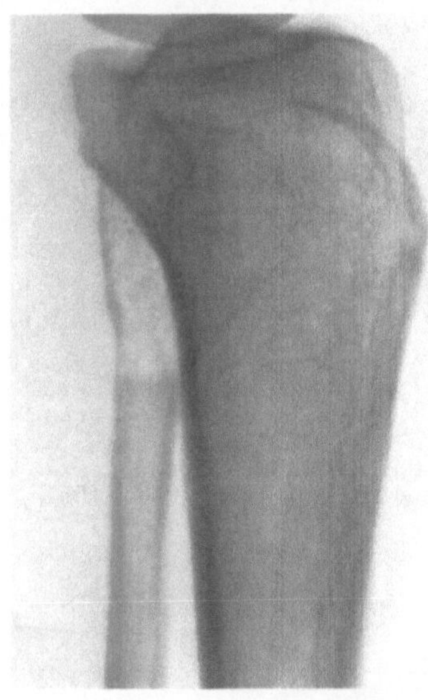

Das 1. Röntgenbild läßt bereits eine zentrale Knochenzerstörung am oberen Wadenbeinende erkennen (zentrales Sarkom).

The first Röntgen picture already shows a central bone destruction at the upper end of the fibula. (Central sarcoma.)

Series 61.

Spindle Cell Sarcoma of the Fibula Head.

A fifty year old woman suffered with pain under the knee, which was first thought to be neuralgia. The first Röntgen picture showed a myelogenic sarcoma, but it was not correctly estimated. The swelling grew rapidly, destroyed the bone and penetrated into the fleshy parts. Amputation was performed.

2.

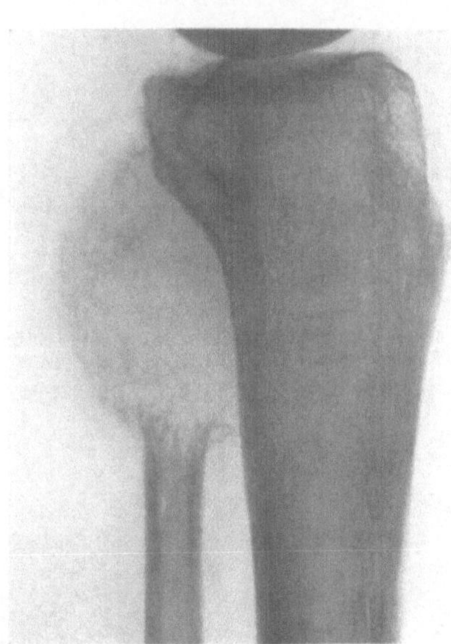

5 Monate später ist das Fibulaende von der sehr viel größer gewordenen Geschwulst vernichtet und ersetzt.

Five months later. The greatly enlarged swelling has entirely destroyed the fibula end and replaced it.

<table>
<tr><td>

Serie 62.

Spindelzellsarkom des Calcaneus.

Der bei dem 40 jährigen Mann schließlich histologisch als „Spindelzellsarkom mit vielen Mitosen" festgestellte Krankheitsprozeß schien sich zunächst — was man als Bestrahlungserfolg zu deuten geneigt war — abzukapseln, wuchs aber in Wirklichkeit unaufhaltsam. Amputation.

</td><td>

Series 62.

Spindle Cell Sarcoma of the Calcaneus.

A man of forty suffered with a complaint histologically diagnosed as "spindle-cell-sarcoma with numerous mitoses". At first the progress of the disease seemed inclined to be arrested, owing, it was thought, to irradiation treatment. Later however, it proved impossible to bring it to a standstill. Amputation.

</td></tr>
</table>

$^2/_3$ n. Gr.   1.   2.

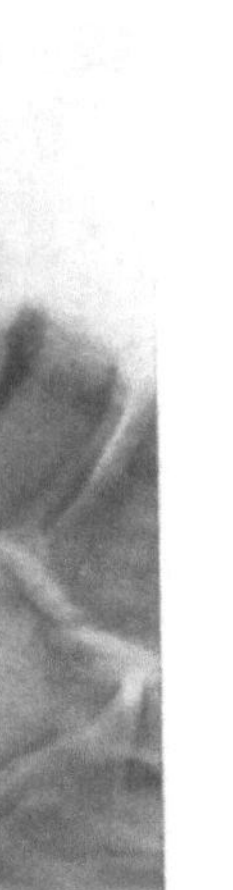 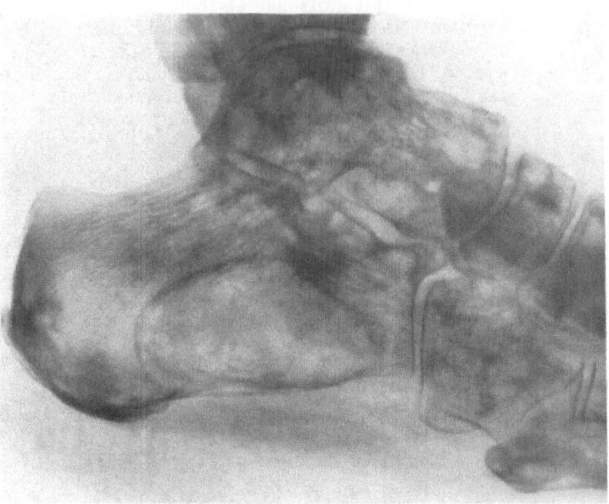

<table>
<tr><td>

Kurz nach Einsetzen der Schmerzen ist ein ovaler Bezirk abgebauten Knochens im Fersenbein zu erkennen.

Shortly after commencement of pain an oval patch of devitalised bone is noticeable in calcaneus.

</td><td>

Nach 3$^1/_2$ Monaten ist eine starke Entkalkung der Fußknochen eingetreten; der Tumor selbst ist größer geworden und erscheint scharf umgrenzt.

After three and a half months the foot-bones have become considerably decalcified. The tumour itself has grown and has a distinct outline.

</td></tr>
</table>

3.

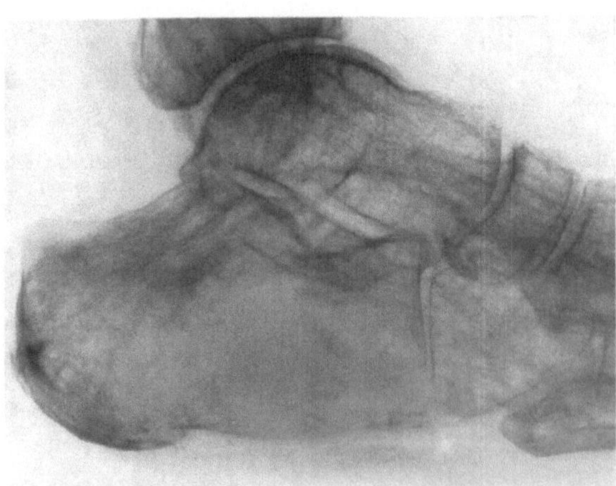

Nach 1 Jahr — regelmäßiger Róntgenbestrahlung — hat der Tumor den größeren Teil des Calcaneus zerstört und dessen Grenzen durchbrochen. — Die Knochenatrophie ist noch hochgradiger.

After one year, during which regular Röntgen irradiation treatment was administered The tumour has destroyed the greater part of the calcaneus and broken through the boundary. The bone atrophy has increased.

Serie 63.
Chondrosarkom der Hüfte.

Der 19jährige Mann litt seit Jahren an unbestimmten Beschwerden in der Hüfte, die in dem letzten halben Jahr unerträglich wurden. Röntgenbestrahlung des Tumors war erfolglos, daher wurde die extrakapsuläre Resektion der Hüfte ausgeführt. — Das Präparat zeigte eine ausgedehnte Zerstörung des Gelenkes und der angrenzenden Beckenknochen bei dichter Durchsetzung mit Knorpelinseln. (Histologisch Chondrosarkom.)

Series 63.
Chondro-Sarcoma of the Hip.

A young man of nineteen suffered with vague pain in the hip, which had become unbearable in the last six months. Röntgen ray treatment was tried but without success. Therefore extracapsular resection was performed. Extensive destruction of joint was found and the neighbouring bones were marbled with cartilage.
(Histologically-chondrosarcoma.)

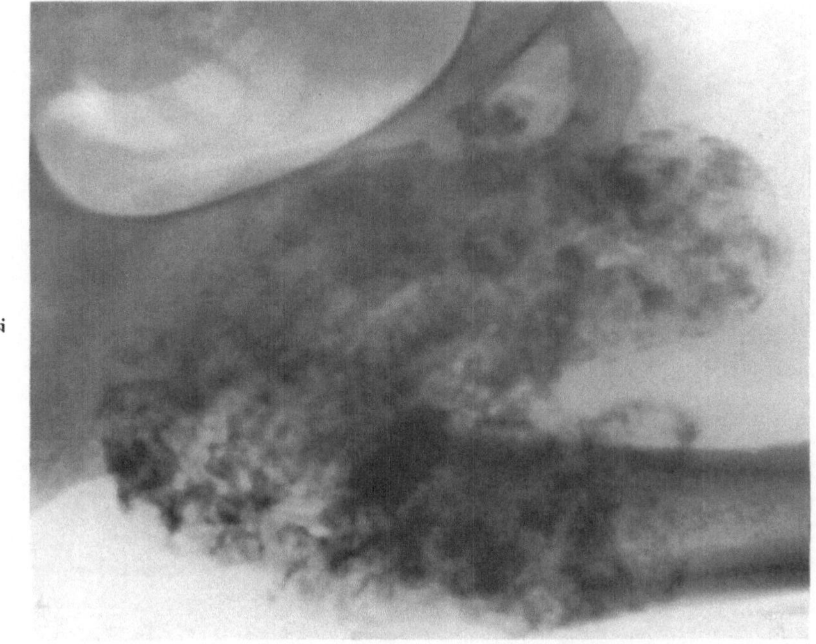

Ein halbes Jahr später ist das Tumorgewebe stärker verkalkt und dichter. Die Konturen des Gelenkes sind nicht mehr erkennbar.

Six months later. The tumour tissue has become more ossified and compact. The outlines of the ioint are no longer recognizable.

Um das Hüftgelenk, dessen Konturen teilweise noch eben erkennbar sind, ist eine schwammartige Knochengeschwulst ausgebreitet, welche zerstörendes Wachstum des Femurendes erkennen läßt.

A spongy bone swelling has spread, around the hip-joint, the outlines of which are still just recognizable. The destruction of the femur is recognizable.

6/10 n. Gr.

Serie 64.

Osteoidsarkom des Oberschenkels.

Der 19jährige Mann bemerkte eine wenig schmerzhafte
Anschwellung am Oberschenkel, deretwegen er 1 Jahr
lang intensiv röntgenbestrahlt wurde, ohne daß die verhältnismäßig ausgereifte Geschwulst (Knochenbildung) in
ihrem Wachstum gehemmt wurde. Amputation.

$^1/_2$ n. Gr.   1.

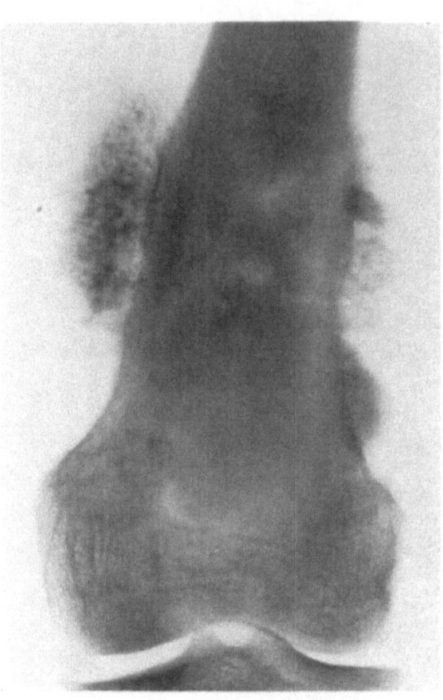

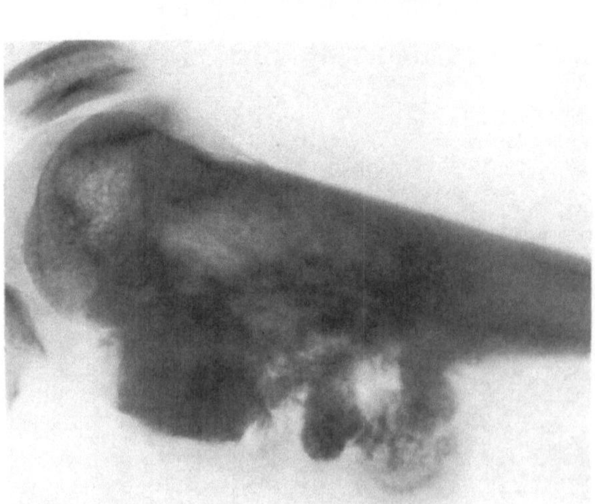

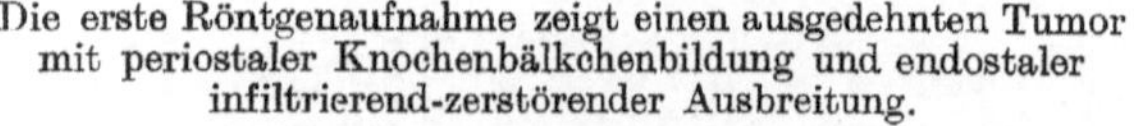

Die erste Röntgenaufnahme zeigt einen ausgedehnten Tumor
mit periostaler Knochenbälkchenbildung und endostaler
infiltrierend-zerstörender Ausbreitung.

The first X-ray picture shows a wide spread tumour with
periosteal bone beam-structure and spreading with endosteal
infiltration.

Series 64.

Osteo-Sarcoma of the Thigh.

A young man of nineteen noticed a slightly painful swelling
in the thigh. The swelling which was a bony growth, and
almost fully developed was not influenced by one years
intensive Röntgen irradiation treatment. Amputation.

2.

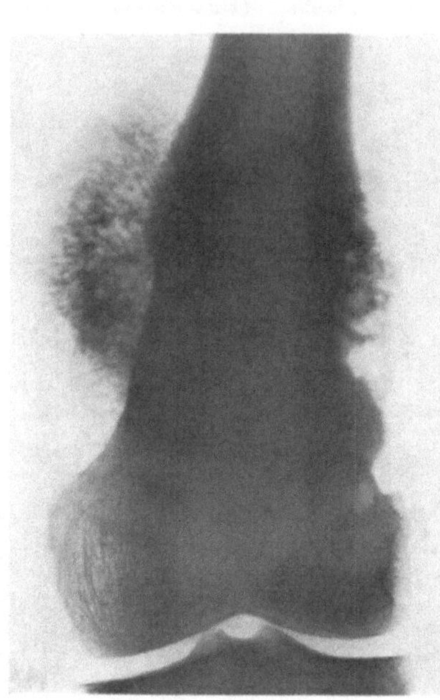

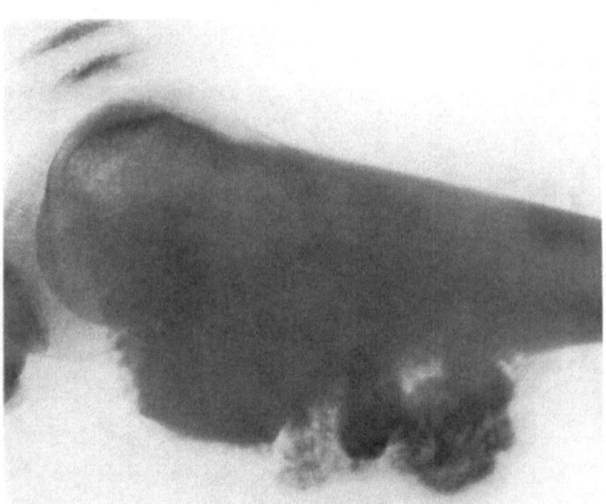

Ein Vierteljahr später ist das Sarkom nach allen Richtunge:
weiter gewachsen.

Three months later. The sarcoma has grown extensivel,
on all sides.

Serie 64.

3.

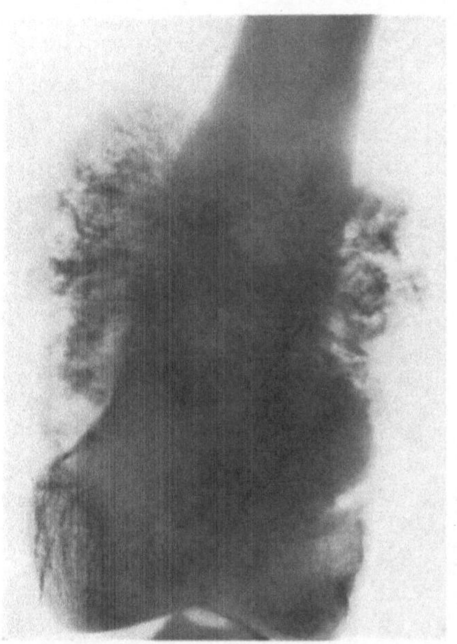

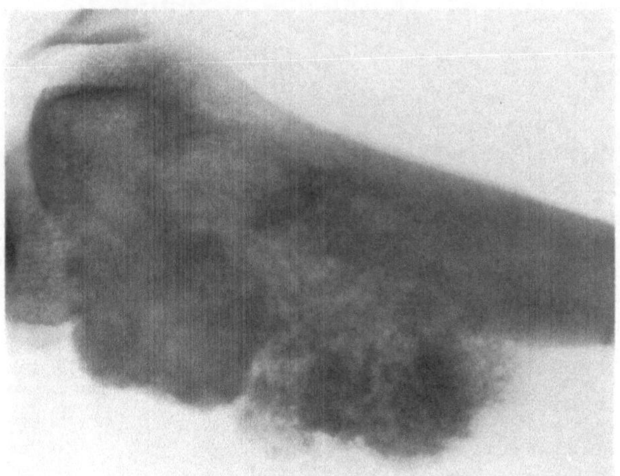

Nach einem Jahr ist die Geschwulst noch viel größer: periostal weiter ossificierend, im Innern stark destruierend.

After one year. The tumour has become much larger, the periosteum is more ossified and the interior is greatly destroyed.

Serie 65.

Osteoidsarkom des Femur.

Bei dem 17 Jahre alten Mann wurde 7 Wochen
nach einem Unfall (Stoß gegen das Knie) durch
das Röntgenbild die Knochengeschwulst festgestellt. Trotz mehrfacher intensiver Röntgenbestrahlungen wuchs sie in wenigen Monaten auf
mehr als die doppelte Größe, so daß die hohe
Absetzung des Beines gemacht werden mußte.
(Histologisch: Osteoidsarkom.)

$^6/_{10}$ n Gr.   1.

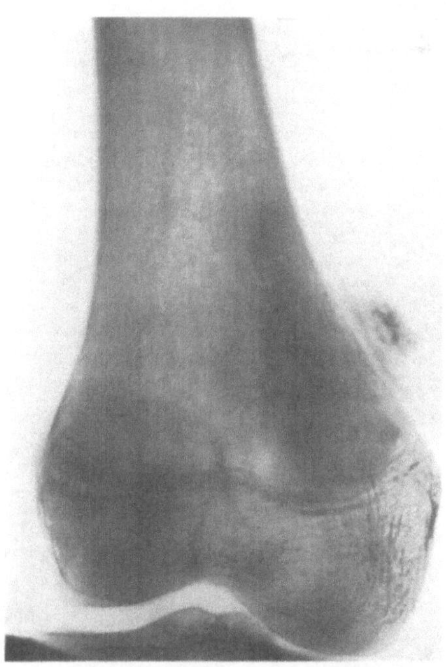

1. Röntgenaufnahme: Periostal wucherndes und
im Knochen infiltrierend wachsendes Sarkom
von schon beträchtlicher Größe.

First X-ray photograph. A growing sarcoma of
considerable size with abundance of periosteum,
is seen penetrating into the bone.

Series 65.

Osteo-Sarcoma of Femur.

A young man of seventeen met with an accident
(blow against the knee). Seven weeks after, an
X-ray photograph was taken in which a swelling
of the bone could be seen. Although treated
several times intensively with X-rays, it doubled
its size within a few months, and necessitated
amputation of the leg.

2.

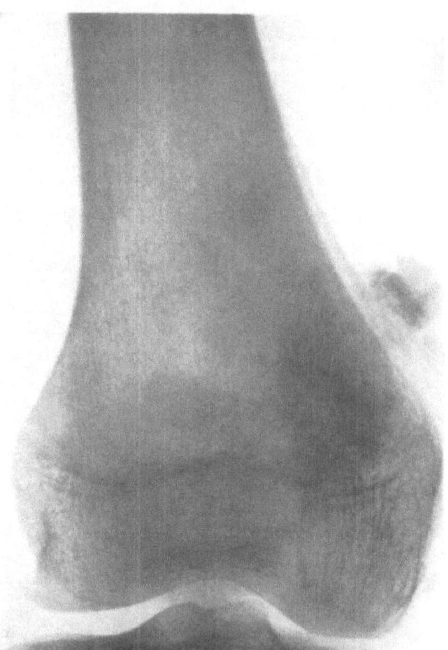

14 Tage später — nach der ersten Röntgenbestrahlung — erschien eine gewisse Rückbildung
des Tumors in seinem endostalen Anteil feststellbar.
Periostal freilich war er bereits größer geworden.

Fourteen days later. After the first X-ray treatment. There seems to be a certain decrease in
the endosteal part of the tumour. The periosteum
has increased.

Serie 65.

3.

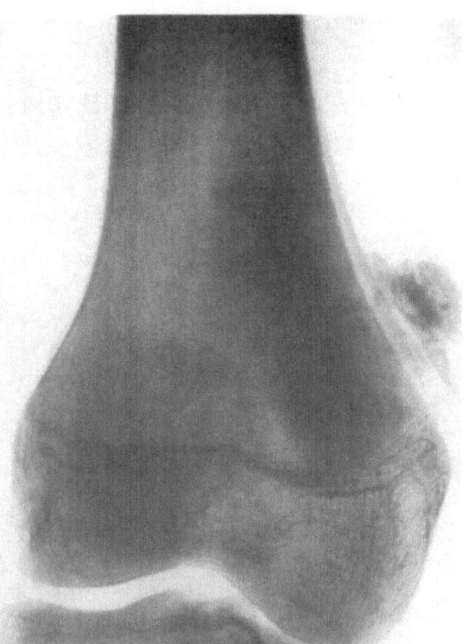

4.

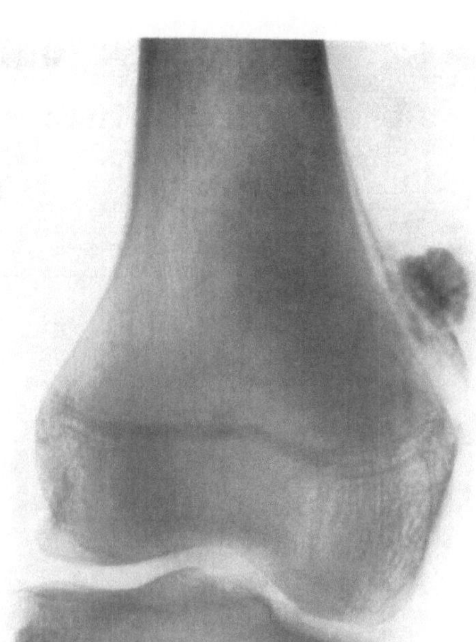

4 Wochen später
hat das expansive Wachstum nach allen Seiten mehr und mehr zugenommen.

Four weeks later. The growth has increased on all sides.

Six weeks later. The same condition.

6 Wochen später

5.

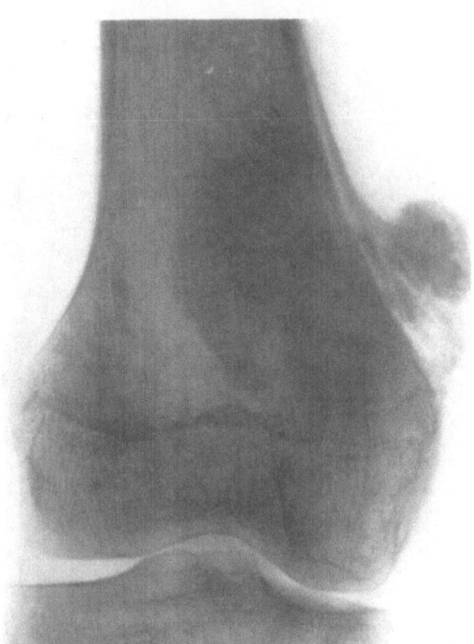

6.

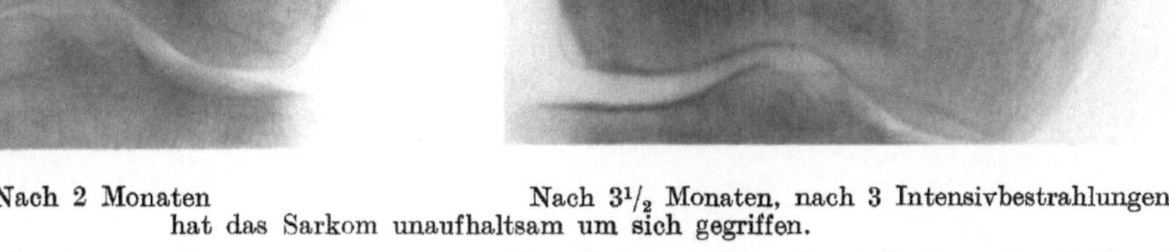

Nach 2 Monaten
hat das Sarkom unaufhaltsam um sich gegriffen.

After two months.

Nach 3½ Monaten, nach 3 Intensivbestrahlungen

After three months and a half. In spite of three intensive courses of X-ray irradiation, the sarcomatous growth continued to progress.

8*

Serie 66.

Oberarm-Metastase eines Bronchialcarcinoms.

Die 54jährige kachektische Frau erlitt kurz vor dem Tode eine Spontanfraktur des Oberarmes infolge osteoklastischer Metastase, welche eine unaufhaltsam fortschreitende Einschmelzung des Knochens verursachte.

$^2/_3$ n. Gr.   1.

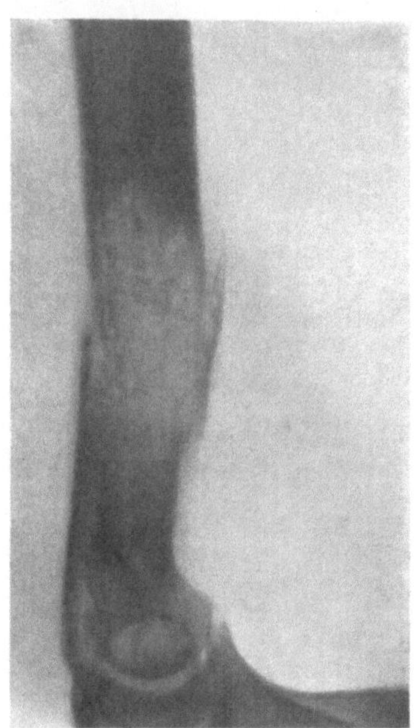

Große umschriebene Knochenzerstörung mit Einbruch der Corticalis.

The cortex is broken in and extensive circumscribed bone destruction has occurred.

Series 66.

Bronchial Carcinoma Metastasis in Humerus.

A fifty year old woman became ill with rapidly developing cachexia. Just before her death she had a spontaneous fracture of the humerus caused by osteoclastic metastasis which caused a progressive destruction of the bones.

2.

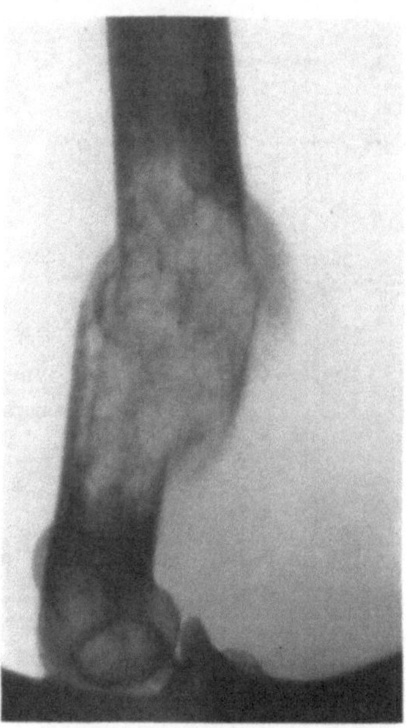

Bereits 12 Tage später ist der Zerfallsherd erheblich größer.

Twelve days later. The destroyed area is already very much larger.

Serie 67.

Osteoplastische Oberarmmetastase eines Mammacarcinoms.

Die 45jährige Frau erlitt 2 Jahre nach einer Operation wegen Brustdrüsenkrebs eine Spontanfraktur des Oberarmes. Der Bruch war nach einigen Monaten konsolidiert, da die ursprünglich rein osteoklastische Metastase nach erfolgter Fraktur osteoplastische Fähigkeit erhielt.

$^2/_3$ n. Gr.   1.

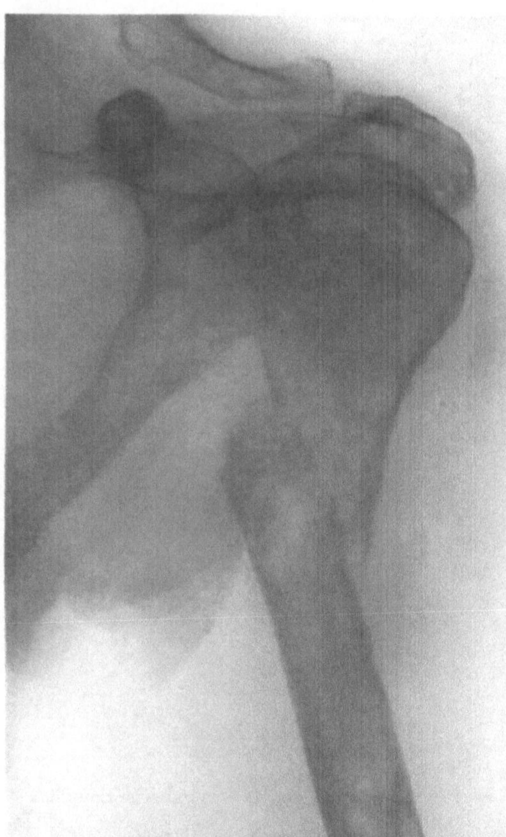

Schulterblatt und Humerus sind hochgradig atrophisch, die frische Spontanfraktur zeigt unregelmäßig angenagte Ränder: außerdem finden sich kleinere fleckförmige osteoklastische Metastasen im Schaft.

The scapula and humerus are exceedingly atrophied. The recent spontaneous fracture shows irregular eroded edges, besides which, there are small patchy osteoclastic metastases in the shaft.

Series 67.

Mammary Carcinoma Metastasis (Osteoplastic) of Humerus.

A woman of forty three had carcinoma of the breast for which she underwent an operation. Two years later at the age of forty five, she had a spontaneous fracture of the humerus. As the original osteoclastic metastasis had retained its osteoplastic ability, the fracture was repaired within a few months.

2.

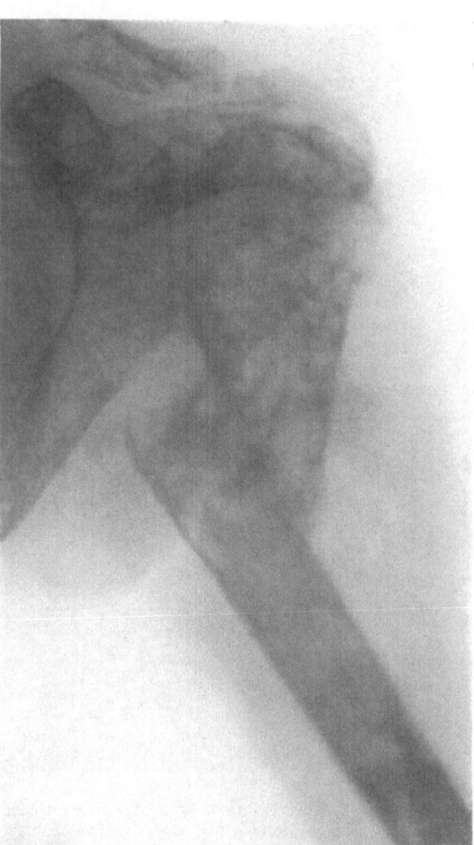

Nach 9 Monaten sind die dislocierten Fragmente deutlich durch Knochenbälkchen verbunden. Außer dieser osteoplastischen Metastase finden sich noch neue osteoklastische Herde.

After nine months. The displaced fragments are clearly joined together by small bone girders. There are new osteoclastic areas as well as those osteoplastic metastases.

Serie 68.

Wirbelmetastase eines Mamma-carcinoms.

Die 56 jähr. Frau wies bei der Operation des Brustdrüsenkrebses bereits Myelocyten im Blutbild auf. 5 Monate später Röntgenaufnahme wegen Rückenschmerzen: geringe Annagung am 3. Lendenwirbel, die im Verlaufe von 8 Monaten zu einer ausgedehnten Zerstörung des Wirbelkörpers führte.

$^7/_{10}$ n. Gr.　　　　1.

Series 68.

Mammary Carcinoma Metastasis in Vertebra.

At the time of operation for mamma-carcinoma, the 56 year old woman already had myelocytes in the blood. 5 months later a Röntgen photograph was taken because of backache. It showed slight corrosion of the 3rd lumbar vertebra, which within 8 months, advanced to extensive destruction of the vertebral-body.

2.

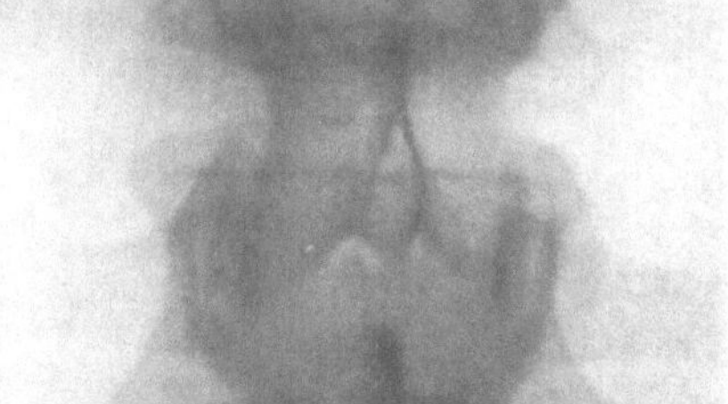

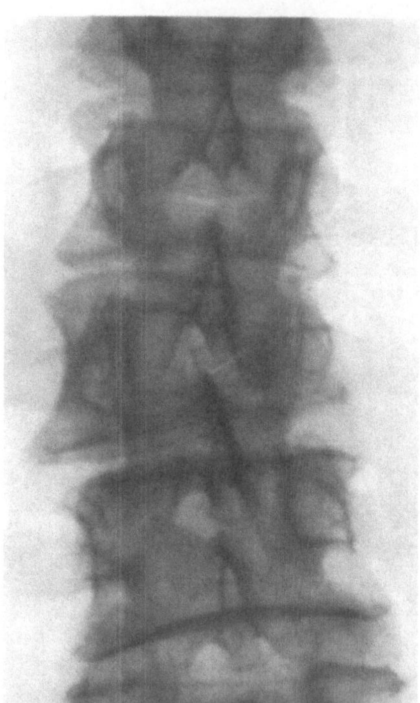

Aufnahme 5 Monate nach Operation des Brustkrebses (geringe Zerstörung der rechten unteren Ecke des 3. Lendenwirbels).

Photograph taken 5 months after operation for mammary carcinoma. (Slight destruction of the right lower corner of the third lumbar vertebra.)

3 Monate später noch ungefähr der gleiche Befund.

3 months later. Condition is practically unaltered.

Serie 68.

3.

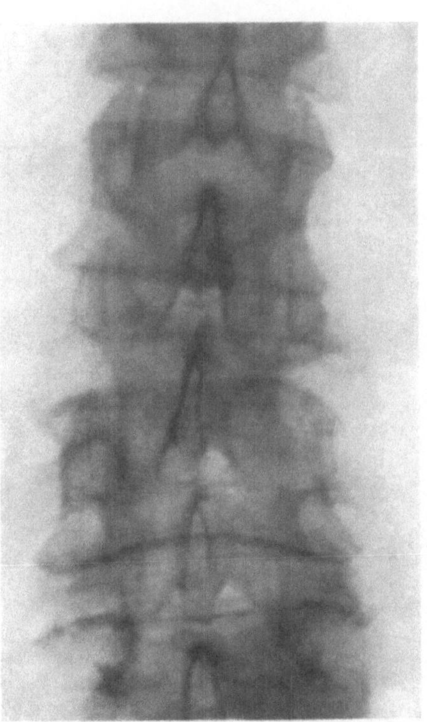

Nach 8 Monaten ist der 3. Lendenwirbel über die Hälfte zerstört, so daß der darüberliegende
in ihn hineinsinken konnte.

After 8 months. More than half of the lumbar vertebra has been destroyed, allowing the one above
to sink into it.

Serie 69.

Beckenmetastase eines Hypernephroms.

Ohne irgendwelche Erscheinungen von seiten des Primärtumors der Niere entstand sehr rasch eine große Geschwulst der Beckenschaufel, die in einer Probeexcision histologisch und bei der Obduction als Hypernephrommetastase erkannt wurde; die ausgedehnte Zerstörung der Beckenschaufel und des Schambeins schritt im weiteren Verlauf — $^3/_4$ Jahre bis zum Tode — nur wenig fort.

$^4/_{10}$ n. Gr. 1.

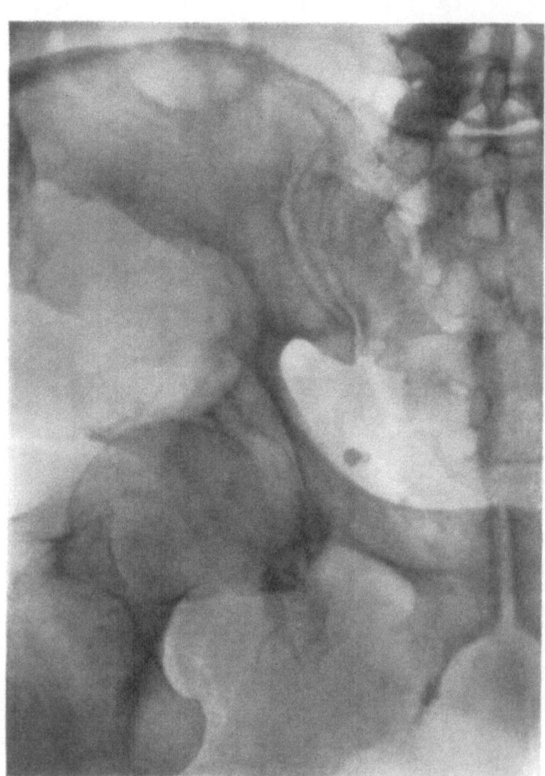

Etwa ein halbes Jahr nach Beginn der Beschwerden hat die riesenhafte Geschwulst den größten Teil der Beckenseite zerstört und ist auch in die Hüftgelenkpfanne eingebrochen.

About six months after onset of complaint. The gigantic tumour had destroyed the greater part of the ilium and had broken into the acetabulum.

Series 69.

Hypernephroma Metastasis in the Innominate Bone.

Without any symptoms from the primary tumour in the kidney, a large swelling suddenly appeared in the ilium which was proved, first by trial excision and later at post mortem, to be a hypernephroma metastasis. The extensive destruction of the os innominatum made little further progress in the nine months before death took place.

2.

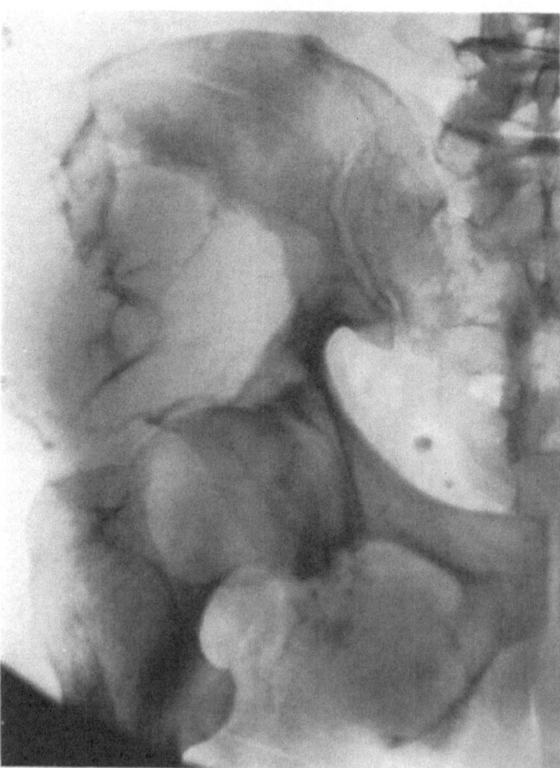

Ein halbes Jahr später ist der Befund wenig verändert, nur darmbeinwärts ist die Geschwulst noch etwas vorgedrungen und zeigt selbst stellenweise Knochenbälkchenstruktur.

Six months later. The condition is scarcely altered. The tumour has advanced slightly towards the hip-joint and shows bone girder structure in some places.

Serie 69.

3.

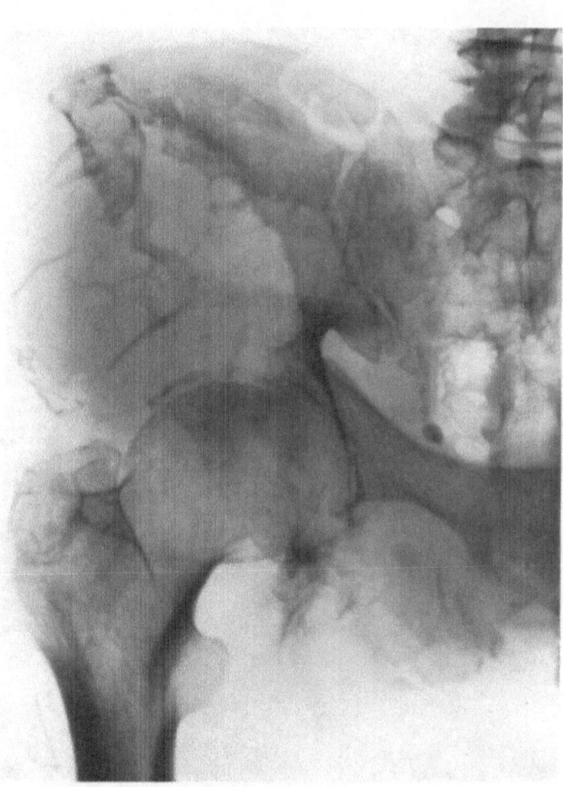

10 Monate später — beim Tode — ist das Sitzbein ganz zerstört, im wesentlichen aber besteht der gleiche Befund.

Ten months later. At death the ischium is entirely destroyed, but apart from this there is no change.

Serie 70 a.
Chondromatose des Skelets.

Vom 20. bis 40. Lebensjahr des Mannes wuchsen die End-
chondrome an den Händen unter dem Einfluß der Funktion
wesentlich stärker als an den Füßen, ohne daß er seine Arbeit
als Figurenschnitzer aufgeben mußte.

Series 70 a.
Chondromatosis of Skeleton.

The enchondromata grew considerably more on the hand
which were continually in use, than upon the feet. T?
patient was a wood-carver and was able to continue h
employment. The pictures show the changes which took pla
between the twentieth and fortieth years of the man's lif

¹/₂ n. Gr.   1.   2.

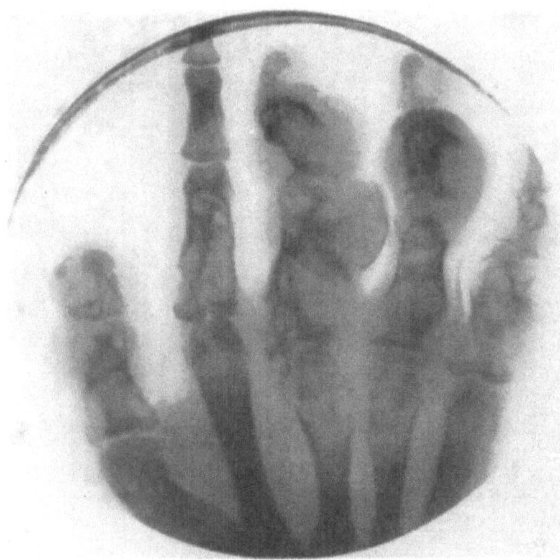

Im Alter von 20 Jahren.
Twenty years of age.

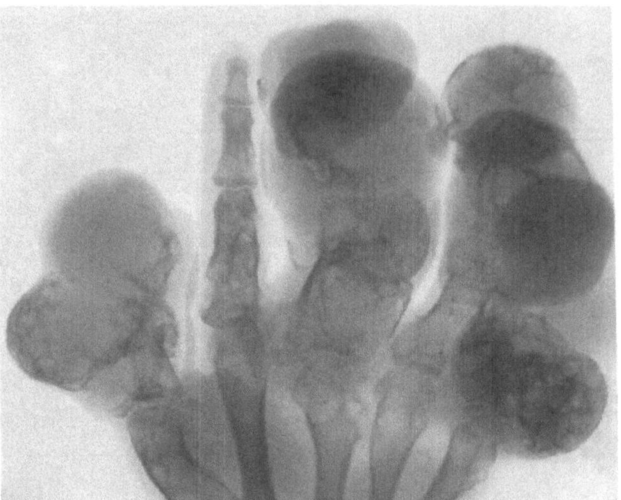

Im Alter von 32 Jahren.
Thirty two years of age.

3.

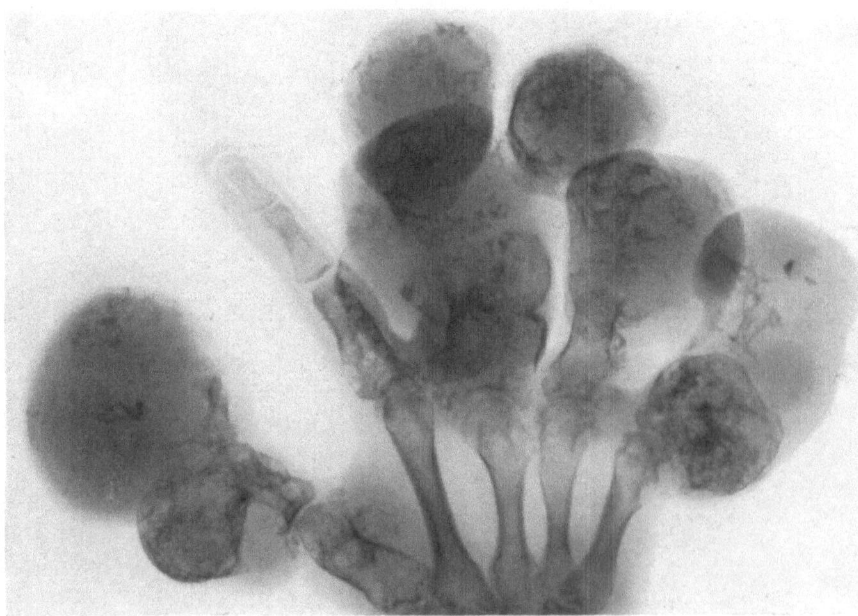

Im Alter von 40 Jahren.
Forty years of age.

Serie 70 b.

$^2/_3$ n. Gr.

1.

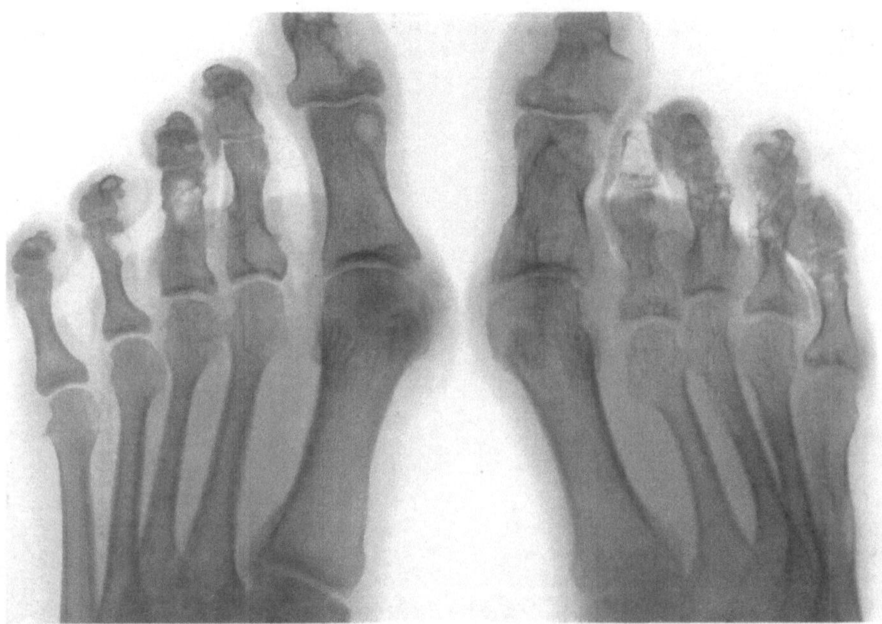

Im Alter von 20 Jahren. — Twenty years of age.

2.

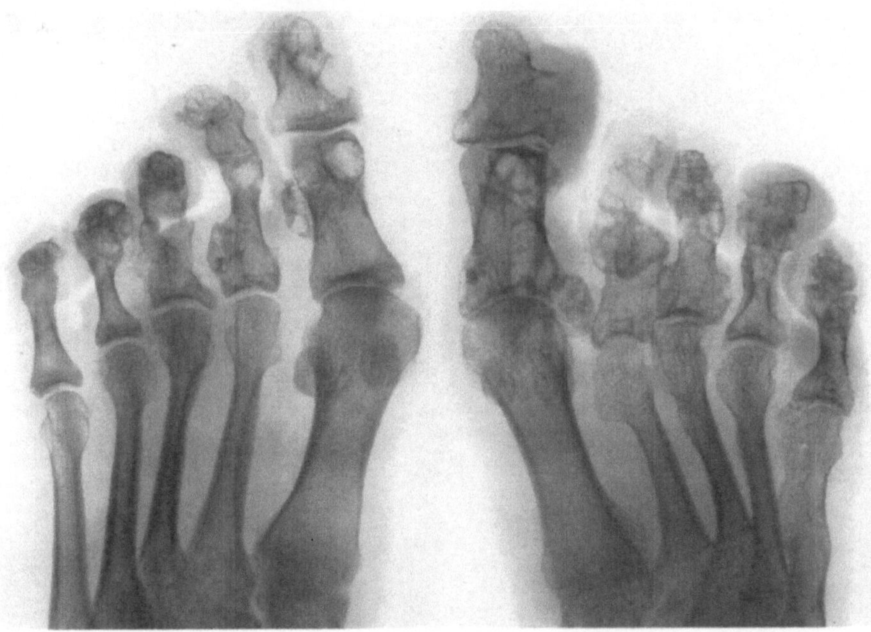

Im Alter von 40 Jahren. — Forty years of age.

Serie 70 c.

Chondromatose.

Außer den Chondromen der Hände und Füße
zeigten sich bei diesem Mann Unregelmäßigkeiten
der enchondralen Ossification an mehreren großen
Wachstumslinien: das Längenwachstum geschah
nicht gleichmäßig im Querschnitt des Röhrenknochens, sondern an einer Seite stärker und mit
einem exostoseartigen Überschuß. Offensichtlich
stehen diese Wachstumsfehler in engster Beziehung
zu den knorpeligen Geschwülsten („Hamartome")
der Finger und Zehen; jedoch wuchsen diese weiter,
jene aber seit dem 20. Lebensjahr nicht mehr.

$^1/_2$ n. Gr.   1.

Series 70 c.

Chondromatosis.

Besides the chondromata of hands and feet, the
man had irregularities of the enchondral ossification
at several large epiphyses. The growth in length
did not correspond to that of the cross-section of
hollow bone; the one side growing more and being
accompanied with exostosis-like superfluity. These
growth disturbances are apparently in close connection with the cartilage excrescences ("hamar-
tomes") of the fingers and toes. The growth of the
latter continued, but after the man reached his
twentieth year the growth of the former ceased.

2.

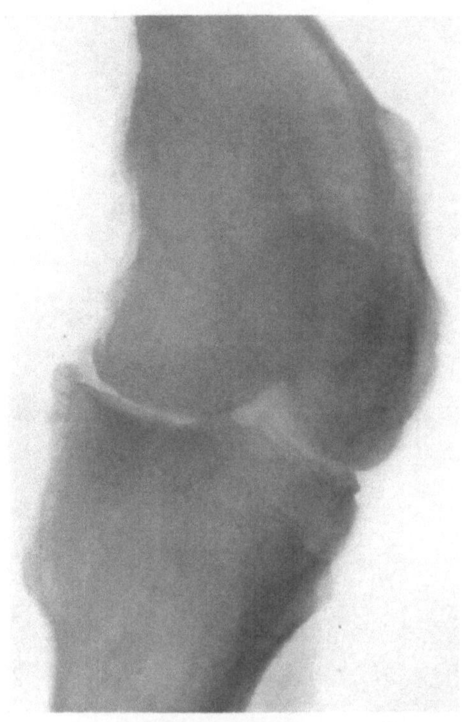

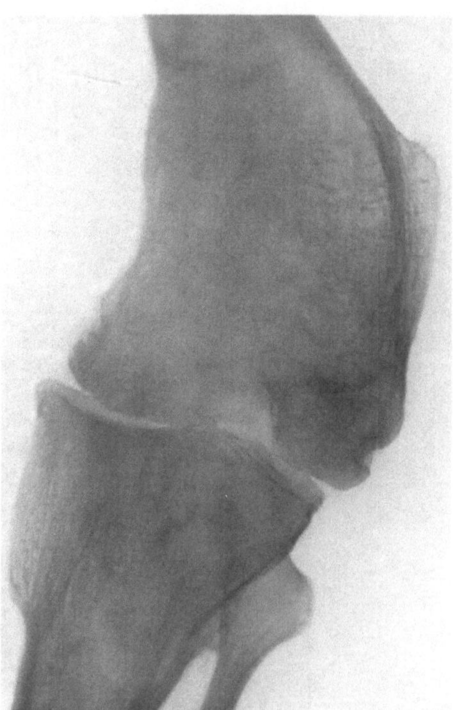

20. Lebensjahr.
Der Femur ist gebogen und trägt an der Außenseite eine flache Exostose; die Epiphysenfuge ist
nicht mehr erkennbar. — An der Innenseite der
Tibia ist gleichfalls eine Exostose.

In the twentieth year.
The femur is curved and there is a flat exostosis
on the outer side. The epiphyseal line is no longer
recognizable. — There is also an exostosis at the
inner side of the tibia.

40. Lebensjahr.
Ein späteres Wachstum ist nicht mehr erfolgt.

In the fortieth year.
There has been no further growth.

Anhang: Hyperplasie, Exostose.   *Supplement: Hyperplasia, Exostosis.*

Serie 71.
Cartilaginäre Exostosen.

Die Exostosen sind bei dem 13jährigen Mädchen, in dessen Familie dieses Leiden sowie Enchondrome mehrfach vorkamen, bis zum 18. Lebensjahr erheblich gewachsen.

Series 71.
Cartilaginous Exostosis.

A girl was affected with exostoses, which grew considerably between her thirteenth and eighteenth year. This condition and also enchondromata were common in the family.

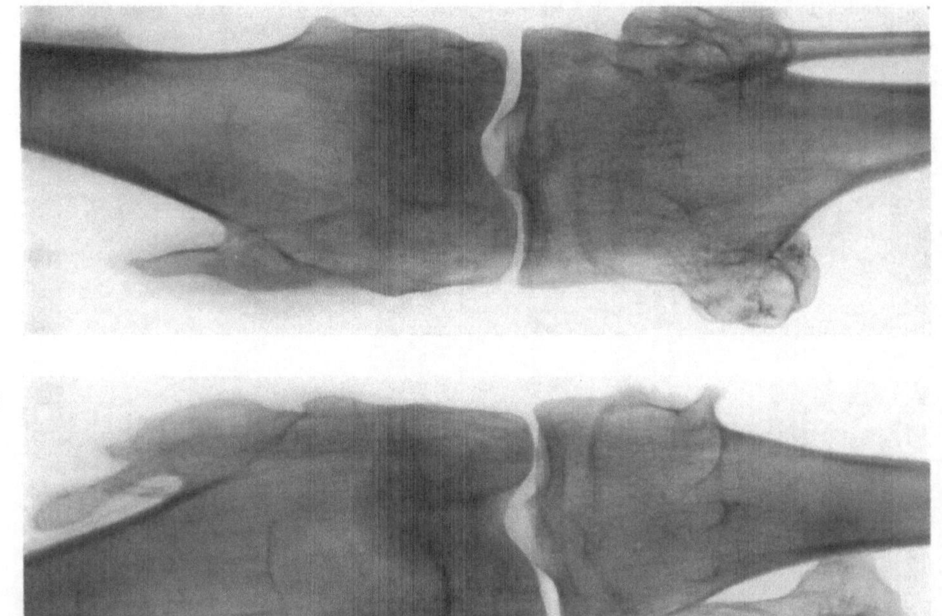

2.

Im Alter von 18 Jahren sind die cartilaginären Exostosen sämtlich sehr viel größer geworden, die Epiphysenfugen bereits geschlossen.

At the age of eighteen the cartilaginous exostoses have all become very much larger and the epiphyseal line is already closed.

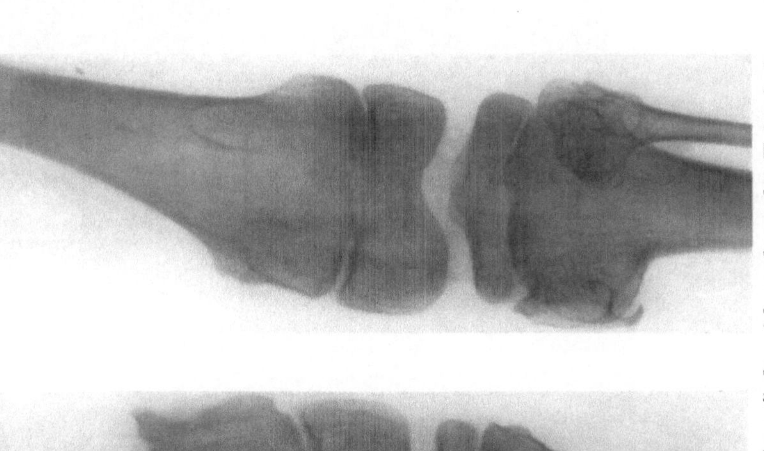

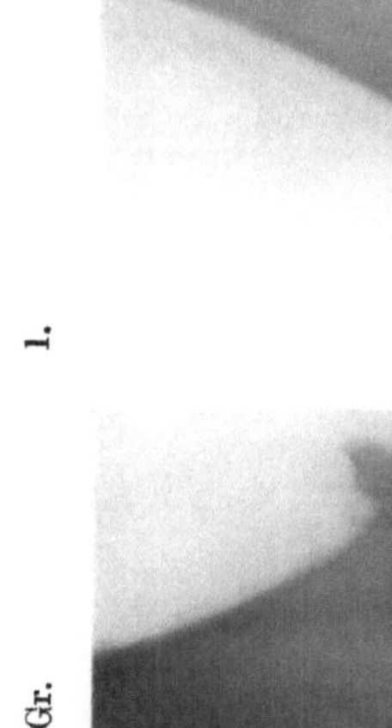

1.

½ n. Gr.

Im Alter von 13 Jahren finden sich rund um das Kniegelenk die Wachstumsexcesse.

At the age of thirteen exostoses are seen in the region of the knee-joint.

Serie 72.

Osteoide Hyperplasie.

Die periostale Knochenwucherung der Tibia zeigte zwar die
für das periostale Sarkom so charakteristischen strahligen
Knochensprossen, war aber dem Wesen nach keine echte
Geschwulst. Dementsprechend war der weitere Verlauf: nach
flacher Abmeißelung entstand kein Rezidiv. Histologisch fand
sich eine gewucherte Periostlage mit osteoidem Gewebe,
welches fleckweise verkalkt war und große Herde von hyalinem
Knorpel enthielt, während das umgebende Knochengewebe
eburnisiert und frei von entzündlichen Prozessen war.

Series 72.

Osteoid Hyperplasia.

The periosteal bone-growth of tibia showed the ray-like bon
process which is distinctive of periosteal sarcoma. It was
however, not a genuine swelling. The further course wa
therefore in accordance and there was no relapse after bein
levelled by chisel. Histologically, there was an abundant laye
of periosteum with osteoid tissue which was calcified i
patches and in which were considerable areas of hyaline carti
lage, while the surrounding tissue was eburnated and free c
inflamed processes.

³/₄ n. Gr.   1.   2.   3.

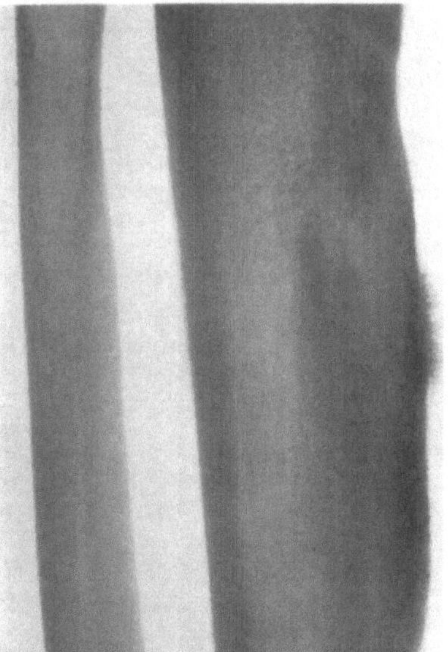

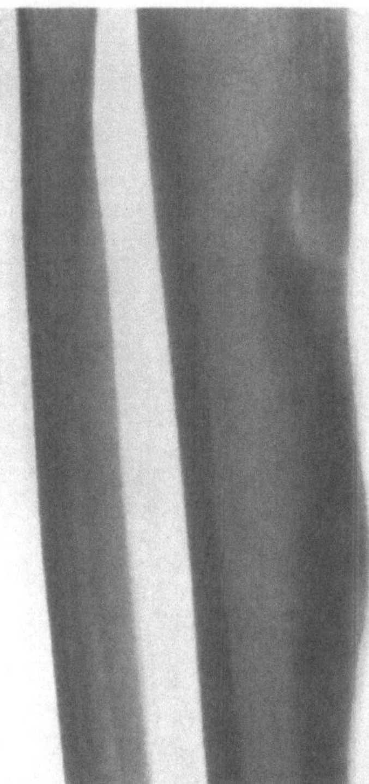

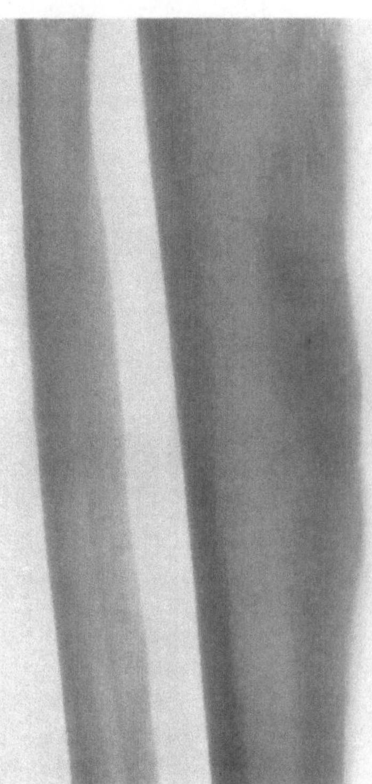

Ausgedehnte periostale Knochenbildung mit
den nadelartigen Knochensprossen, wie
sie das Sarkom zeigt.

Extensive periosteal bone growth with
needle-like processes, such as are usually
seen in sarcomata.

2 Monate nach der Abmeißelung ist die
Operationswunde noch erkennbar, eine
erneute Wucherung nicht eingetreten.

Two months after removal by chisel. The
wound caused by operation is still recognizable. No new growth has set in.

Nach 1¹/₂ Jahr ist der Prozeß beruhigt

After one year and a half. The condition
has disappeared.

Serie 73.

Exostose.

Der histologisch als „spongiöse Exostose" bezeichnete Knochentumor war nach einem leichten Stoß entstanden, indem wahrscheinlich ein Bluterguß verkalkte und verknöcherte. Dem Wesen nach keine echte Geschwulst — nur im Röntgenbild als solche erscheinend — war sie lediglich durch Abmeißelung dauernd beseitigt.

Series 73.

Exostosis.

The bone tumour, known histologically as "spongy exostosis" developed after a slight knock. Probably there was a blood effusion, which later became calcified and then ossified. According to its species, it is not a genuine tumour — it only appears to be solid in the X-ray photograph. It was chiselled away and did not reappear.

$^{7}/_{10}$ n. Gr.   1.   2.

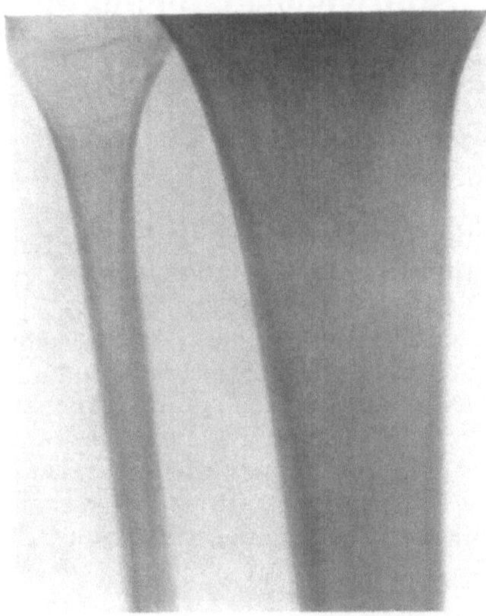

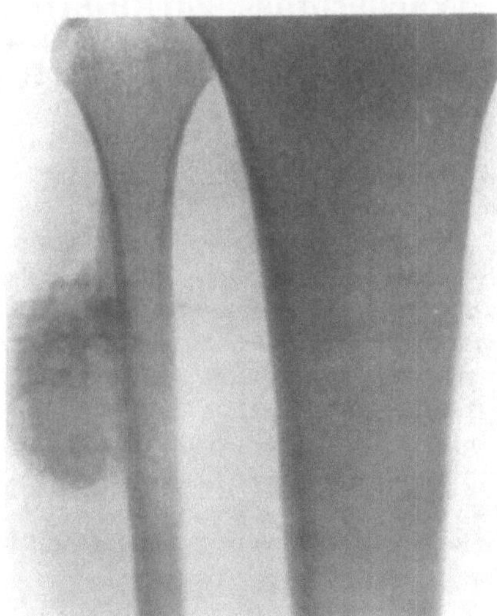

4 Wochen nach dem Unfall ist röntgenologisch ein krankhafter Befund am Knochen nicht vorhanden, zu einer Zeit, als eine derbe Schwellung deutlich tastbar war.

Four weeks after accident. At this time nothing unusual could be seen in the Röntgen picture although an obvious swelling could be felt.

6 Wochen später zeigt das Röntgenbild einen periostalen Knochentumor der Fibula.

Six weeks later. The Röntgen picture shows a periosteal bone tumour of the fibula.

3.

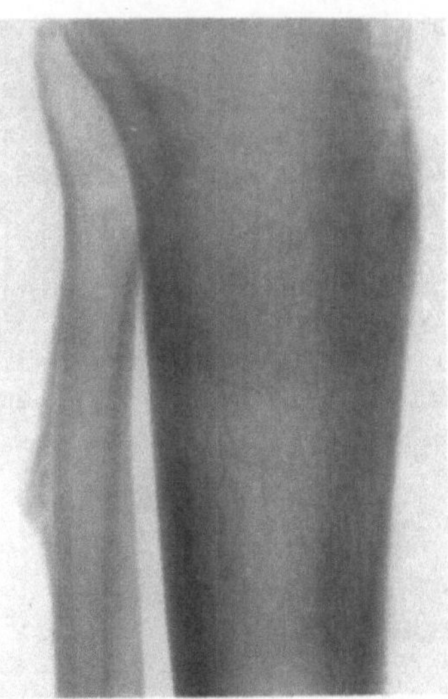

2 Jahre nach einfacher Abmeißelung ist ein Rezidiv nicht entstanden.
Two years after the removal by chiselling, recurrence had not occurred.

IV. Kapitel.

Wachstums-, Zirkulations- und Stoffwechselstörungen.

A. Primäre Wachstumshemmungen.

Die *Chondrodystrophie* (Serie 74) ist eine *angeborene Störung der enchondralen Ossification:* der Wachstumsknorpel verknöchert vor der Zeit und führt dadurch zum Zwergwuchs.

Die *Osteogenesis imperfecta* (Serie 75) und die *Osteopsathyrosis* (Serie 76) stellen verschiedene Grade der gleichen Entwicklungsstörung dar, einer *mangelhaften Ausbildung von Knochensubstanz durch Mark und Periost während der Fetalzeit. Die Folge ist abnorme Brüchigkeit der Knochen.* Bei der schweren Form — Osteogenesis imperfecta — kommen die Kinder bereits mit zahlreichen Knochenbrüchen zur Welt und sterben schon im Laufe des ersten Lebensjahres an einer interkurrenten Krankheit. Bei der Osteopsathyrosis erleiden die Menschen während des ersten und zweiten Lebensjahrzehntes bei geringfügigen Ursachen immer wieder Frakturen, bis sich das Leiden nach Abschluß des Wachstums allgemein bessert. — Die Knochenbrüche selbst werden in normaler Zeit fest und heilen mit dem Mindestmaß von Callus.

Chapter IV.

Disturbances of growth.

A. Primary Growth Interception.

Chondrodystrophia (Series 74) is a congenital disturbance of endochondral ossification. The growing cartilage becoming prematurely ossified, leads to stunted growth.

Osteogenesis imperfecta (Series 75) and Osteopsyarthrosis (Series 76) are different degrees of the same developmental disturbance — that is, a deficient development of bone substance from marrow and periosteum during the foetal period. As a result, the bones are extremly brittle. Osteogenesis imperfecta is the more serious condition. Affected children are born with numerous broken bones and die in the course of the first twelve months from an intercurrent disease. People afflicted with osteopsyarthrosis are liable to repeated fractures from the slightest possible causes. This is commoner during the first and second decades; the liability ending with the cessation of growth. The fractures heal with the least possible callus and within the normal time.

Serie 74.

Chondrodystrophie.

Die angeborene Störung der enchondralen Ossification (die Knorpelverknöcherungsstörung) führt zu einem frühzeitigen Schluß der Wachstumsfugen und somit zum Zwergwuchs.

$^6/_{10}$ n. Gr.   1.

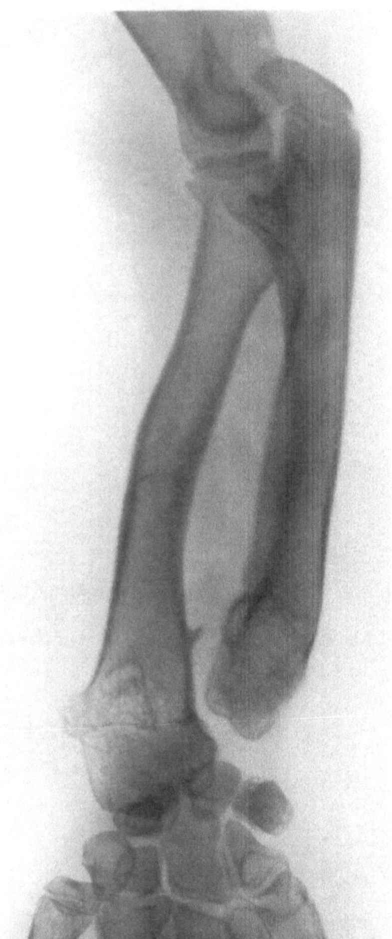

Alter: 13 Jahre. Die Epiphysenfugen der plumpen Knochen sind zum Teil bereits geschlossen.

Thirteen years of age. The epiphyseal lines of the larger bones are already partly closed.

Series 74.

Chondro-Dystrophy.

A child was born with a disturbance of ossification (cartilage bone disturbance). It led to a premature closing of the epiphyseal line and the child remained small.

2.

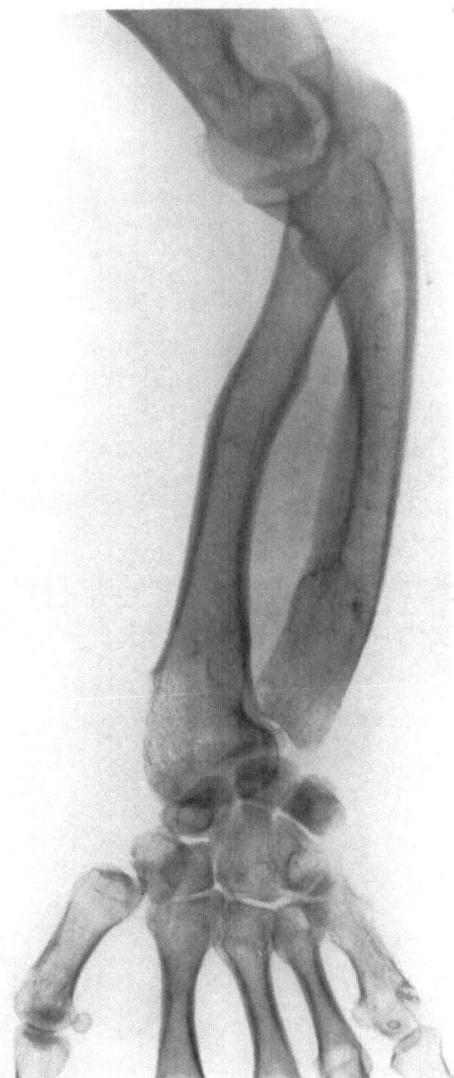

Alter: 34 Jahre. Ein Längenwachstum hat seit dem 13. Lebensjahr nicht mehr stattgefunden.

Thirty four years of age. No growth in length has taken place since the thirteenth year.

Serie 75.
Osteogenesis imperfecta.

Infolge der während der fetalen Entwicklung auftretenden Skeleterkrankung — einer mangelhaften Ausbildung von Knochensubstanz durch Mark und Periost — kam es noch in utero zu zahlreichen Knochenbrüchen, die bei der Geburt des Kindes bereits deutlich Callus zeigten und sich in den nächsten Monaten „auswuchsen".

Series 75.
Imperfect Osteogenesis.

During foetal development, a child was afflicted with a skeletal disease which constituted an unsatisfactory development of bone from the marrow and periosteum. Due to this, several fractures occurred while still in utero. A birth, callus could be plainly seen, but after a few months was levelled.

$^6/_{10}$ n. Gr.   1.

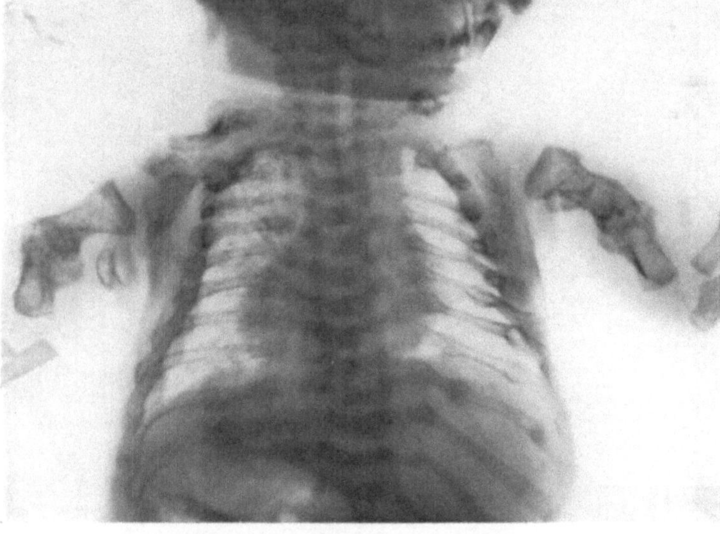 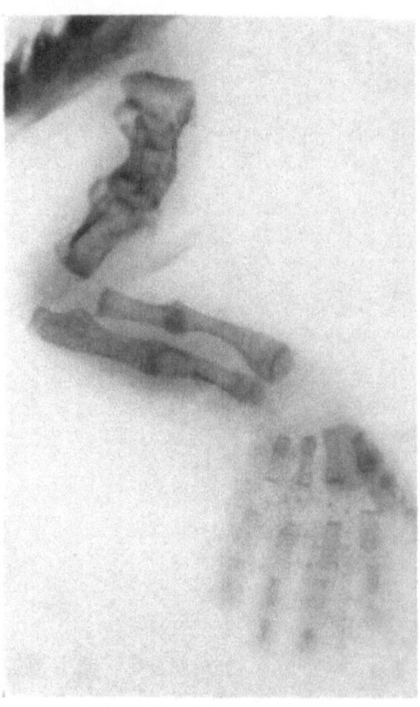

14 Tage nach der Geburt ist an den zahlreichen Knochenbrüchen der Rippen und der Gliedmaßen bereits reichlich Callus vorhanden.

Fourteen days after birth, considerable callus is already present at the site of the numerous fractures of the ribs and limbs

2.

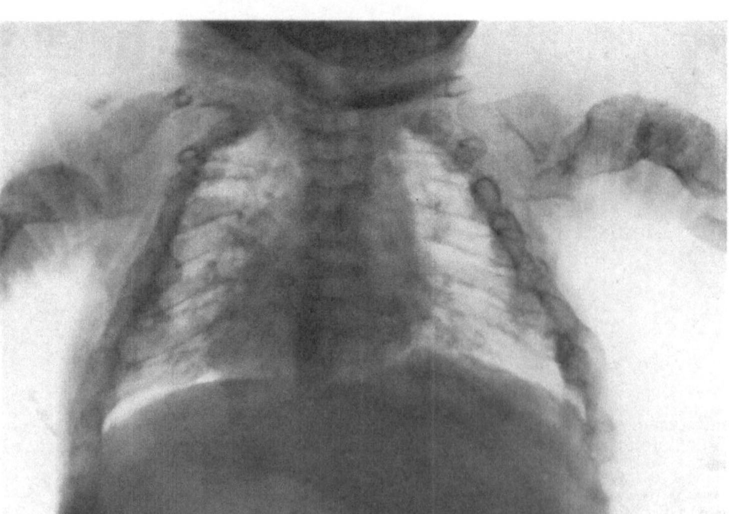 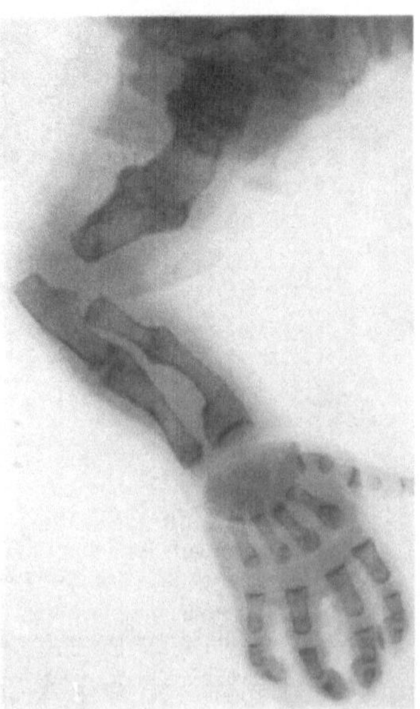

4 Wochen nach der Geburt ist die Bruchheilung deutlich weiter fortgeschritten.
Four weeks after birth, the healing of the fractures has clearly progressed.

Serie 75.

3.

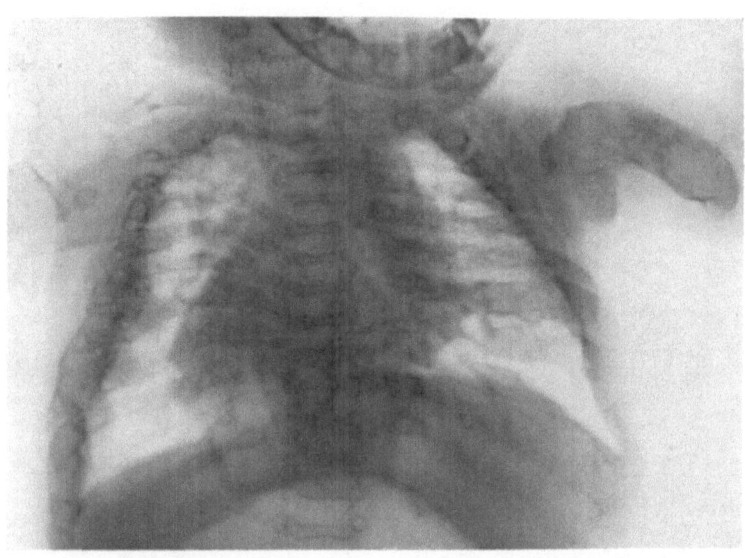 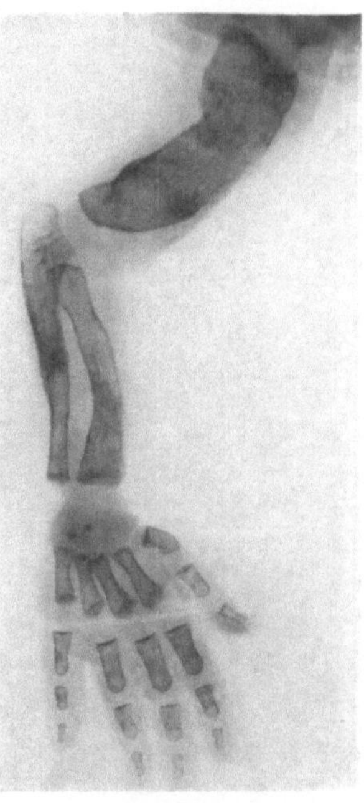

Im Alter von $^1/_2$ Jahr — als der Tod des Säuglings an Bronchopneumonie erfolgte — waren die Knochenbrüche kaum noch erkennbar, durch das Wachstum ausgeglichen.

At the age of six months, when the baby died of bronchopneumonia, the fractures are hardly recognizable, having been almost obliterated by growth.

Serie 76.

Osteopsathyrosis.

Der zarte, aus gesunder Familie stammende Knabe mit „blauen Skleren" hat bis zu seinem 9. Lebensjahre über 20 Knochenbrüche erlitten, meist aus geringfügigen Ursachen. Diese heilten in normaler Zeit, aber entsprechend dem Wesen des Leidens — einer mangelhaften Ausbildung der Knochensubstanz — mit dem Mindestmaß regeneratorischer Leistung.

Series 76.

Osteopsathyrosis.

A delicate boy with blue sclerae, of healthy family, had had more than twenty fractures before he was nine years of age, mostly resulting from slight causes. They healed in the normal time but with unsatisfactory deposition of bone substance and the smallest measure of regenerative efficiency, corresponding to the nature of the malady.

$^{6}/_{10}$ n. Gr.   1.   2.   3.

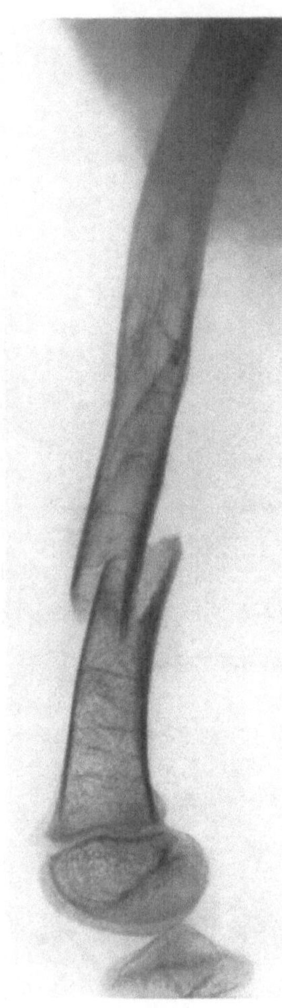

Frischer Bruch des dünnen, porösen Oberschenkelknochens.

Recent fracture of thin porous femur.

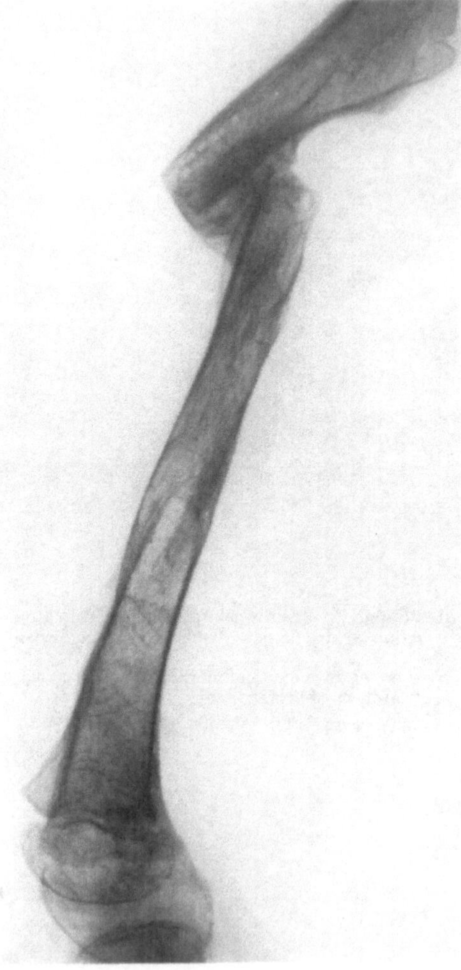

Nach 10 Monaten ist *der gut adaptierte* (distale) Knochenbruch *ohne Callus* geheilt, *ein zweiter stark dislozierter* (proximaler) Bruch in 7 Wochen *durch den eben notwendigen Callus* verwachsen.

After ten months *the well adapted* (distal) fracture has healed *without callus*. The second fracture [proximal] was considerably out of alignment and healed within seven weeks, with only just the necessary amount of callus.

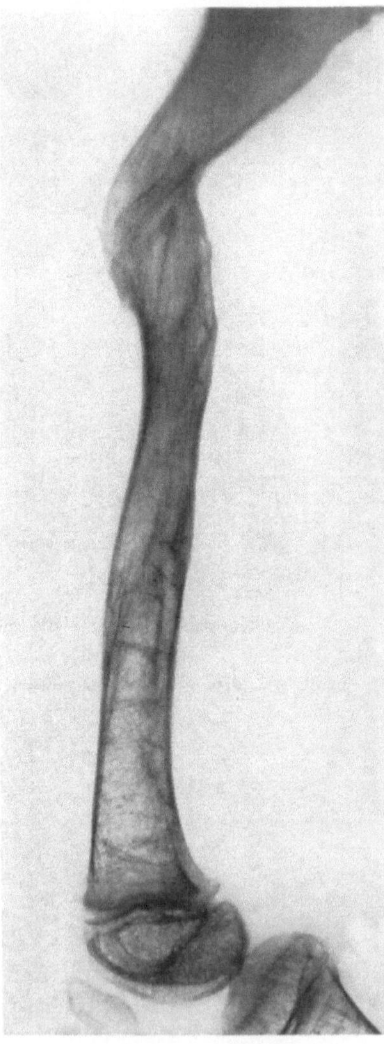

Nach 1½ Jahren ist die Callusüberbrückung strukturell ausgebaut und in das Bälkchensystem des Oberschenkelknochens eingefügt, die Verkrümmung weitgehend durch das Wachstum ausgeglichen.

After one year and a half the callus bridge has developed and united with the beam system of the femur, the crookedness to a very great extent righting itself by growth.

Anhang.

Serie 77.

Finger-Mißbildung.

Die Verkrüppelung des Fingers beruht auf
angeborener Fehlbildung.

$^2/_3$ n. Gr.   1.

Supplement.

Series 77.

Finger Deformity.

The deformity of the finger was of congenital
origin.

2.

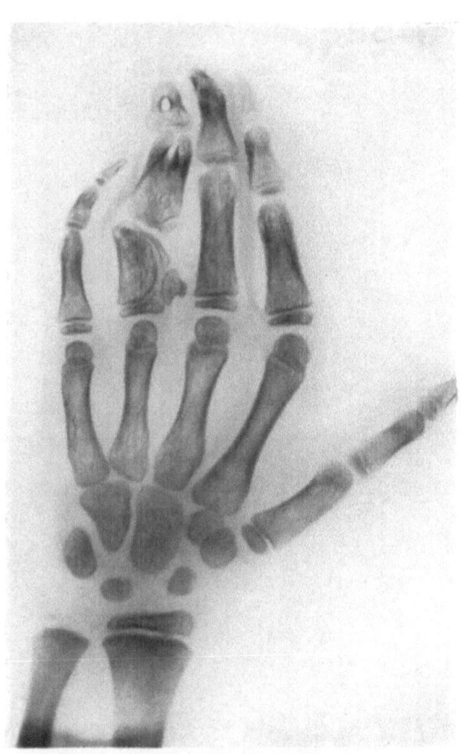

Lebensalter: 11 Jahre. Sämtliche Glieder des
4. Fingers weisen Anzeichen einer Doppelbildung
bzw. Teilung auf.

Eleven years of age. All portions of the fourth
finger show signs of double formation or division.

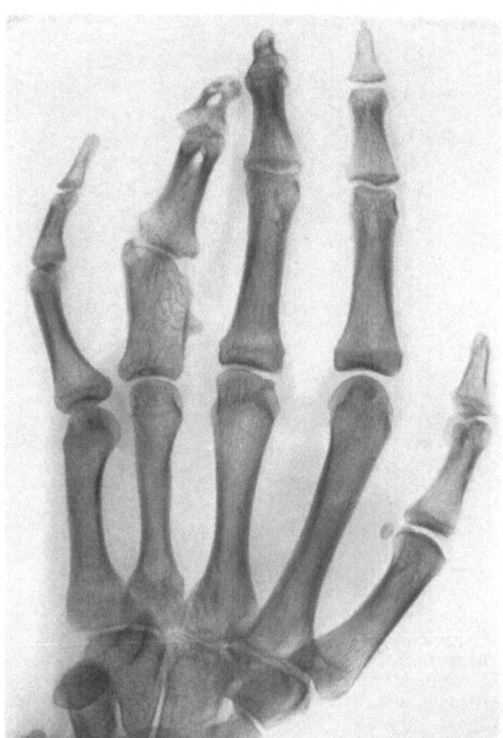

Lebensalter: 19 Jahre. Nach Schluß der Wachstumsfugen bestehen verschiedene Unregelmäßigkeiten: loch-
artige Substanzdefekte, ungleichmäßige Gelenkflächen
und eine Exostose, die aus der überzähligen Epiphyse
hervorgegangen ist.

Nineteen years of age. After closing of the epiphyseal
lines, various irregularities exist. There are hole-like
defects in the bone substance, irregular joint surfaces
and an exostosis caused by the superfluous epiphysis.

Anhang.

Supplement.

Serie 78.

Series 78.

Congenitale Pseudarthrose.

Congenital Pseudarthrosis.

Die Mißbildung erwies sich histologisch als eine
fetale Osteodystrophia fibrosa mit schwersten
Folgen für das spätere Wachstum.

This condition was histologically shown to be a
foetal osteodystrophia fibrosa with serious
disturbance of subsequent growth.

²/₃ n. Gr. 1.   2.   3.

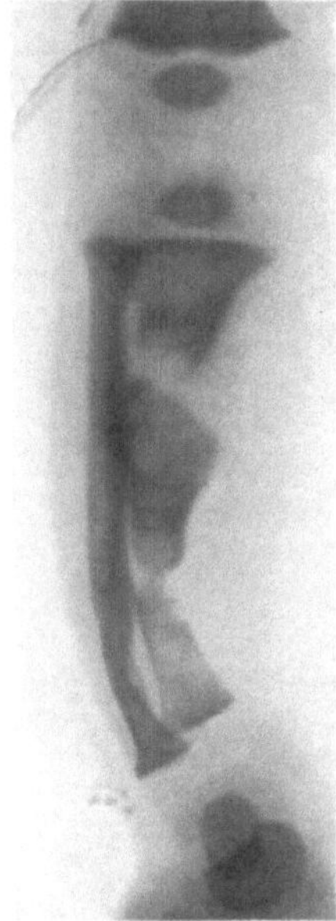

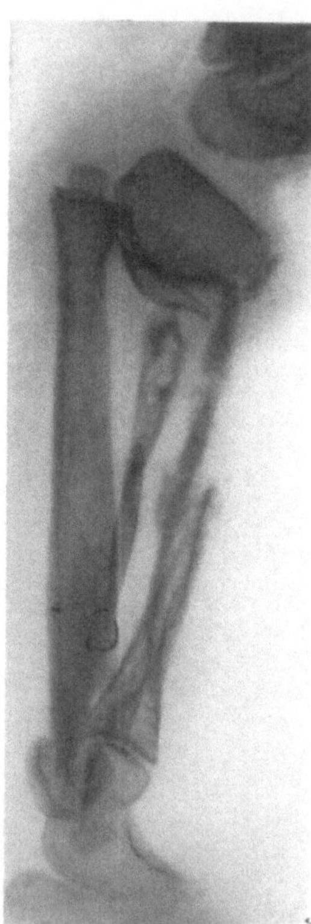

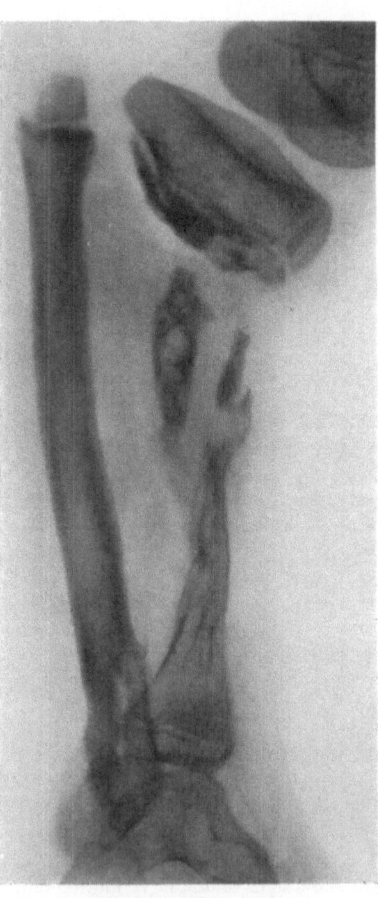

Lebensalter: 8 Wochen.
Der knöcherne Schien-
beinschaft ist an 2
Stellen durch fibröses
Gewebe unterbrochen.

Age eight weeks.
The bony tibial shaft
is interrupted in two
places by fibrous
tissue.

Lebensalter: 5 Jahre.

Fifth year.

Lebensalter: 9 Jahre.
Lediglich von der distalen Epiphysenfuge
erfolgt ein Längenwachstum. Die Fibula
ist vikariierend erstarkt; transplantierte
Knochenspäne sind teilweise resorbiert.

Ninth year.
Longitudinal growth has only occurred
from the distal epiphysis. The fibula has
undergone compensating strengthening.
The transplanted bone shavings have
been partly resorbed.

B. Sekundäre Wachstumshemmungen.

Bei dem endemischen *Kretinismus* entsteht infolge der Hypothyreosis eine allgemeine Entwicklungsstörung, die am Skelet ein *Zurückbleiben der Entwicklung* und Zwergwuchs mit unproportioniertem Körperbau zur Folge hat. Hier wie bei dem *Myxödem* ist das verspätete Auftreten der Knochenkerne und der gehemmte Verschluß der Epiphysenfuge charakteristisch. — In dem Fall der Serie 79 gelang es durch fortgesetzte Organtherapie — Verabreichung von Schilddrüsensubstanz — in erstaunlich kurzer Zeit den Rückstand einzuholen und die weitere Entwicklung normal zu gestalten.

B. Secondary Growth Interception.

Endemic cretinism, by means of hypothyroidism causes a general disturbance of development. The growth of the skeleton is retarded and stunted growth and disproportionate body structure results. As in myxoedema, the late appearance of the bone centres and interference with the closing of the epiphyseal lines are characteristic. In the case shown in series 79, the retarded growth etc. was counteracted and the further development became normal in an incredibly short time, by the continuous use of thyroid therapy.

Serie 79.

Myxödem.

Das 7 jährige, aus gesunder Familie stammende Mädchen war nur 73 cm lang, überhaupt in der Entwicklung stark zurück und bot das ausgesprochene Bild des Myxödems. In erstaunlich kurzer Zeit gelang es, den durch (angeborenen) Ausfall des Schilddrüsenhormons bedingten Entwicklungsrückstand durch entsprechende Organtherapie einzuholen (Geh. Rat Prof. Dr. SIEGERT). Auch die Weiterentwicklung konnte auf normaler Kurve gehalten werden.

Series 79.

Myxoedema.

A girl seven years of age from a healthy family was only 73 cm long and very backward in development. A genuine case of myxoedema. In a remarkably short time, by the use of the necessary organo-therapy, the backward development, which was caused by the missing thyroidhormone, was cured. (Geh. Rat Prof. Dr. SIEGERT.) The further development remained normal.

$^2/_3$ n. Gr. 　　　　1. 　　　　　　　　　　2.

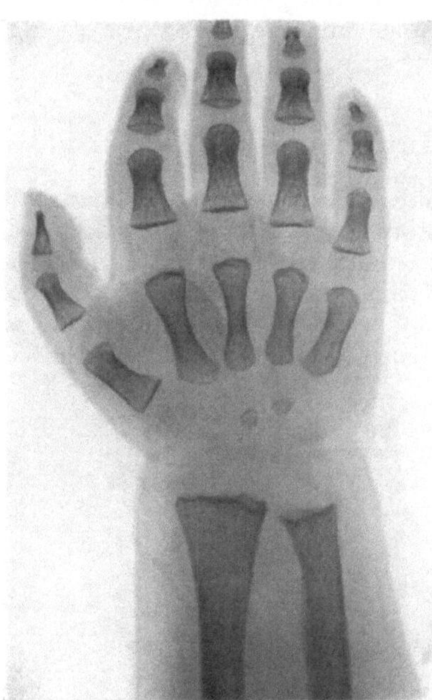

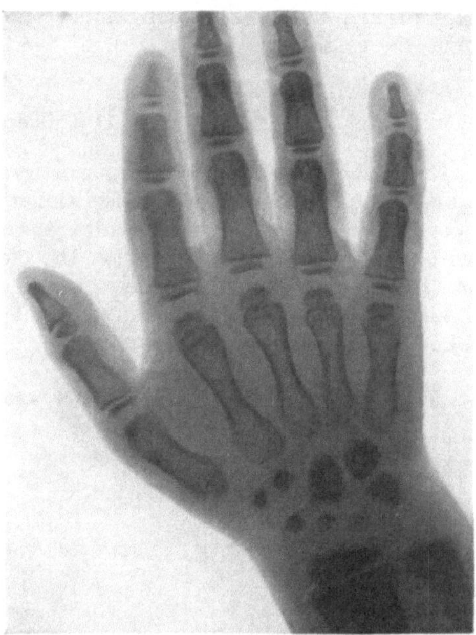

Im Alter von **7 Jahren** steht das Skelet auf der Entwicklungsstufe eines Kindes von *etwa 4 Monaten*: alle Epiphysen und die Handwurzelkerne bis auf zwei (Os capitatum und hamatum) lassen die Ossification vermissen.

At the age of seven, the skeleton was on a par with that of a child of *four months*. The epiphyses and the hand base centres, with the exception of two (os capitatum and hamatum), showed no ossification.

$^3/_4$ *Jahr später*, nachdem die Schilddrüsen-Organtherapie so lange durchgeführt war, *entspricht die Entwicklung des Handskeletes dem wirklichen Alter*: die Epiphysen sämtlicher Finger, des Radius und 5 Handwurzelkerne sind aufgeschossen.

Nine months later, during which time the thyroid treatment had been carried out, the development of the hand skeleton corresponded to the child's age. The epiphyses of all the fingers, the radius and five basal centres in the hand have developed.

Serie 79.

3.

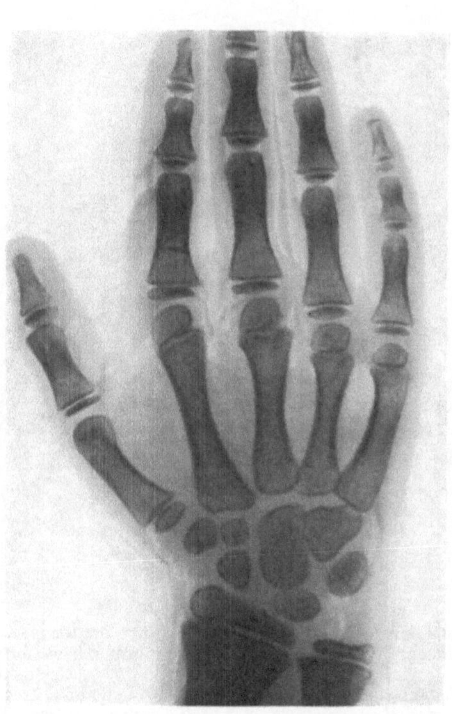

Im 14. Lebensjahr ist das Mädchen in normaler Weise weiterentwickelt.

In the fourteenth year. Normal development continued.

Serie 80.

Endemischer Kretinismus.

Das 5³/₄ Jahre alte Mädchen bot den charakteristischen kretinen Habitus und war in der Entwicklung des Skeletes um etwa 2 Jahre zurückgeblieben.

²/₃ n. Gr.   1.

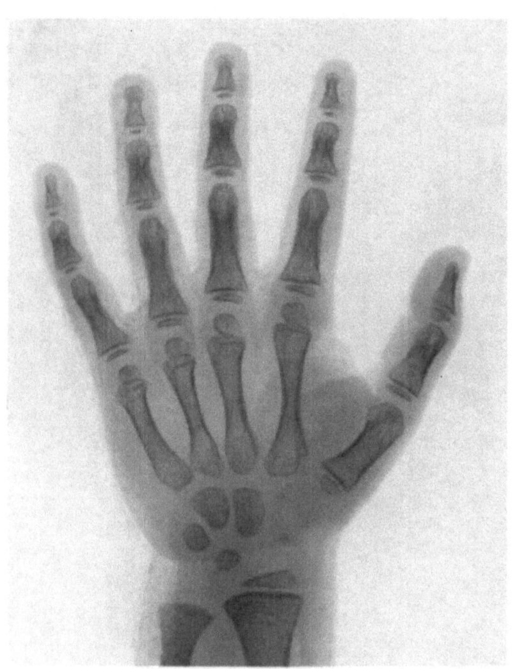

Im 6. Lebensjahr des Mädchens sind erst 6 Handwurzelknochen und die Radiusepiphyse ossifiziert.

6 years of age. Only six wrist bones and the radial epiphysis have ossified.

Series 80.

Endemic Cretinism.

The girl of 5³/₄ showed the characteristic symptoms of cretinism. The development of the skeleton was also retarded.

2.

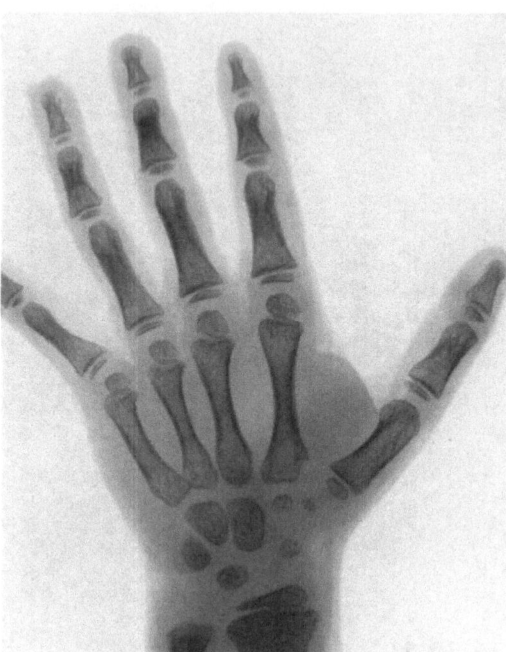

2 Jahre später ist auch der Knochenkern des Os multangulum majus aufgetreten, die distale Ulnaepiphyse aber noch nicht.

Two years later. The bone centre of the os magnum has appeared, but so far no signs of the distal ulnaepiphysis.

C. Örtliche Zirkulations- bzw. Wachstumsstörungen.

1. Aseptische Epiphysennekrosen.

Die Wachstumsstörungen im späten Kindesalter werden als Folge einer subchondralen aseptischen Knochennekrose aufgefaßt. Jedenfalls wird *ein gestörter Umbau durch einen unbekannten Faktor* ausgelöst, bei dem die Apposition hinter der Resorption zurückbleibt. Der Prozeß zieht sich über Jahre hin und tritt am häufigsten am Hüftgelenk auf. *Hier geht er, wie die Serie 81 zeigt, auch bei günstigstem Verlauf nicht ganz spurlos über das Gelenk hinweg. Oft ist der Endzustand eine schwere Wachstumshemmung und Deformierung* (Serien 82—84). Dabei ist die statische Belastung nächst der primären umschriebenen Ernährungsstörung die wichtigste Ursache der Defektheilung. — Kleinere derartige Störungen an Stellen, die gar nicht oder weniger statisch belastet werden, brauchen keine Deformierung zu hinterlassen (Serien 88—90).

1. Aseptic Epiphyseal Necrosis.

In the latter years of childhood, growth disturbances are considered to be the result of a subchondral aseptic bone necrosis. Some unknown factor causes a hindrance in construction, and deposition of bone does not keep pace with resorption. The process is protracted for many years. The hip-joint is most often attacked and traces are left behind in the joint even when the course has been most favourable (Series 81). Deformity and serious interference with growth very often results (Series 82 bis 84). Next to the primary circumscribed nutritional disturbance, the most important cause of defective healing is the statical burden. Smaller but similar disturbances of parts which are not subjected to, or only slightly subjected to strain, do not necessarily cause deformation (Series 88—90).

Serie 81.

Osteoarthritis def. juvenilis coxae.

Die Erkrankung des Knaben begann im Alter von 5 Jahren mit Hinken und Schmerzen in der Hüfte. Eine besondere Behandlung wurde nicht durchgeführt, er ging zur Schule. Die Wachstumsstörung heilte mit unbehinderter Funktion und gutem anatomischen Endzustand aus, hinterließ aber doch eine gewisse Abflachung des Kopfes und Verkürzung des Schenkelhalses.

$^2/_3$ n. Gr.   1.

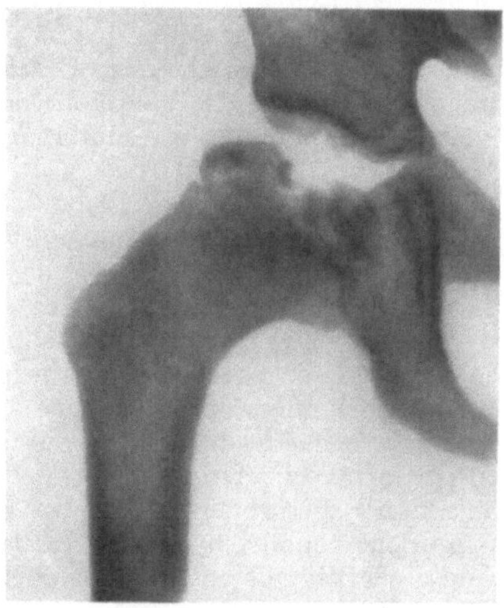

Im Alter von 5 Jahren: Fragmentation und hochgradiger Umbau der Kopfkappe, der die Epiphysenfuge überschreitet, bereits wenige Wochen nach Auftreten der Beschwerden.

5 years of age: Fragmentation and excessive alteration of head cap and penetration of the epiphyseal line which took place some weeks after commencement of illness.

Series 81.

Juvenile Osteo-Arthritis Def. of the Hip.

The boy's illness began when he was 5 years of age with lameness and pain in the hip. No particular treatment was carried out, and he continued to go to school. The condition healed with unhindered function and good anatomical result, leaving the surface of the head somewhat flat and the neck of femur shortened.

2.

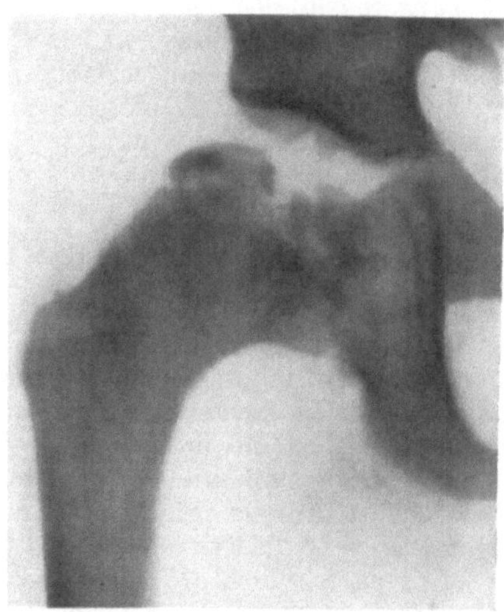

Im Alter von 7 Jahren: Der Umbauprozeß ist noch im Gange.

7 years of age: The process is still progressing.

Serie 81.

3.

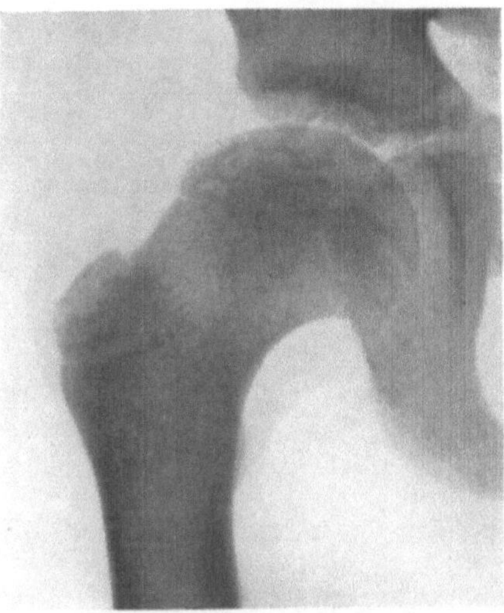

4 a.

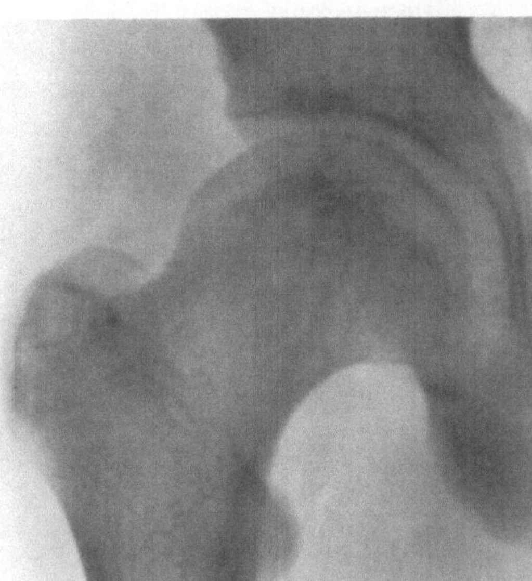

Im Alter von 9 Jahren: Die Wachstumsstörung ist beendet; der Schenkelkopf hat
wieder Kugelform angenommen und die
innere Bälkchenstruktur ist wiederhergestellt.

9 years of age: The condition has come to
a standstill. The head of femur has regained
its roundness, and the inside beam structure
has regenerated.

Im Alter von 16 Jahren: Entsprechend gewachsen, eine
leichte Abflachung des Kopfes und Verkürzung des Halses
wurde nicht mehr ausgeglichen.

16 years of age: Adequate growth, a slight flattening of
head and shortness of neck remaining.

4 b.

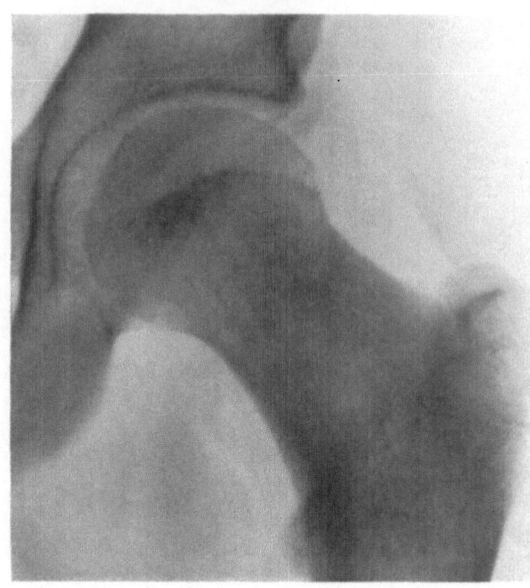

Ungestörtes Wachstum der anderen Hüfte.

Undisturbed growth of the other hip.

Serie 82.

Osteoarthritis def. juven. coxae.

Bei dem 9jährigen Knaben lief die juvenile Wachstumsstörung der Hüfte, die etwas später auch die andere Seite befiel, in charakteristischer Weise ab: der im Gleichgewicht gestörte Wachstumsumbau, bei dem die Apposition stark hinter der Resorption zurückblieb, führte zu Nachgiebigkeit des Knochens, so daß dieser durch die statische Belastung deformiert wurde; das Wachstum des Schenkelhalses blieb zurück. Auch funktionell erfolgte eine Defektheilung.

Series 82.

Juvenile Osteo-Arthritis Def. of the Hip.

A boy nine years of age suffered with infantile growth disturbance of the hip. Somewhat later the other hip was also attacked. The disturbed growth equilibrium (apposition remaining far behind resorption), led to yielding of the bone so that it became deformed and the growth of femur neck ceased. A disturbance in function also remained.

$^6/_{10}$ n. Gr.　　　　1.　　　　　　　　　　2.

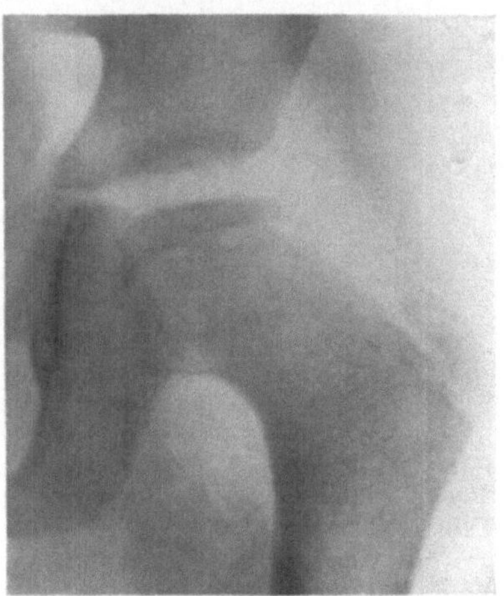

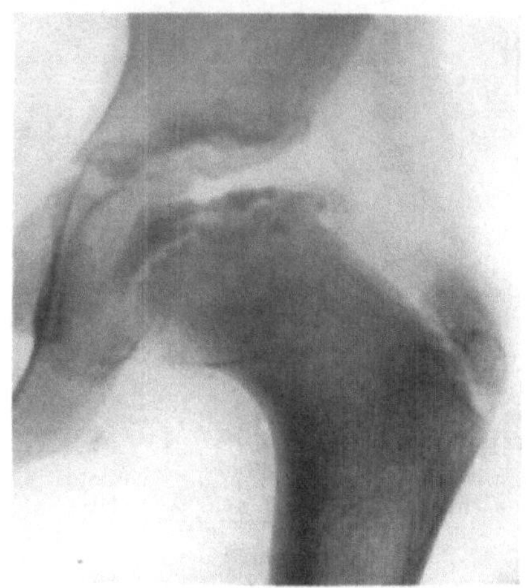

Etwa $^1/_4$ Jahr nach Beginn der Beschwerden ist die Kopfkalotte bereits abgeflacht.

About three months after commencement of complaint, the head-calotte is already levelled.

$^3/_4$ Jahr　　　　　und hat die Zerklüftung der Kopfepiphyse

Nine months and one year and a half later, the cleft

5.

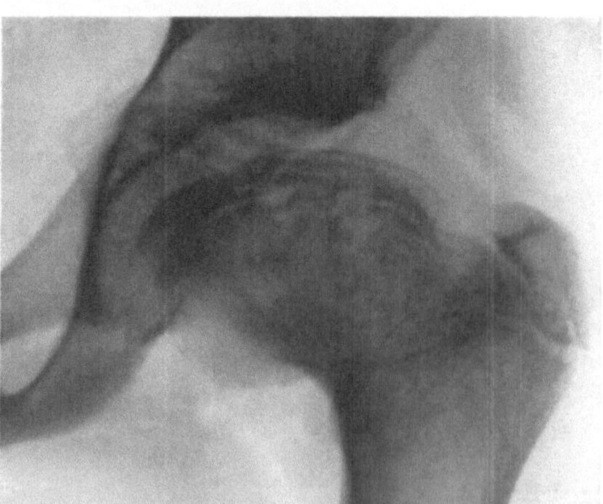

Nach 4 Jahren ist der Endzustand erkennbar: Schenkelkopf und Schenkelhals sind ein kurzer, abgeflachter Knochenstumpf.

After four years, the final condition is recognizable. Head and neck of femur are shortened into a flattened bone stump.

Serie 82.

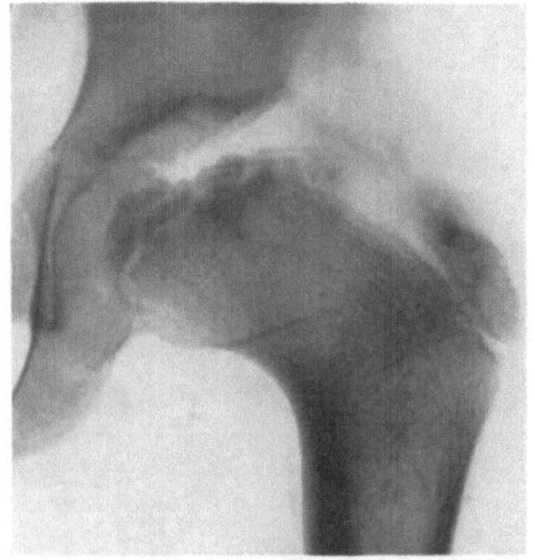

3.

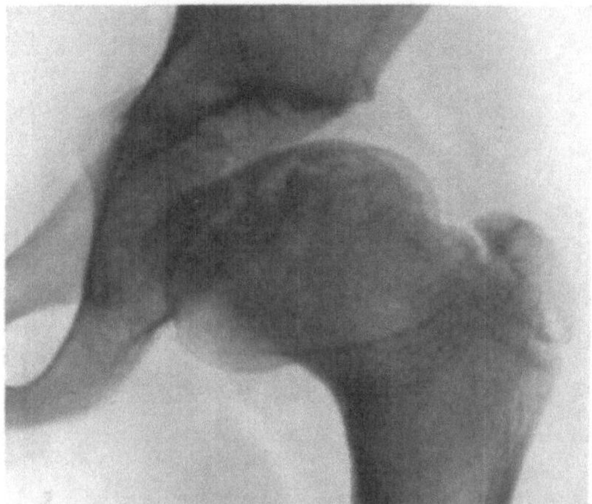

4.

1¹/₂ Jahr später
mehr und mehr zugenommen.

in the epiphyseal head has greatly increased.

Nach 2¹/₂ Jahren ist das floride Stadium überwunden.
Die Kopfkalotte stellt wieder ein breites Band dar.
Freilich ist eine Wachstumshemmung und Deformierung
schon sehr deutlich.

After two years and a half, the flourishing stage has
been overcome. The head-calotte shows again as a wide
ligament but the growth disturbance and deformity are
already very distinct.

Serie 83.

Osteoarthritis deformans juvenilis coxae.

Die Wachstumsstörung der Hüfte begann im 11. Lebensjahr und war nach 6 Jahren trotz der 9 Monate durchgeführten statischen Entlastung im Gehgipsverband mit sehr erheblicher Wachstumshemmung und Deformierung ausgeheilt.

$^6/_{10}$ n. Gr.

Series 83.

Juvenile Osteo-Arthritis Def. of the Hip.

The growth disturbance in the hip began in the eleventh year and although it had been relieved from statical strain by being placed in a walk-permitting plaster of Paris bandage, it took six years to heal. There was very considerable interference with growth and deformity.

1. 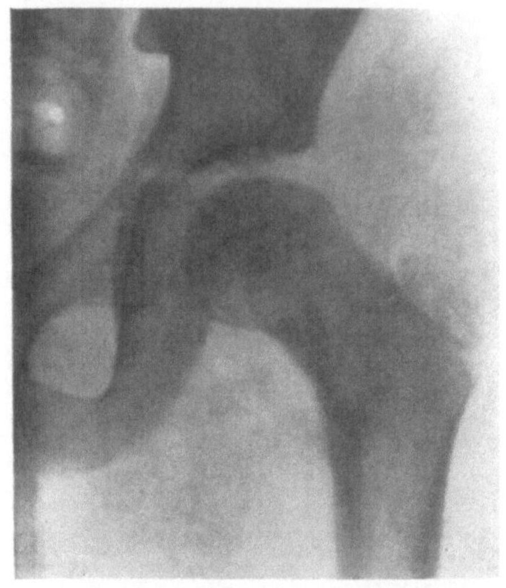

Im 11. Lebensjahr zu *Beginn* der Beschwerden besteht noch ein normaler Röntgenbefund.

In the eleventh year when the disease commenced, the X-ray picture was normal.

2. 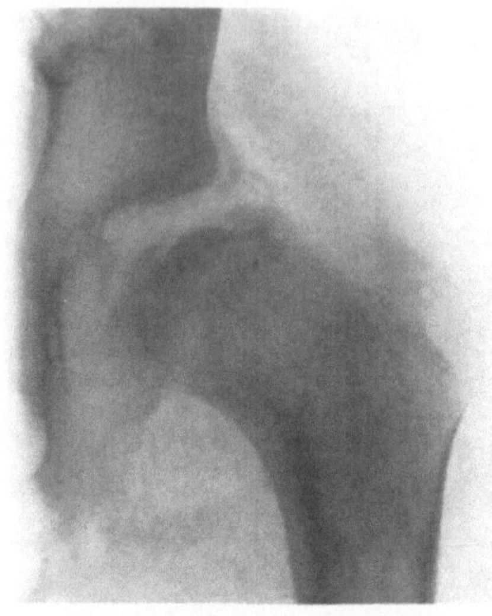

1 Jahr später *florides Stadium:* Umbau und Deformierung der Kopfepiphyse.

One year later, *flourishing stage.* Alteration and deformity of epiphyseal head.

3. 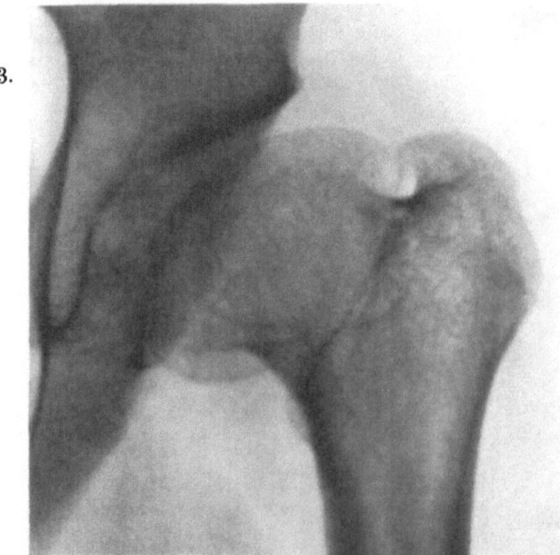

Endzustand nach 6 Jahren: Abflachung des Schenkelkopfes und der Pfanne; sehr kurzer Schenkelhals.
Final condition after six years. Flattened femur-head and cup. Very short neck of femur.

Serie 84.

Osteoarthritis deform. juvenilis coxae.

Auch in diesem Fall ist das Ergebnis des durch die „subchondrale Knochennekrose" gestörten Umbaues und der mechanischen Belastung eine schwere Gelenkdeformierung.

$^6/_{10}$ n. Gr.   1.

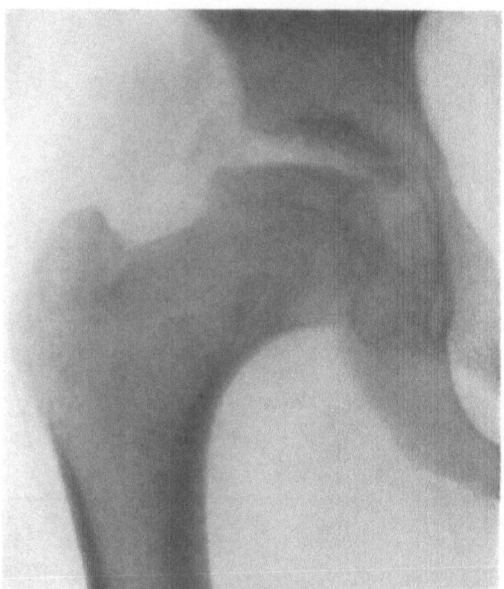

Bei Beginn der Beschwerden — im 12. Lebensjahr — ist lediglich eine leichte Abflachung der Kopfepiphyse feststellbar.

At the commencement of complaint — when patient was in the twelfth year — only a slight flattening of the epiphyseal head was found.

Series 84.

Juvenile Osteo-Arthritis Def. of the Hip.

A severe joint deformation was in this case also the result of disturbed reconstruction and mechanical burden, caused by "subchondral bone-necrosis".

2.

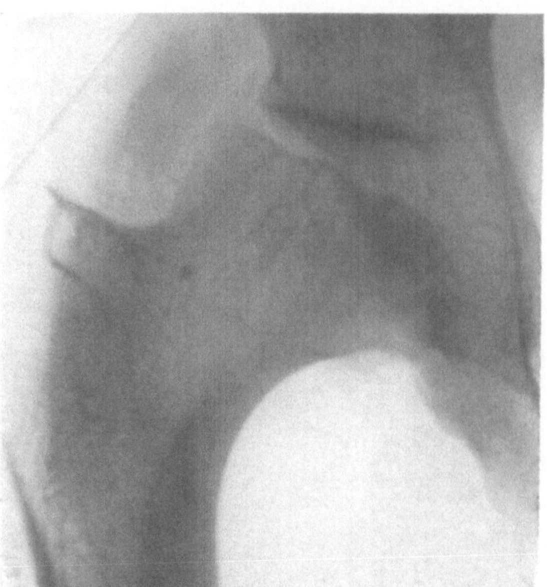

6 Jahre später ist das Kopf-Halsstück im Wachstum zurückgeblieben und hochgradig deformiert, und zwar ist die obere Hälfte des Gelenkkopfes entsprechend der stärkeren Belastung dieser Stelle am meisten abgeflacht.

Six years later. The head-neck portion is backward in growth, very much deformed and, because of the greater burden to this part, the upper half of the joint-head is much flattened.

Serie 85.

Osteoarthritis deformans juvenilis coxae.

Das Leiden wurde wegen des Röntgenbefundes – „Herd" am unteren Pfannenrand — zuerst als tuberkulöse Hüftgelenkentzündung aufgefaßt, und deswegen trug der 11 jährige Knabe ³/₄ Jahr lang einen entlastenden Gipsverband. Danach war er sehr bald beschwerdefrei bei nahezu voller Beweglichkeit der Hüfte. Der Verlauf aber — die charakteristische Gelenkdeformität — zeigte, daß es sich in Wirklichkeit um die juvenile Wachstumsstörung handelte, bei welcher *der gestörte Umbau in der Pfanne begonnen* hatte.

⁶/₁₀ n. Gr.   1.

Series 85.

Juvenile Osteo-Arthritis Def. of the Hip.

The „area" at the lower acetabular edge was at first thought, from the X-ray photograph, to be a tuberculous inflammation of the hip-joint. The patient, a boy of eleven, was forced to wear a plaster of Paris bandage for nine months and he soon recoverd almost the full use of the hip. The course of the disease and also the characteristic deformity of the joint showed however, that the condition was really a juvenile growth interruption, which had commenced in the acetabulum.

2.

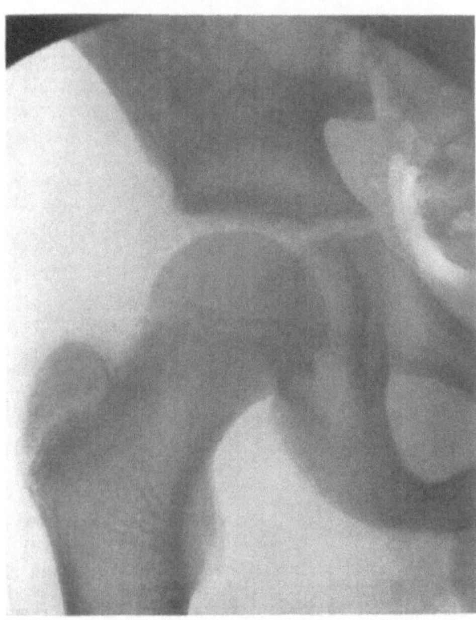

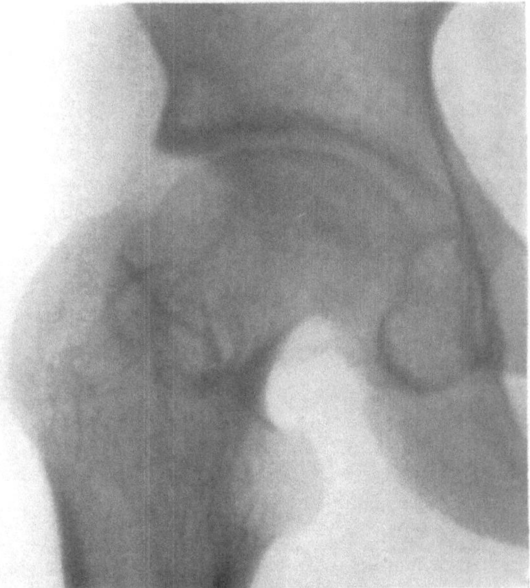

Am unteren Rand der Hüftpfanne ist eine umschriebene Strukturunregelmäßigkeit vorhanden; Schenkelkopf und -hals erscheinen normal.

There is a limited irregularity in the structure of the lower edge of the hip socket. The head and neck of the femur appear normal.

6 Jahre später — im 17. Lebensjahr — zeigt die Hüfte den *Endzustand der juvenilen Wachstumsstörung:* der Schenkelkopf ist pilzförmig abgeflacht, der Hals abnorm kurz und jene Stelle der *Gelenkpfanne — gleichfalls ein Bezirk gestörten Umbaues —* entsprechend gewachsen.

Six years later — in the seventeenth year. The hip shows the *result of the juvenile growth interruption;* the femur-head is shaped like a mushroom, the neck abnormally short and that part of joint socket which also shows an area of interrupted development, has grown accordingly.

Serie 86.

Coxa vara adulescentium.

Die Wachstumsstörung führte schleichend im 13. Lebensjahr des Mädchens zu hochgradiger Deformierung und Fraktur des Schenkelhalses, heilte dann aber unter längerer Extensionsbehandlung verhältnismäßig schnell aus unter weitgehendem Ausgleich der 2. Deformität.

Series 86.

Adolescent Coxa Vara.

A girl suffered with slowly progressing disturbance of growth. By the time she attained her thirteenth year, the femur-neck was extremely deformed and fractured. Extension treatment was carried out for a long time; she was fairly quickly cured and the deformity to a very great extent was compensated.

1.

⁶/₁₀ n. Gr.

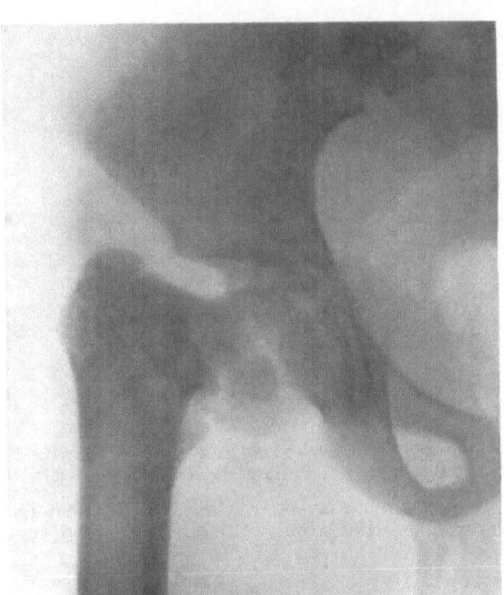

Das Kopf-Halsstück des Femur hat sich gesenkt und ist eingebrochen.

The head and neck of the femur has broken and has sunken.

2.

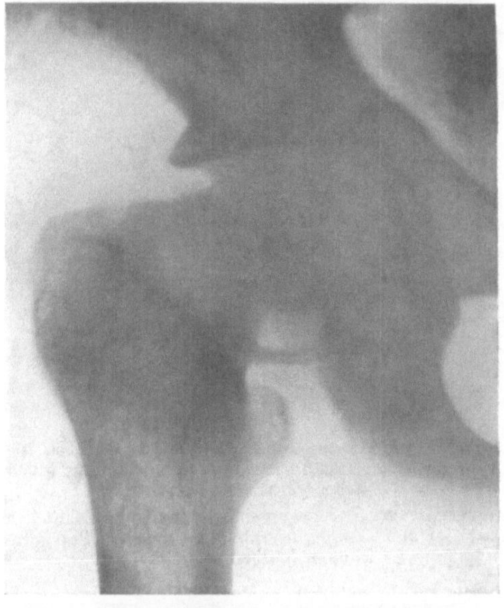

1¹/₂ Jahre später besteht wieder ein *solider Knochenbau*, der Neigungswinkel ist *aufgerichtet* und der Knochen ist *gewachsen*; auch eine stützende Knochenspange hat sich gebildet.

Eighteen months later, a solid bone structure again exists. The angle of declination is raised and the bone has grown. A supporting bridge of bone has also appeared.

10*

Serie 87.

Coxa vara adulescentium.

Das 16jährige wohl entwickelte Mädchen verspürte
erst seit 14 Tagen — ohne daß ein Unfall vorher-
gegangen war — Schmerzen in einer Hüfte und
hinkte. Nach mehrwöchiger Krankenhausbehandlung
(Streckverband) war die Kranke beschwerdefrei und
blieb es seitdem.

$^6/_{10}$ n. Gr.

Series 87.

Adolescent Coxa vara.

For about 14 days a well developed girl of 16, without
any former accident, had pain in one hip and limped.
After several weeks treatment in a hospital (extension
bandage) the invalid was without complaint and has
remained so.

1 a.
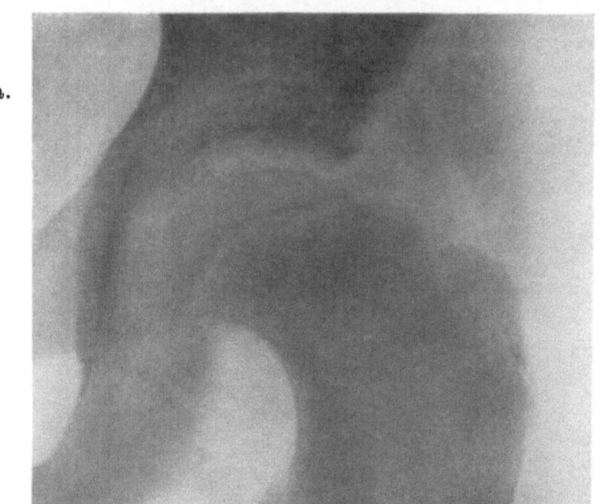

2.
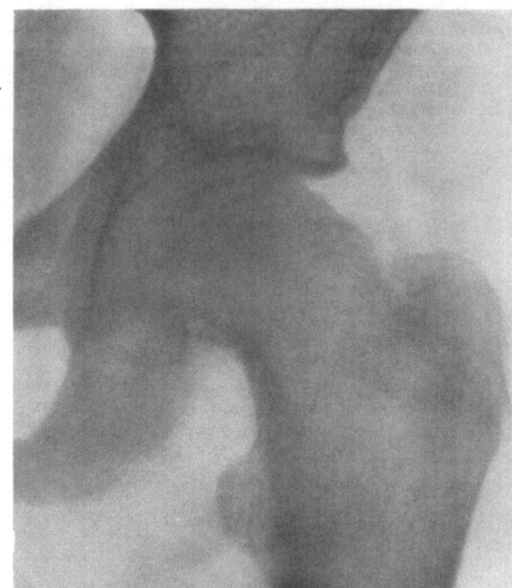

14 Tage nach Beginn der Beschwerden ist die Kopfkappe abgeflacht und verschoben, das Gelenk überhaupt atrophiert.

Fourteen days after commencement of complaint, the
head-cap is flattened and out of place. The joint
is completely atrophic.

Nach $3^1/_2$ Monaten — bei der Entlassung aus dem
Krankenhaus — ist die Knochenatrophie beseitigt.

After $3^1/_2$ months — at the time of leaving the
hospital — the atrophy of the bone has disappeared.

1 b.
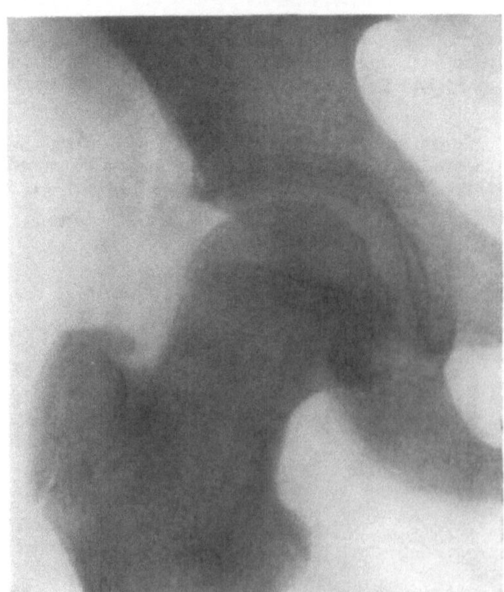

(Die gesunde Seite zum Vergleich.)

The healthy side for comparison.

Serie 87.

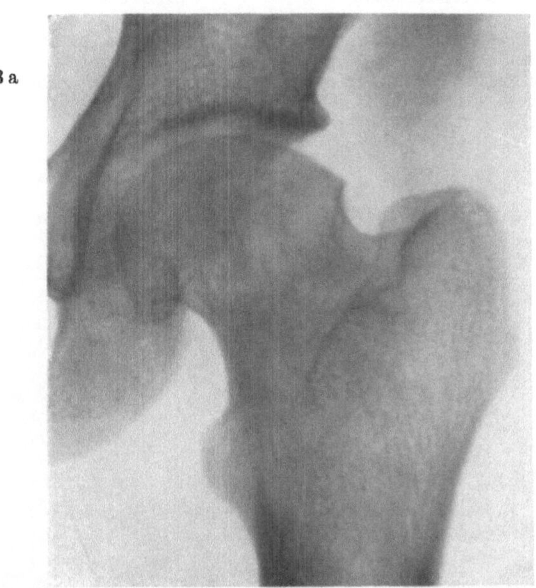

3 a

$4^1/_2$ Jahre später (am Ende des Wachstums) ist *die seit der Epiphysenlösung eingetretene Entwicklungs-hemmung am Schenkelkopf und -hals sehr deutlich,* ohne daß Beschwerden bestehen.

$4^1/_2$ years later — when she had finished growing. The interruption of development in the femur-head and neck, which took place after the epiphysis had loosened, is very plain though there was no complaint of any kind.

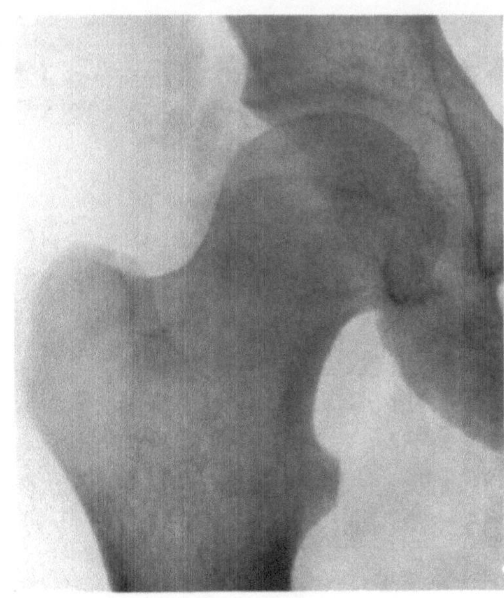

3 b.

Serie 88.

SCHLATTERsche Krankheit.

Der 15jährige Knabe bekam — ohne vorherigen Unfall — ziehende Schmerzen am Knie, als deren Ursache die Wachstumsstörung der Tibiaapophyse erkannt wurde. Die Beschwerden verloren sich nach einigen Monaten von selbst.

$^2/_3$ n. Gr.   1.

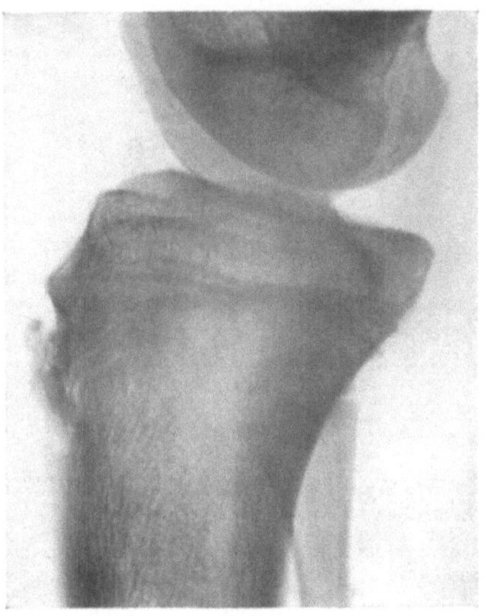

Im 15. Jahr Zerklüftung der Tibiaapophyse.

In the 15th year, cleavage of the tibia-apophysis.

Series 88.

SCHLATTERs Disease.

A boy 15 years of age had — without any former accident — drawn-out pain in the knee, caused by the growth impediment of the apophysis of tibia. The pain ceased after a few months.

2.

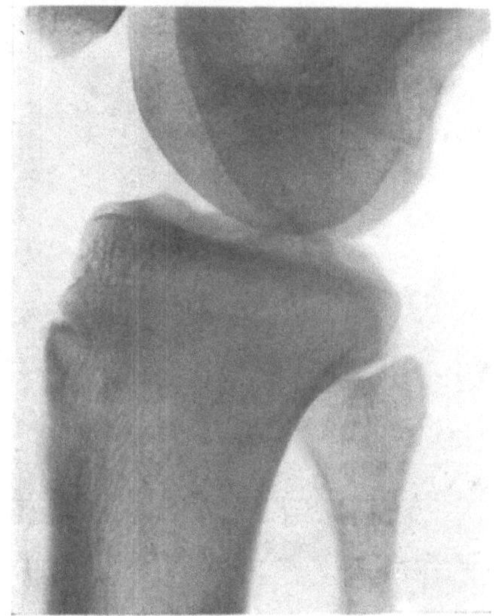

Im 22. Jahr ist noch eine kleine Kerbe als Zeichen der überstandenen Wachstumsstörung erkennbar.

In the 22nd year there is still a slight depression noticeable showing the past growth disturbance.

Serie 89.

Köhlersche Erkrankung
des Os naviculare.

Die Wachstumsstörung des kindlichen Kahnbeines wurde im 6. Lebensjahr des Knaben an einer schmerzhaften Anschwellung bemerkt. Eine besondere Behandlung geschah nicht und nach 2 Jahren war das Leiden „ausgewachsen".

$^7/_{10}$ n. Gr.   1.

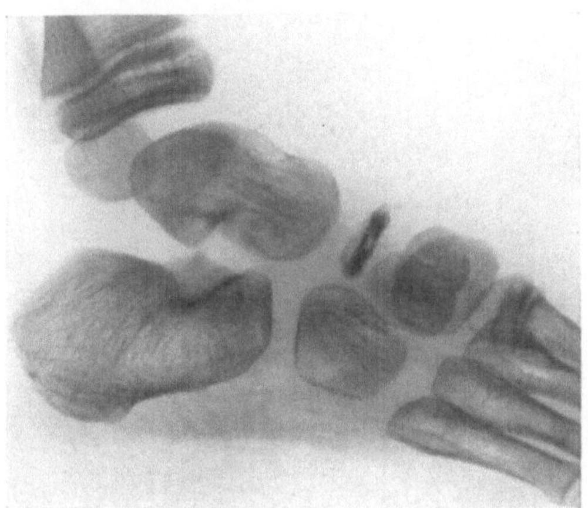

Lebensalter: 6 Jahre. Der Knochenkern des Kahnbeines ist hochgradig komprimiert, seine Struktur verdichtet, bzw. zerstört.

Six years of age. The bone centre of the os naviculare is seriously compressed. Its structure is dense and is in places destroyed.

Series 89.

Koehlers Disease
of the Os Naviculare.

The growth disturbance of the navicular bone was discovered in the boy's sixth year by the presence of a painful swelling. No special treatment was advised and the condition disappeared within two years.

2.

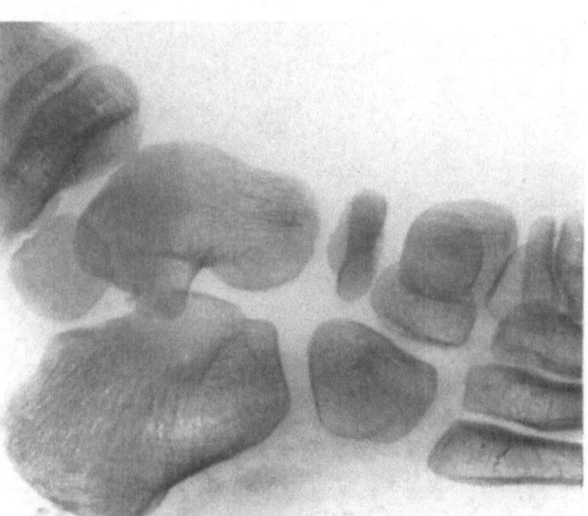

Lebensalter: 8 Jahre. Das Os naviculare ist gewachsen und seine innere Bälkchenstruktur weitgehend wiederhergestellt. *Die Störung ist zum größten Teil ausgeglichen.*

Eight years of age. The navicular bone has grown and the inner beam structure has regenerated to a great extent. *The disturbance is almost compensated.*

Serie 90.

„Epiphyseonecrosis" vertebrae.

Die Ossificationsstörung an der Wirbelsäule — im Lendenteil — heilte mit der anatomischen Restitutio ad integrum und dem Aufhören der Schmerzen.

$^6/_{10}$ n. Gr.   1.

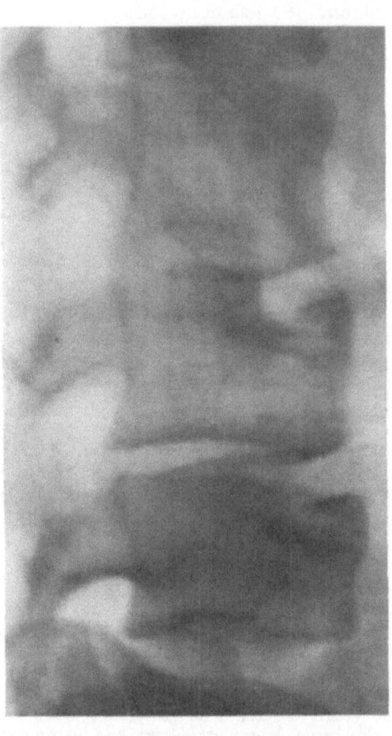

Im 16. Lebensjahr sind die oberen Epiphysen des 3. und 4. Lendenwirbels abgeglitten, die Fugen unregelmäßig.

In the sixteenth year. The upper epiphyses of the third and fourth lumbar vertebrae have slipped off. The joints are irregular.

Series 90.

"Epiphyseonecrosis" Vertebrae.

The ossification disturbance of the dorsal and lumbar portions of the spine healed with anatomical restitutio ad integrum and cessation of pain.

2.

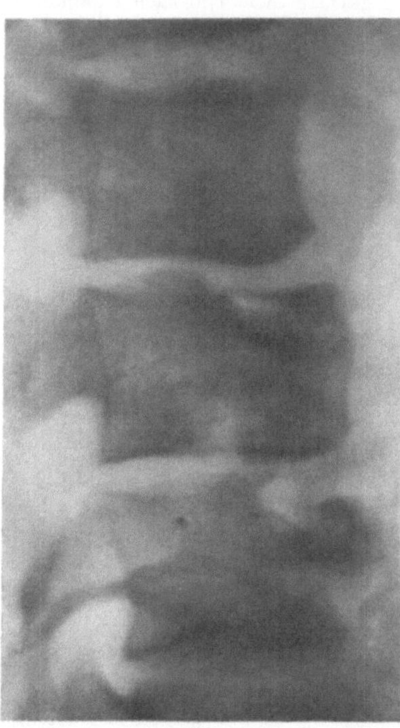

$^3/_4$ Jahr später erscheint die Epiphyse des 3. Lendenwirbels schon angeglichen, am 4. aber besteht die Unregelmäßigkeit noch.

Nine months later. The epiphysis of the third lumbar vertebra already appears to be regular, but the fourth still shows irregularity.

Serie 90.

3.　　　　　　　　　　　　　　4.

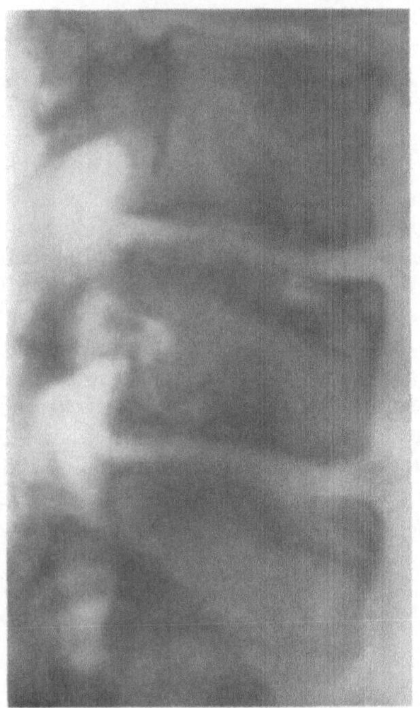

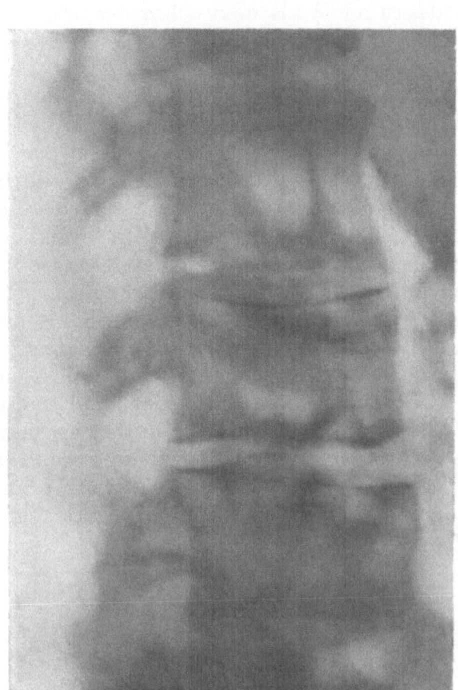

Nach 1¹/₄ Jahren ist auch am 4. Lendenwirbel
die Reparation im Gange.

After one year and three months. Reparation of
the fourth lumbar vertebra is now taking place.

Nach 2 Jahren ist die ebenmäßige Form der
Wirbelkörper wiederhergestellt.

After two years. The vertebral bodies have now
regained their symmetrical shape.

2. Ostitis fibrosa. — Osteochondritis dissecans.

Die *Ostitis fibrosa* wird jetzt Osteodystrophia fibrosa genannt. Das Wesen des Krankheitsprozesses und seine Prognose ist erst in den letzten Jahren richtig erkannt worden. Wurde sie doch früher wegen des histologischen Bildes („Riesenzellentumor") als eine echte bösartige Geschwulst aufgefaßt; deswegen bestand die Behandlung auch immer in einer radikalen Operation (Amputation, Resektion). Heute wissen wir, daß es sich dabei um ein *Granulationsgewebe* handelt. *Die Reihen dieses Buches zeigen, daß der ernährungsgestörte Knochenbezirk nach einem spontanen Einbruch oder einer einfachen Auskratzung ausheilt. Freilich erfolgt eine Defektheilung* (Serien 91—93). Keineswegs aber beruhen selbst wiederholte Frakturen unbedingt auf einer Progredienz des Leidens oder gar auf destruktivem Geschwulstwachstum, sondern auf der durch die Narbe bedingten verminderten mechanischen Festigkeit. Echte, nach Jahren auftretende wirkliche maligne Degeneration, wie ich sie einmal gesehen habe, gehört zu den allergrößten Seltenheiten; sie war in dem Einbruch in die Weichteile als solche erkennbar. Immerhin ist der Prozeß nicht in allen Fällen gleichwertig; an der Tibia (Serie 91) erscheint er als eine Art Infarkt, der gesetzmäßige Folgen nach sich zieht, aber selbst längst beendet ist; bei dem Schädel (Serie 94) sehen wir einen über Jahre sich erstreckenden primären Krankheitsablauf.

Ebenfalls eine umschriebene Ernährungsstörung des Skeletes ist die *Osteochondritis dissecans*. Sie tritt ausgesprochen an einer Prädilektionsstelle auf (Serie 96) und erinnert an das Ulcus ventriculi bzw. duodeni. Ein Knorpel-Knochenstück wird mehr oder weniger sequestriert, kann dann als freier Gelenkkörper gelöst werden, scheint aber meist wie ein Infarkt organisiert zu werden (Serie 96 u. 97).

2. Ostitis fibrosa. — Osteochondritis dissecans.

Osteitis fibrosa is now called osteodystrophia. The nature and the prognosis of the condition has only been correctly recognized within the last few years. Until then, on account of the histological picture (giant cell tumour), it was thought to be a genuine malignant growth and was therefore treated by amputation or resection. Now we know that it consists of granulation tissue. The pictures in this book show that a bone area which has suffered from a nutritional disturbance, heals after a spontaneous fracture or a simple scraping, though of course defective healing results (Series 91—93). Repeated fractures do not necessarily mean that the disease is becoming worse or that they are necessarily caused by a destructive tumour growth. They are due to the lessened mechanical strength caused by the scar. Genuine malignant degeneration appearing after many years, is extremly rare. I have seen only one case myself, and it was recognized when the soft parts were incised. The process does not always run the same course. It appeared in the tibia as a sort of infarct which healed, leaving behind natural results (Series 91). In the skull (Series 94), we see the final stage of the primary disease which had lasted for many years.

Osteochondritis dissecans is also a circumscribed nutritional disturbance of the skeleton. It appears at a predisposed place (Series 96) and reminds one of an ulcer of the stomach or duodenum. A piece of bony cartilage may become more or less sequestrated or may also be quite free. Usually it resembles an infarct (Series 96 and 97).

Serie 91.

Ostitis fibrosa tibiae.

Die Knochencyste wurde bei dem 11 jährigen Knaben erst bemerkt, als die Spontanfraktur geschehen war. — Der Bruch heilte rasch und seitdem war der Kranke wieder völlig beschwerdefrei. Der Krankheitsprozeß selbst — die Ernährungsstörung und ihre unmittelbare Auswirkung (Osteodystrophia fibrosa) — war rasch abgelaufen; dennoch wurde die Höhle im Laufe der Jahre größer, weil das Wachstum den Knochen streckte.

Series 91.

Osteitis Fibrosa of the Tibia.

A boy eleven years of age had a spontaneous fracture and only then was the bone-cyst observed. The fracture healed rapidly and the patient had no further disorder. The progress of the malady itself — nutriment disorder and its immediate result (osteo-dystrophia fibrosa) was soon brought to an end, but in the course of time the cavity became larger as growth caused lengthening of the bone.

$^2/_3$ n. Gr.　　　　1.　　　　　　　　　　　　2.

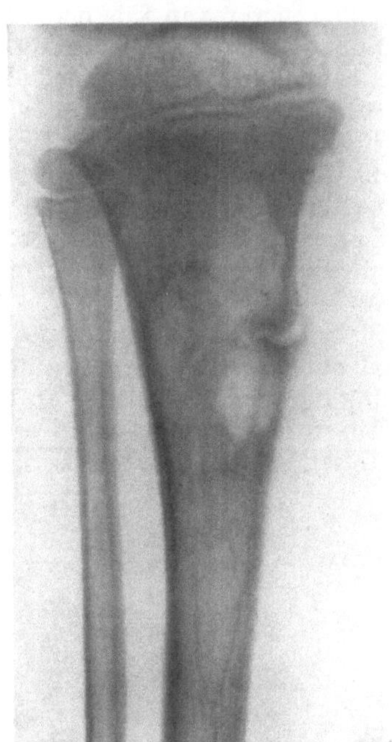 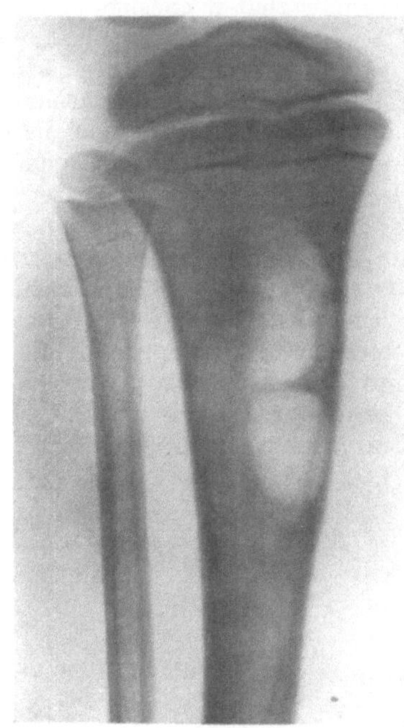

Knochencyste der Tibia mit Spontanfraktur.

Bonecyst of the tibia with spontaneous fracture.

1 Jahr später　　　　　　　und
ist an der Bruchstelle eine Callusbrücke vorwachstum entsprechend

One year and two years later, at the fractured cavity has become larger

Serie 91.

3.

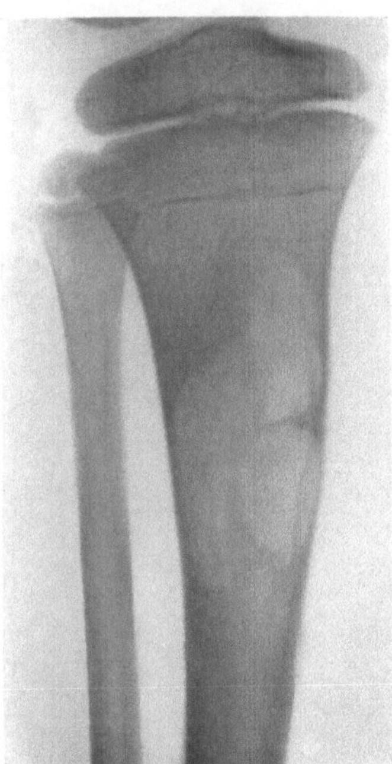

2 Jahre später
handen; die Knochenhöhle ist dem Knochen-
größer geworden.

point a callus bridge is to be seen. The bone
with the growth of the bone.

4.

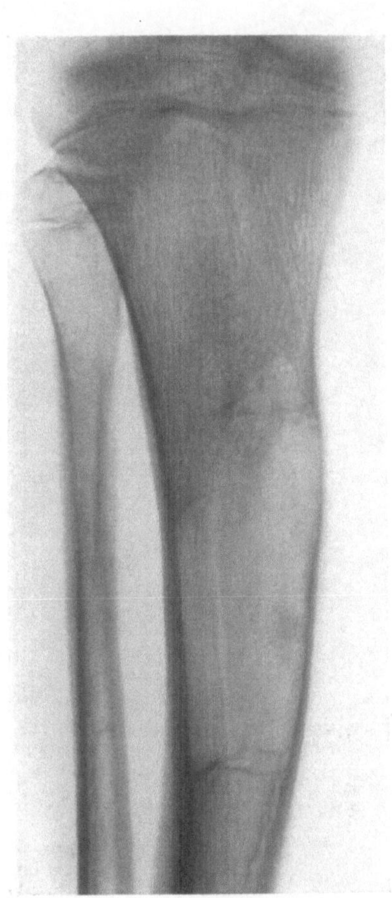

Nach 9 Jahren ist mit dem Knochen auch die
Höhle gewachsen und nach der Mitte zu abgerückt.

After nine years, the bone and the cavity are larger
and the latter has moved towards the middle.

Serie 92.

Ostitis fibrosa humeri.

Bei dem 16jährigen Mädchen ereignete sich bei einer harmlosen Bewegung die Spontanfraktur des Oberarmes. Die Behandlung bestand lediglich in einem Schienenverband. Der Knochenbruch heilte wie an einem gesunden Knochen und verursachte dem Mädchen keine Beschwerden mehr.

Series 92.

Fibrous Osteitis of the Humerus.

A 16 year old girl after quite a casual movement had a spontaneous fracture of the upper arm. It was put into a splint and bandaged. The fracture healed like a healthy bone and the girl had no further complaint.

²/₃ n. Gr.   1.   2.   3.

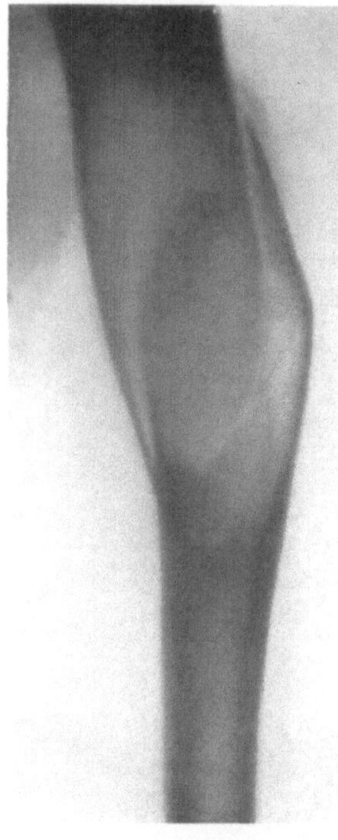

Große Knochencyste mit Spontanfraktur.

Large bone cyst with spontaneous fracture.

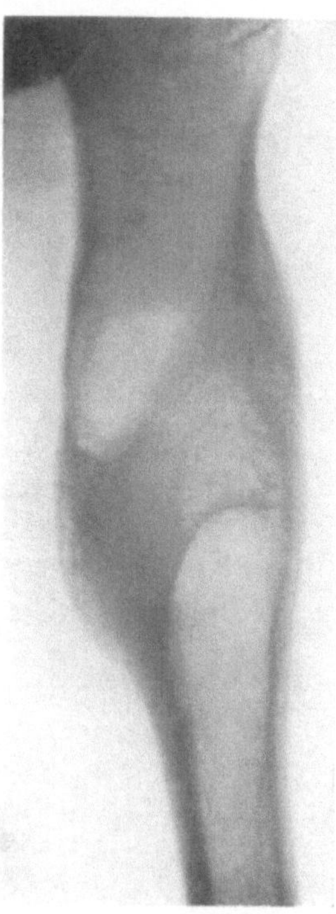

Nach 8 Monaten besteht eine breite Callusbrücke quer durch die Cyste, nachdem die Fraktur bereits nach 6 Wochen fest war.

After 8 months a wide bridge of callus passes across the cyst although the fracture had already become firm after 6 weeks.

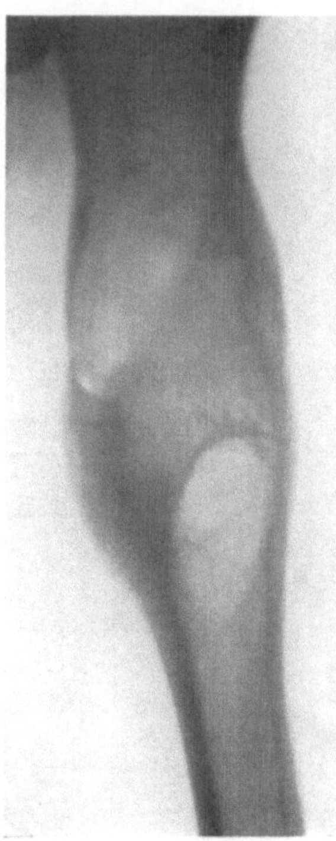

Nach 1 Jahr ist die Knochenbrücke noch dichter.

After 1 year the bridge of bone is still thicker.

Serie 92.

4.

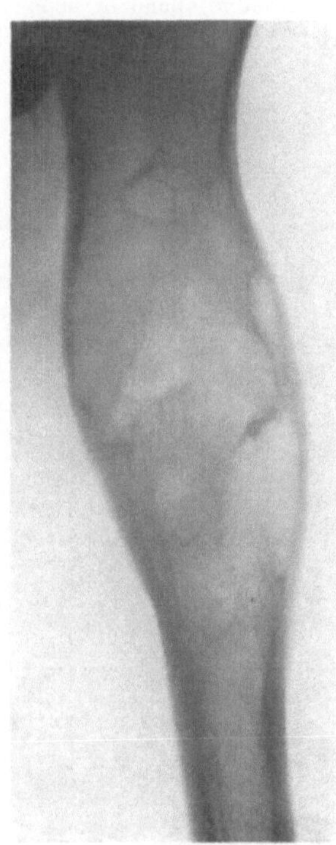

Nach 3¹/₂ Jahren ist die durch den Knochen
ziehende Callusbrücke resorbiert.

After 3¹/₂ years the callus bridge which passes
through the bone is resorbed.

5.

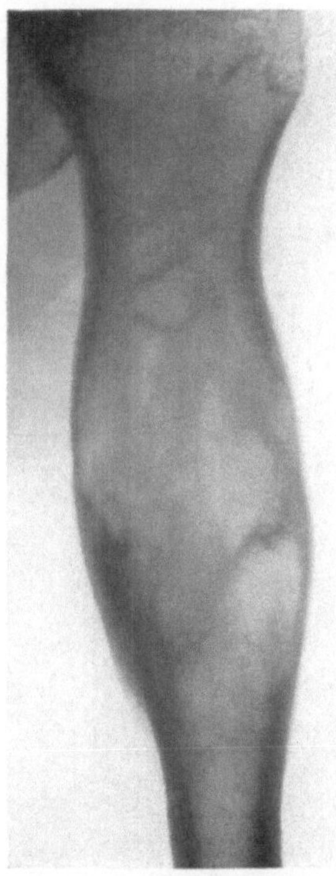

Nach 5 Jahren ist die Knochenstruktur etwas
dichter, die Form aber unverändert, *der Krankheitsprozeß narbig ausgeheilt.*

After 5 years the bone structure is somewhat
thicker, but the shape unaltered. The healing
process left a scar.

Serie 93.
Ostitis fibrosa humeri.

Der Degenerationsbezirk des Humerus — eine für die Osteodystrophia fibrosa typische Stelle — erfuhr infolge der verminderten mechanischen Festigkeit, nicht etwa durch Fortschreiten des Krankheitsprozesses, wiederholte Frakturen. Auf diesem Wege aber entstand durch reaktive Knochenwucherung eine Festigkeitsvermehrung des Humerus und die narbige Ausheilung.

Series 93.
Fibrous Osteitis of the Humerus.

This portion of humerus, most liable to undergo degeneration — typical for osteo-dystrophia — was fractured repeatedly. The fractures were not caused by the advancing process but through decreased mechanical solidity. The reactive abundant bone-growth resulted in an increased strengthening of humerus and scarry healing.

$^2/_3$ n. Gr.   1.   2.   3.

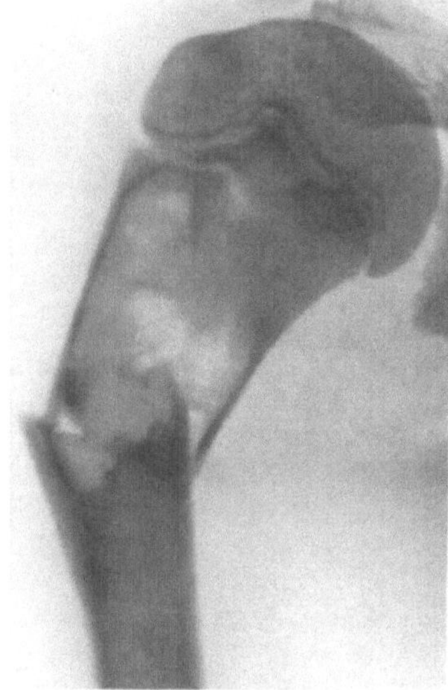 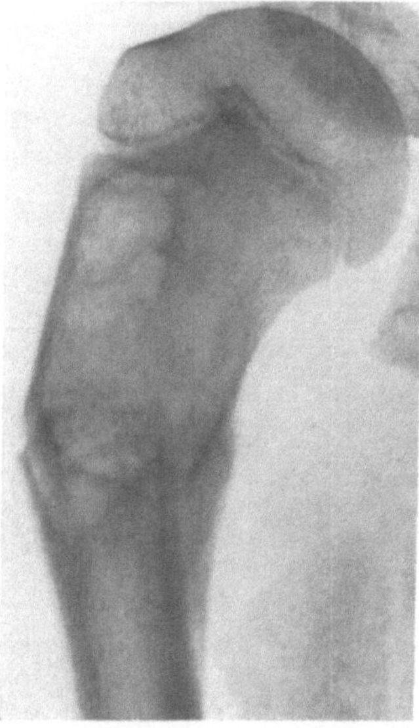 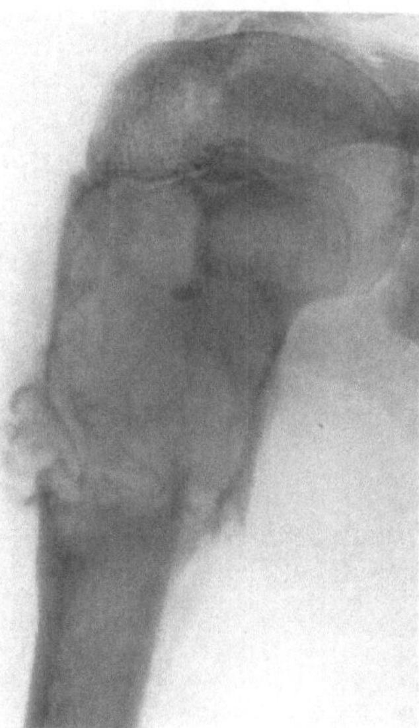

Die große Knochencyste hat die Corticalis stark verdünnt und zur Spontanfraktur am peripheren Ende geführt. (17 jähriger Arbeiter.)

The large bone cyst has caused great thinning of the cortex and led to a spontaneous fracture of the peripheral end (workman seventeen years of age).

Nach $^1/_4$ Jahr ist der Knochenbruch mit deutlichem periostalem Callus geheilt; auch im Inneren ist ossale Verdichtung erkennbar.

After three months, the fracture has healed with distinct periosteal callus; osteal compactness in the interior is also recognizable.

Nach $^1/_2$ Jahr ist der Humerus an derselben Stelle *zum zweitenmal gebrochen.*

After six months, the humerus is fractured for the *second time* in the same place.

Serie 93.

4.

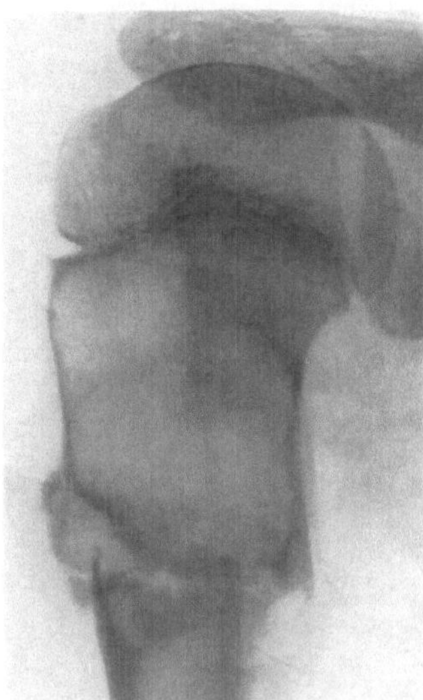

Die Knochenhöhle nach operativer
Auskratzung.
The bone cavity after having been
scraped out.

5.

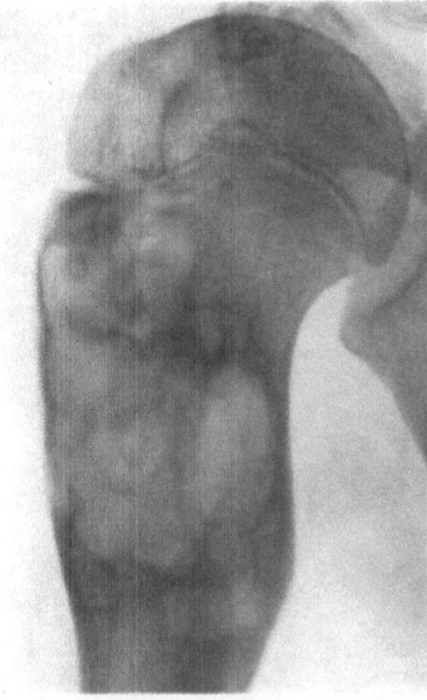

Nach einem weiteren Vierteljahr ist
die Bruchstelle wieder verwachsen,
im Inneren aber nur wenig Knochen
gebildet.
After another three months, the
fractured part has grown together
again but very little bone has grown
in the interior.

6.

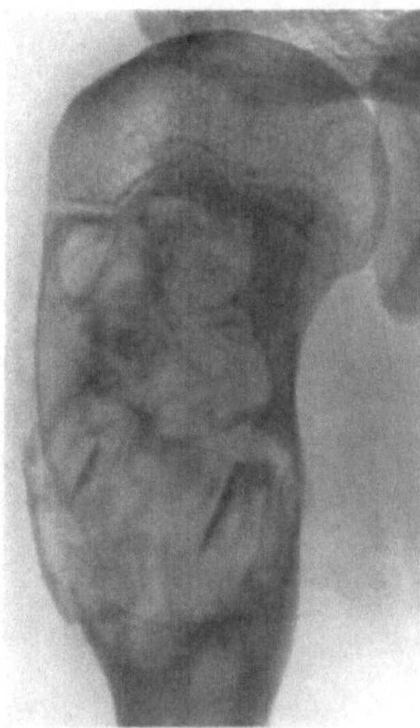

7 Monate nach der Auskratzung
geschah *die 3. Fraktur.*
The *third fracture* occurred seven
months after operation.

9.

7.

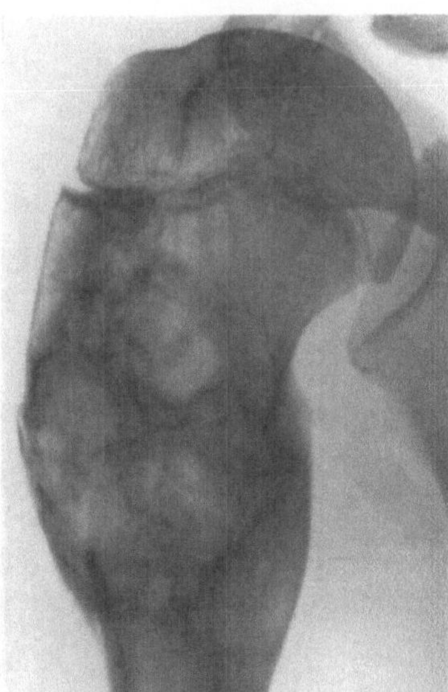

6 Wochen später ist der Bruch wieder
knöchern fest und die Höhle mehr
ausgefüllt.
Six weeks later, the fracture is again
firm and cavity somewhat more
filled out.

8.

½ Jahr später ist wieder ein Umbau
erkennbar.
Six months later, reconstruction is
again noticeable.

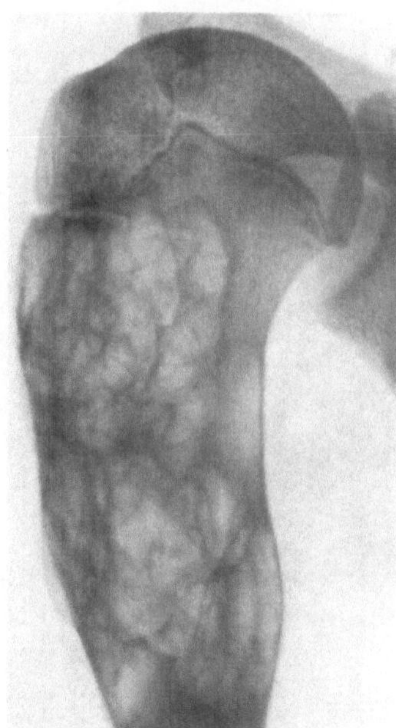

1 Jahr nach der 3. Fraktur ist die
Struktur mehr differenziert: *in der
Rindenschicht verstärkt.*
One year after third fracture, the diffe-
rentiation of *structure* has advanced
and the cortical part is strengthened.

<table>
<tr><td>

Serie 94.

Ostitis fibrosa des Schädels.

Die auf den Schädel beschränkte Knochenerkrankung wurde im 35. Lebensjahr des Mannes erkannt, nachdem schon seit etwa 20 Jahren die Größe des Kopfes aufgefallen war. Er klagte über dumpfe Schmerzen. Wa.R. neg. — Der an sich ungeklärte Knochenumbauprozeß zeigte im Laufe der nächsten Jahre die Tendenz der Ausheilung.

</td><td>

Series 94.

Fibrous Osteitis of the Skull.

The bone disease, which was confined to the skull, was only recognized when the patient was in his thirty-fifth year, although the unusual size of the head had been noticeable for twenty years. He complained of dull pains. W.R. neg. — The unexplained reconstruction process of the bone showed a tendency to heal in the course of the following years.

</td></tr>
</table>

$^4/_9$ n. Gr.

1 a.

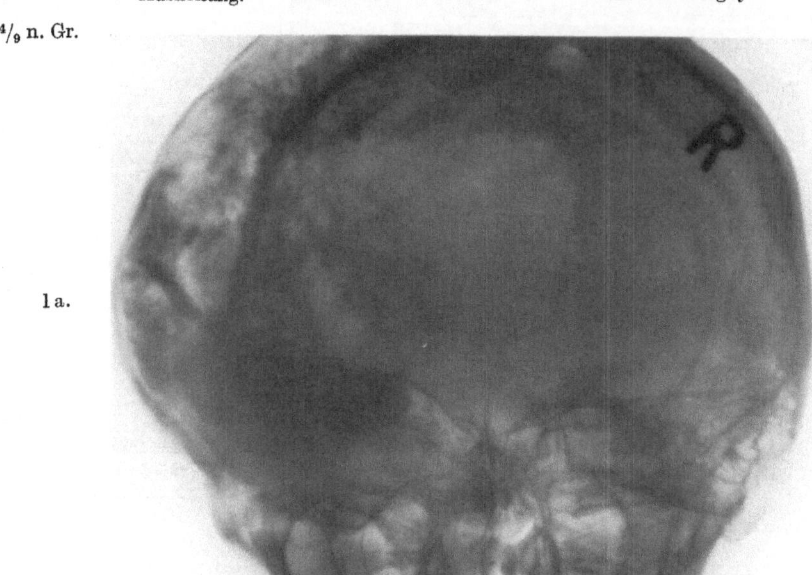

1 b.

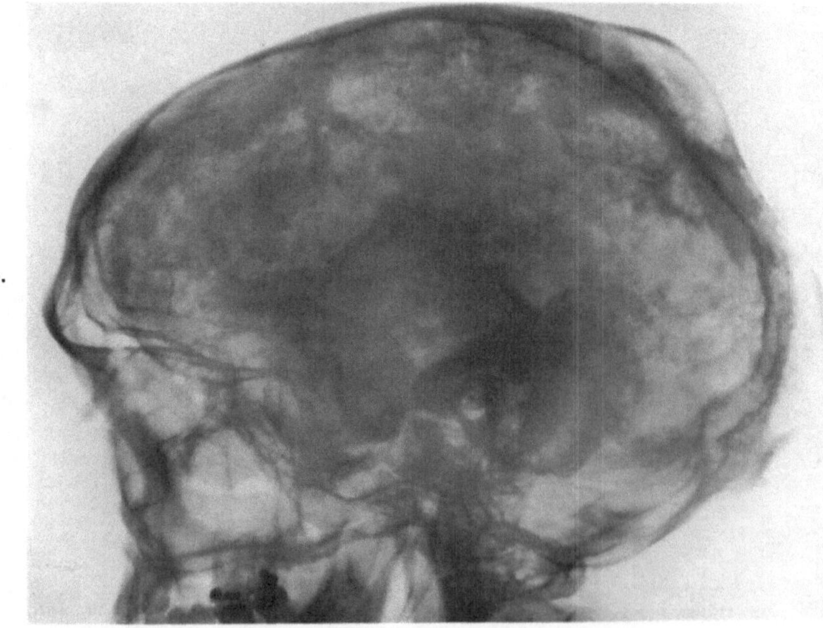

Im Alter von 35 Jahren treten die resorptiven Vorgänge des Umbaues stark hervor, wie die flächenhaften Aufhellungen der Schädelknochen zeigen.

At thirty-five years of age the resorption change is strongly noticeable. This is seen in places by the lighter shade of the skull bone.

Serie 94.

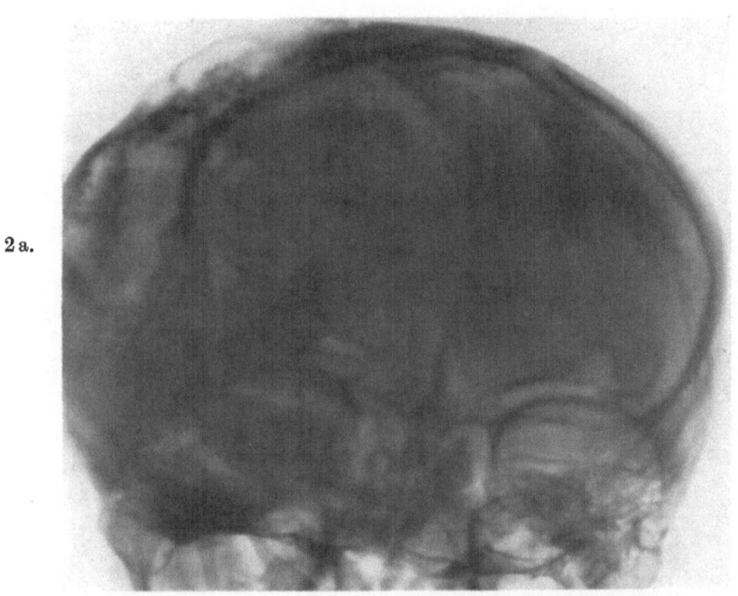

2a.

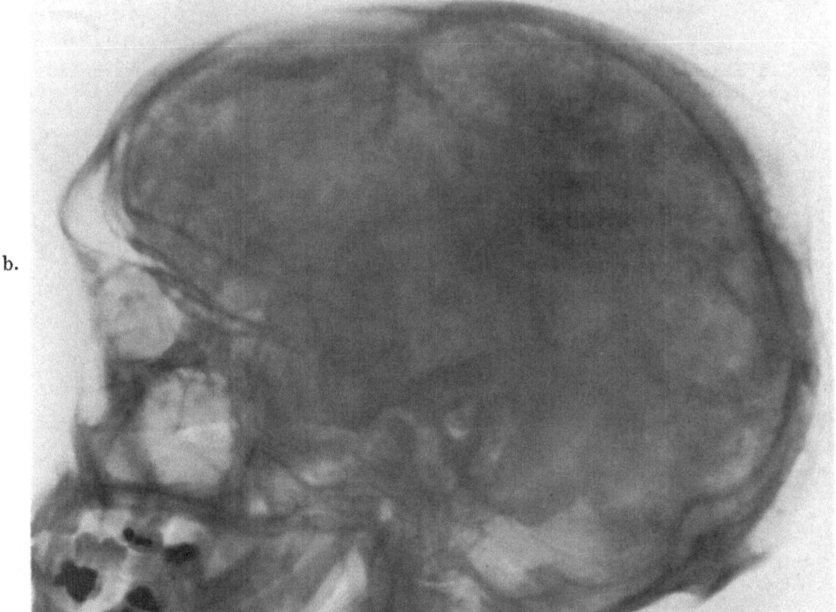

2b.

Im Verlauf der nächsten 4 Jahre ist allenthalben wieder Knochensubstanz angesetzt worden; das Schädeldach ist erheblich dichter.

In the course of the next four years bone substance is deposited all over; the skull roof is more compact.

<table>
<tr><td>

Serie 95.

Ostitis fibrosa generalisata.

Die degenerative Systemerkrankung des Skeletes blieb im 2. und 3. Jahrzehnt des Lebens nicht ganz stationär, vielmehr traten — bei einer Schwangerschaft — vereinzelt neue Herde auf und in den alten vollzog sich langsam ein Umbau. — Die Beschwerden waren verhältnismäßig gering.

</td><td>

Series 95.

Generalized Osteitis Fibrosa.

The degenerative generalized disease of the skeleton did not remain stationary in the second and third decades. Indeed, during pregnancy, new isolated areas formed and the old ones slowly underwent a change. The patient was not greatly inconvenienced.

</td></tr>
</table>

$^1/_2$ n. Gr.   1.

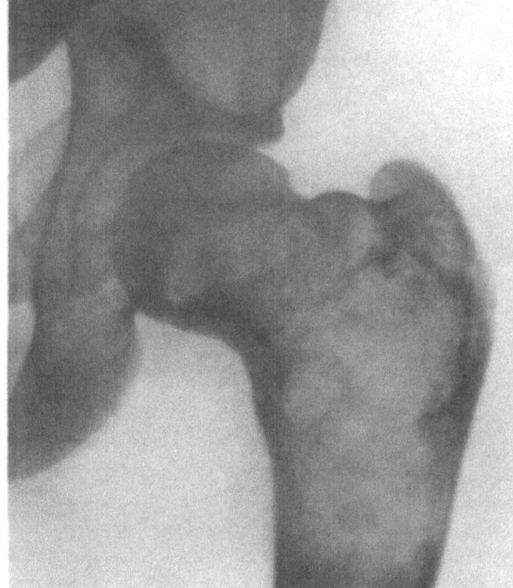

Lebensalter: 15 Jahre.
Große strukturlose Knochenhöhle im Femur, die bis in den Schenkelkopf reicht; eine zweite im Darmbein.

At the age of fifteen, a large structureless bone cavity in femur which reaches into femur head is seen. A second is seen in the ilium.

2.

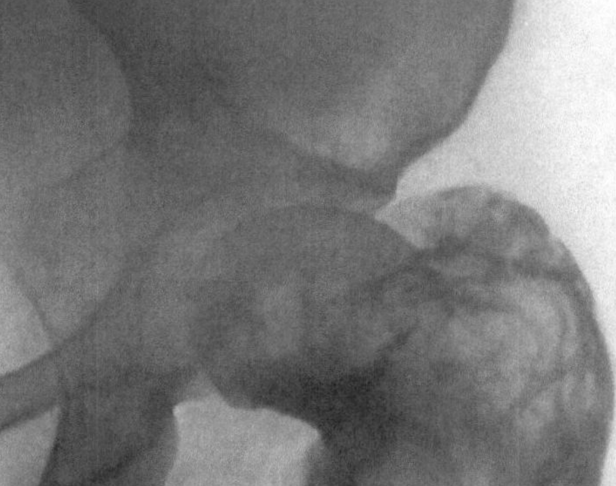

Lebensalter: 21 Jahre.
Der cystische Bezirk ist nicht größer geworden, aber im Inneren differenzierter strukturiert.

Twenty-one years of age. The cystic portion is not enlarged but the interior structure is more differentiated.

Serie 95.

3.

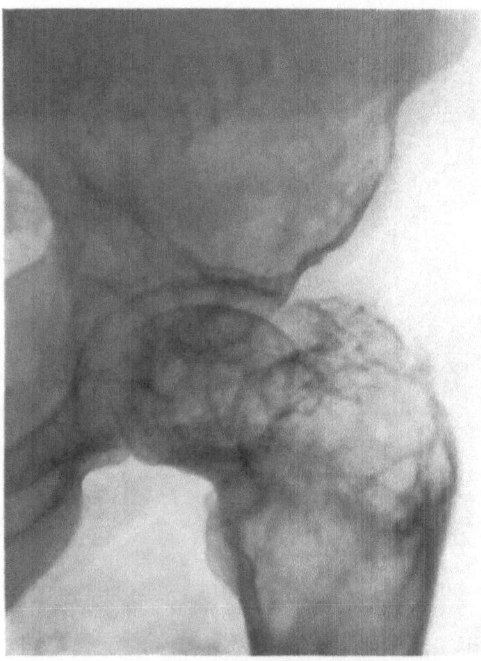

Lebensalter: 28 Jahre
(während der Schwangerschaft).
Der Prozeß ist weiter in den Schenkelkopf vorgedrungen, hat eine stärkere Wabenstruktur ausgebildet und das Femurende aufgetrieben.

Twenty-eight (during pregnancy). The process has
advanced further into femur head, formed a distinct
honeycomb structure and inflated the end
of the femur.

4.

Lebensalter: 32 Jahre.
Der anatomische Zustand hat sich an dieser Stelle
inzwischen nicht verändert.

Thirty-two years of age. The anatomical condition
in the meantime has remained unchanged
in this situation.

Serie 96.

Osteochondritis dissecans des Knies.

Bei dem 24 jährigen Mann heilte die umschriebene „Ernährungsstörung" des Knochens bei Durchführung des Berufes in etwa $1^1/_2$ Jahren, indem der Nekroseherd organisiert wurde.

$^6/_{10}$ n. Gr.   1.

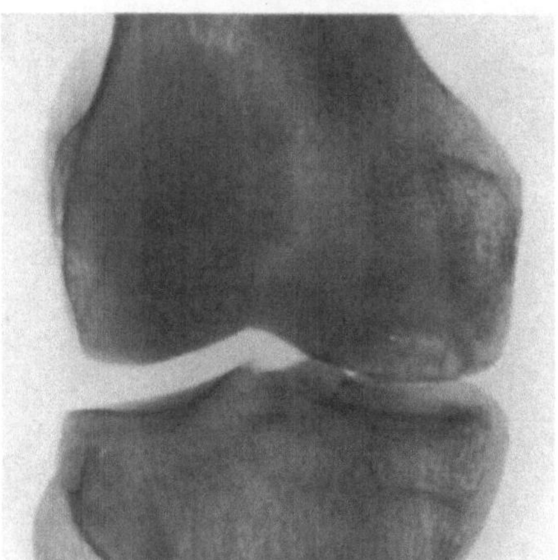

Der charakteristische Befund der Osteochondritis dissecans an der bevorzugten Stelle, dem medialen Femurcondylus.

Characteristic osteo-chondritis dessicans at the medial condyle of the femur — the seat of predilection.

Series 96.

Osteo-Chondritis Dessicans of the Knee.

A young man of twenty four who suffered from a disturbance of bone nutrition, was completely cured without any interruption his work.

2.

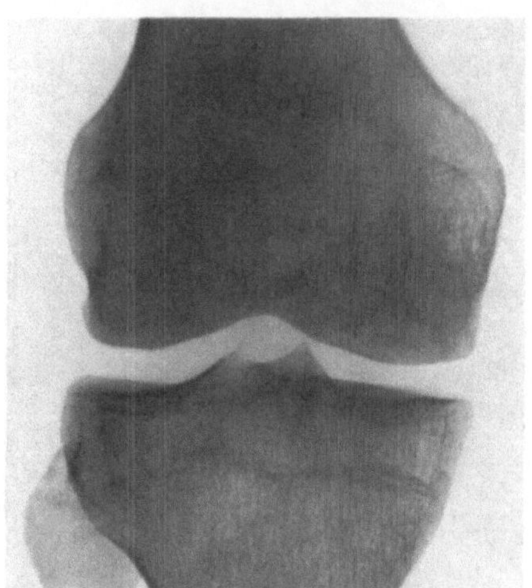

Nach $1^1/_2$ Jahren ist der subchondrale Nekroseherd organisiert, kaum noch erkennbar.

A year and a half later the sub-chondral necrosis has become reorganized and is hardly noticeable.

Serie 97.

Osteochondritis dissecans des Fußgelenkes.

Der osteochondritische Prozeß dieser selteneren Lokalisation wurde bei dem 58jährigen Mann zufällig — anläßlich einer Fersenquetschung am Unfalltage — festgestellt. Seine weitere Entwicklung zeigt deutlich das *spontane Heilbestreben*.

Series 97.

Osteo-Chondritis Dessicans.

The osteo-chondritic process in this unusual locality was found accidentally. The patient was a man, fifty-eight years of age, and he was being treated for a contusion of the heel. The further development shows plainly the *spontaneous healing effort*.

$^6/_{10}$ n. Gr.   1.

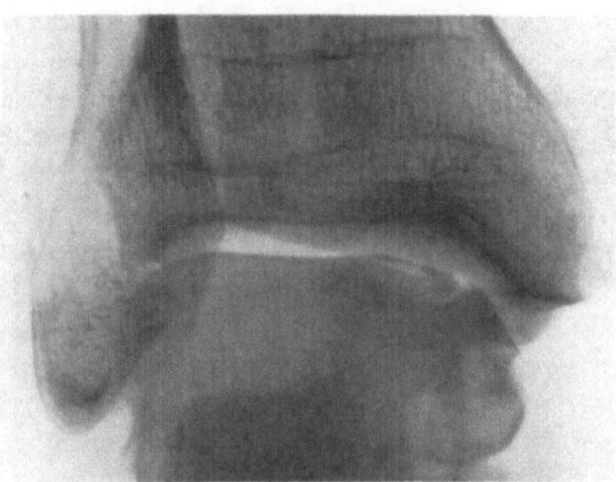

Die Gelenkfläche des Talus ist auf der medialen Seite an umschriebener Stelle unterminiert und zum Teil abgelöst.

The joint surface of the talus on the medial side at circumjacent part is undermined and partly loosened.

2.

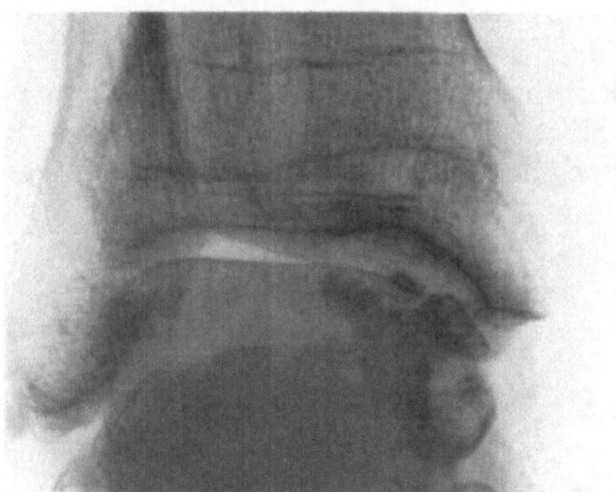

Nach 10 Monaten ist der Bezirk im *Umbau* begriffen.

After ten months. The *re-building* of the area is taking place.

3.

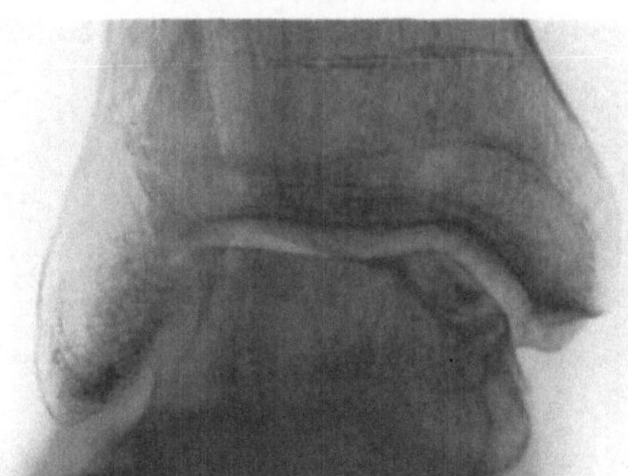

Nach 16 Monaten ist eine glatte Talusoberfläche wieder hergestellt, subchondral befindet sich — mehr am Rande — ein „Sequester" in Resorption.

After sixteen months. The smooth talus surface has been renewed. Subchondrally, near the edge, a sequestrum is about to be resorbed.

D. Stoffwechselstörungen.

Die Rachitis ist eine Erkrankung des wachsenden Skeletes auf der Grundlage einer *Avitaminose*; sie führt zu einer *Störung der endchondralen und periostalen Verknöcherung, indem bei Vermehrung des Knochenwachstums die Verkalkung zurückbleibt.* Das *floride Stadium* ist bei der Früh- wie bei der Spätform durch gemischte vitaminreiche Kost *in wenigen Wochen zu heilen* (Serien 98—101). Da aber die Spätrachitis häufig eine durch die ganze Kindheit geschleppte Schädigung des Skeletes darstellt, bestehen mehr oder weniger schwere *statische Deformitäten.* Auch diese werden unter dem Einfluß der zugeführten Vitamine *durch das Wachstum noch teilweise ausgeglichen*; Verkrümmungen (Serie 102) strecken sich, der Neigungswinkel des Schenkelhalses (Serie 100) richtet sich noch etwas auf. In anderen Fällen muß *operativ korrigiert* werden (Serie 101).

Auch bei der MÖLLER-BARLOW*schen Krankheit* (Serie 103), einer Avitaminose mit besonderer Färbung, die auf den Ausfall des Vitamins-C zurückgeführt wird, gelingt es durch vitaminreiche Kost, *in kurzer Zeit den schweren Zustand zu überwinden,* und *erstaunlich ist der spätere Ausgleich.*

Anhang.

Die echte *Gicht*, eine Störung des Purinstoffwechsels, läßt am häufigsten im Knorpel Urate ausfallen. In dem schweren Fall der Serie 104 entstanden auch im Knocheninneren derartige Ablagerungen, welche die Knochensubstanz abbauten.

Die *Kalkgicht* wird als eine Anomalie des Kalk- und Phosphatstoffwechsels aufgefaßt; in dem Fall der Serie 105 entwickelten sich *schwerste Gelenkdeformierungen*; die generalisierten paraartikulären Kalkablagerungen traten erst mehrere Jahre nach Beginn des Leidens auf.

D. Metabolic Disturbances.

Rickets is a disease affecting the growing skeleton; the fundamental cause being an avitaminosis. Disturbance of the endochondral and periosteal ossification result because calcification fails to keep pace with bone growth. By the use of a mixed diet, rich in vitamines, the flourishing stage of both early and late forms may be cured within a few weeks (Series 98—101). Usually more or less severe statical deformities exist with the late form, because of the effect on the skeleton during childhood. Under the influence of vitamin diet and growth, these deformities are partly compensated. Crookedness (Series 102) is made straight and the declination angle of the neck of the femur (Series 100) is rendered somewhat more obtue. Some cases can only be corrected by operation (Series 101).

Möller-Barlow's disease (Series 103), a particular type of avitaminosis, which is thought to be due to a deficiency of "C" vitamines, can also be cured by the correct diet. Within a short time this serious condition is overcome and the subsequent compensation is astonishing.

Supplement.

Genuine gout — a purin metabolic disturbance, causes the deposition of sodium urate, usually in the cartilages. In the severe case depicted in series 104, the deposits were also found in the interior of the bone causing a disturbance of the bone substance.

Chalk gout is considered an anomaly of chalk and phosphate metabolism. Very serious joint deformities developed in the case shown in series 105. Thegeneralised periarticular chalk deposits only appeared years after the onset of the disease.

Serie 98.

Osteomalacische Frührachitis.

Bei dem 8 Monate alten Knaben, dessen Eltern in ärmlichsten Verhältnissen lebten, bestand eine Rachitis schwersten Grades, die auf eine gemischte, vitaminreiche Kost (Vigantolgaben) in wenigen Wochen heilte.

Series 98.

Osteomalacial Rickets in Infants.

A boy of eight months, whose parents lived in very poor circumstances suffered with a severe form of rickets. By putting him upon a mixed diet, rich in vitamines, (doses Vigantol) he was cured within a few weeks.

$^6/_{10}$ n. Gr.   1.   2.   3.

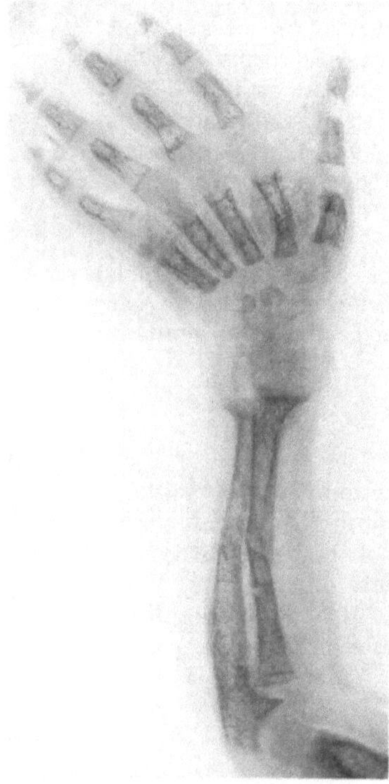 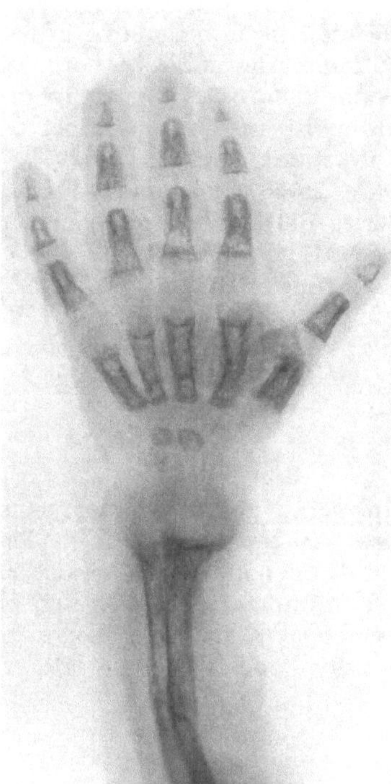 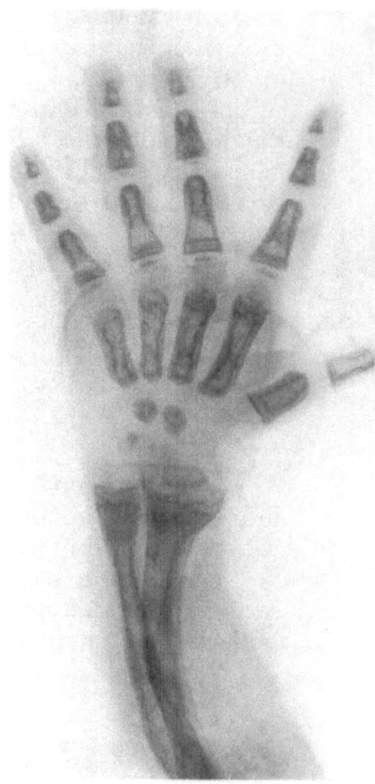

Extreme Kalkverarmung des Skelets; Infraktion des Radius; verbreiterte, unscharfe und ausgefranste Epiphysen.

Extreme decalcification of the skeleton; infraction of radius with widened, indistinct and jagged epiphysis.

Nach 14 Tagen *antirachitischer Behandlung* ist eine Kalkanreicherung der Knochen schon deutlich.

After fourteen days of *anti-rickets treatment*, an increase of chalk in the bones can be seen.

Nach 30 Tagen tritt die Corticalis wiede hervor; zahlreiche Knochenkerne sine aufgeschossen.

After thirty days, the cortex ha become plain again and numerous bone centres have developed.

Serie 98.

4.

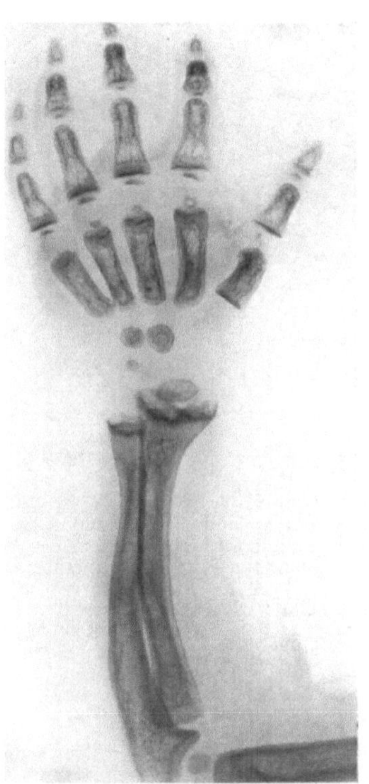

Nach 7 Wochen ist die rachitische Störung
am Skelet ausgeheilt.

After seven weeks the rachitic disturbance
of the skeleton is cured.

5.

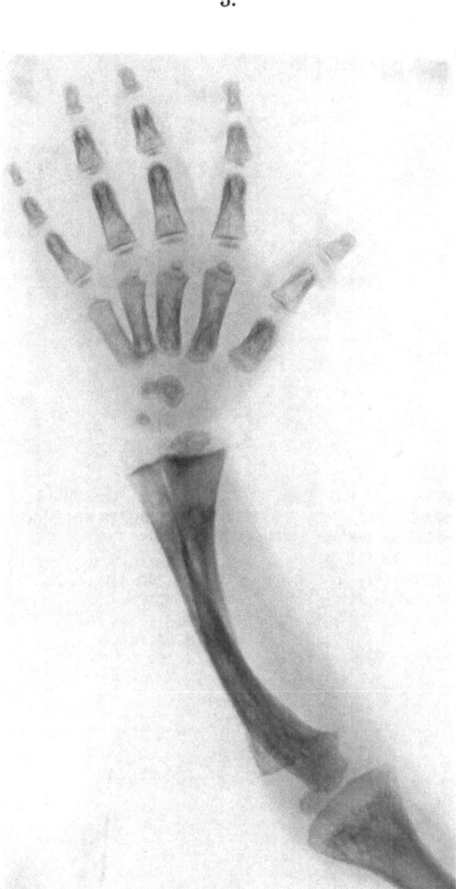

Nach 4 Monaten ist normale Beschaffenheit und normales Wachstum der Knochen festzustellen; eine Verkrümmung des Unterarmes besteht noch, ist aber nach
1 Jahr wesentlich geringer.

After four months the growth and condition of the
bones have become normal. The forearm is still crooked
but a year later considerably less so.

Serie 99.   Series 99.

Frührachitis.   # Infantile Rickets.

Durch vitaminreiche, gemischte Kost waren die rachitischen Knochenschäden des 9 Monate alten Kindes in 6 Wochen geheilt und ein normales Wachstum angebahnt.

The damage to the bones of a child of nine months, due to rickets, was cured in six weeks by the use of a mixed diet, rich in vitamines. A normal growth ensued.

$^3/_4$ n. Gr.   1.   2.

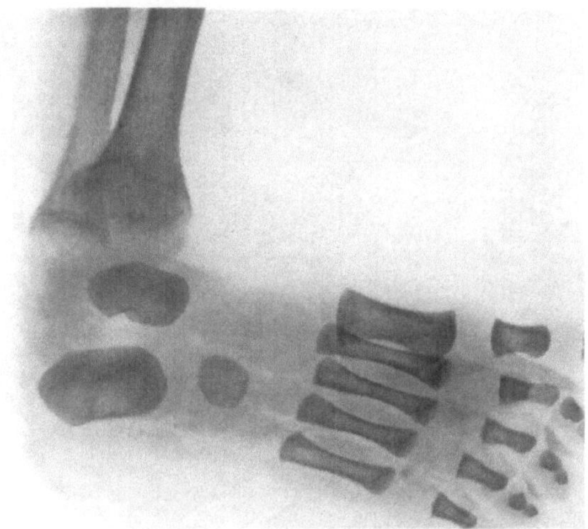

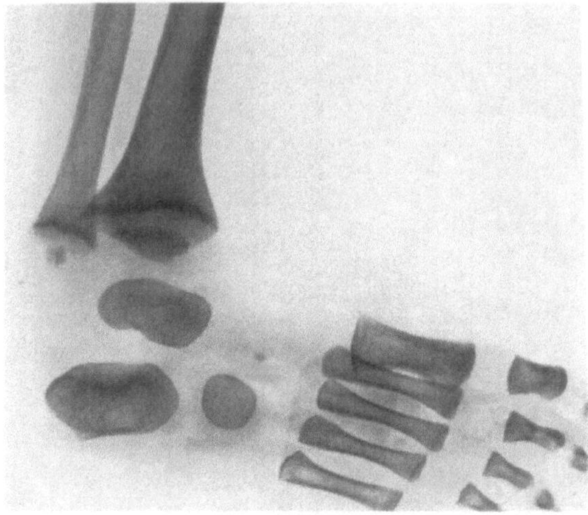

Florides Stadium: die Knochen sind kalkarm, die Metaphysen verbreitert und aufgelockert. Die präparatorische Verkalkungszone tritt nicht hervor.

Flourishing stage. The bones are poor in chalk, the metaphyses widened and loosened.

6 Wochen später — behandelt — *geheilt:* der Knochen ist dichter, Tibia und Fibula sind scharf begrenzt und lassen ihre Epiphysenkerne sowie einen Saum inzwischen gebildeten Knochengewebes erkennen.

Six weeks later. Treated — cured. The bone is more compact. The tibia and fibula show distinct outlines and epiphyseal centres are recognizable.

3.

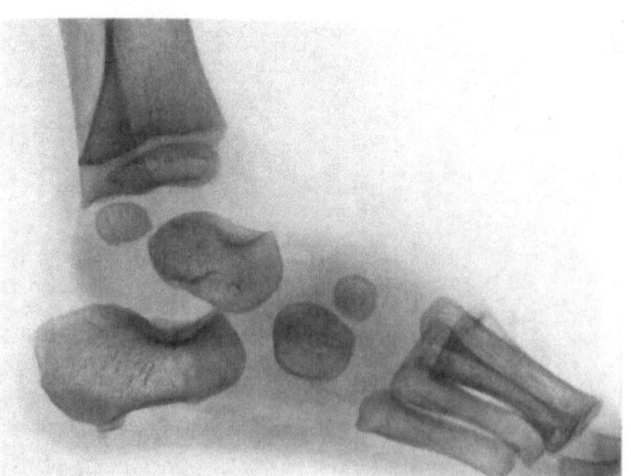

Nach $1^1/_4$ Jahr ist der Knochen in normaler Weise weiterentwickelt.

After fifteen months; the bone has developed normally.

Serie 100.	Series 100.

Spätrachitis.   # Late Rickets.

<table>
<tr><td>

Spätrachitis.

Die rachitische Wachstumsstörung nahm im 6. Lebensjahr des Mädchens schlimme Formen an, überwand aber unter vitaminreicher Kost das floride Stadium und erfuhr auch einen weitgehenden Ausgleich der Deformitäten.

</td><td>

Late Rickets.

The growth of a little girl was severely disturbed in her sixth year by rickets. The acute stage was overcome by the continual use of a diet rich in vitamines and the deformities were, to a very great extent, compensated.

</td></tr>
</table>

$^1/_2$ n. Gr. 1.

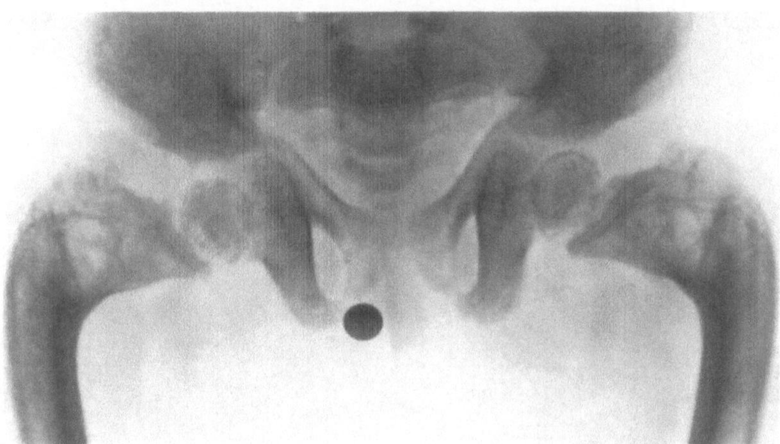

Florides Stadium: Die Knochen sind kalkarm und die Epiphysenfugen unscharf; im Schenkelhals finden sich beiderseits an seinem Ansatz große „Umbauzonen". Der Beckenring ist — wie bei der Osteomalacie — eingedrückt und der Schenkelhals hat sich gesenkt.

Flourishing stage. The bones are decalcified and the growth areas are indistinct. Large "alternating areas" are found in the neck of femur on both sides. The pelvis-ring is compressed as in osteomalacia and the femur-neck has sunk.

2.

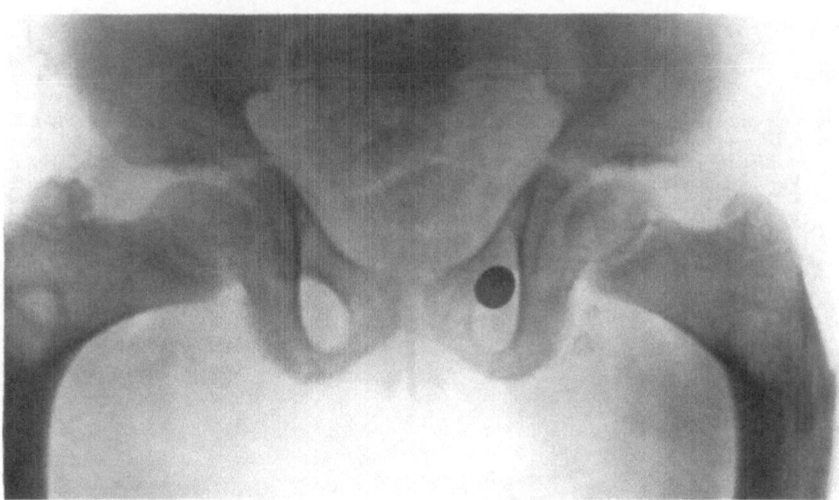

Nach 1 Jahr ist das Skelet erheblich kalkreicher; das osteoide Gewebe der „Umbauzonen" ist rechts ganz, links weitgehend kalkhaltiger Knochen geworden. — Der Neigungswinkel des Schenkelhalses ist etwas aufgerichtet, die Eindellung des Beckenringes ausgeglichen und das Wachstum fortgeschritten.

After one year. The skeleton has become considerably richer in chalk. The osteoid tissue of the "changing areas" on the entire right side has become calcified bone and to a very great extent on the left side also. The inclination angle of the neck of femur is somewhat elevated, the compression of the pelvis ring compensated and growth has advanced.

Serie 101.

Spätrachitis.

Die lang hingezogene Wachstumsstörung des Skeletes
führte zu Belastungsdeformitäten und exacerbierte im
5. Lebensjahr des Knaben. Durch vitaminreiche Kost
wurde rasch der Kalkmangel behoben; die Deformitäten
wurden operativ korrigiert.

$\frac{1}{2}$ n. Gr.   1.

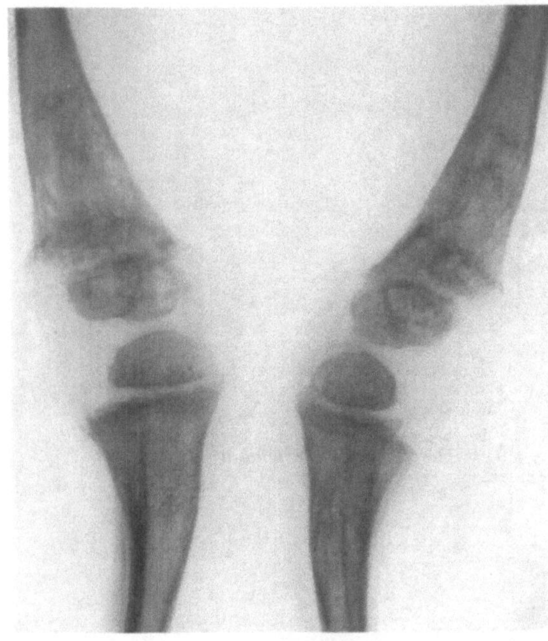

Über die verbreiterten und aufgefaserten Metaphysen hin-
aus besteht ein *ungleichmäßiger Aufbau des kalkarmen
Knochens bis tief in die Diaphyse* der Oberschenkel. —
Starke Verbiegung aller Knochen.

The construction of the chalk impoverished bone above the
widened and frayed metaphysis and *far into the diaphysis
of the femur is irregular.* All bones are very crooked.

Series 101.

Late Rickets.

Deformities and exacerbations were the result of long
drawnout growth disturbance of the skeleton. After five
years, the boy was given a diet rich in vitamines. The
chalk deficiency was quickly made good and the deformities were corrected by operation.

2.

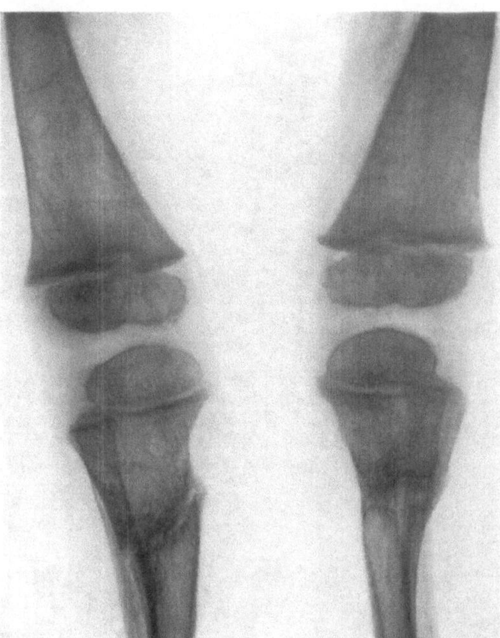

Nach $\frac{1}{4}$ Jahr ist *das floride Stadium überwunden:*
Die Knochen sind kalkreicher, gleichmäßig strukturiert
und scharf gerandet; ein neuer Saum ist angelegt.
Die vor 5 bzw. 3 Wochen ausgeführten Osteotomie-
wunden beider Schienbeine sind mit wenig Callus
geheilt bzw. in Heilung begriffen.

After three months. *The flourishing stage has been
overcome.* The bones have become richer in chalk
and of proportionate structure and distinct outline.
Of the two osteotomy wounds which had been made
in the tibiae, three and five weeks previously, one has
healed with a little callus the other is making progress.

Serie 101.

3.

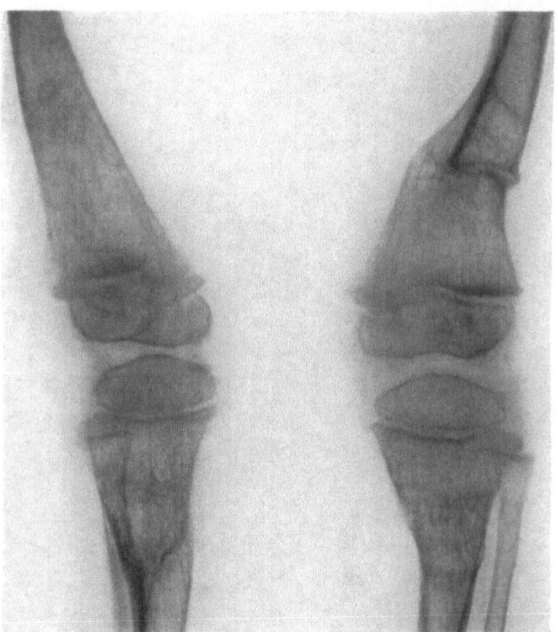

Nach ¹/₂ Jahr besteht — als Folge der Eingriffe — eine Knochenatrophie. — Die Knochenwunden beider Schienbeine sind strukturell weitgehend ausgeglichen, die Oberschenkelosteotomie ist auch schon knöchern fest.

After six months. Bone atrophy exists as a result of the operation. The structure of the bone wounds of both tibiae is considerably reformed and the osteotomy site in the femur has again become solid bone.

Serie 102.	Series 102.
## Rachitische Beinverkrümmungen.	## Leg-Deformity due to Rickets.
Die auf dem Boden der Rachitis entstandene Belastungsdeformität der Unterschenkel hat das Wachstum unter dem Einfluß normaler Ernährung und zeitweiser Gaben von Phosphorlebertran gestreckt.	The deformity of the lower legs which was caused by rickets, was corrected by normal nourishment and temporary doses of phosphorous cod-liver-oil.

1.

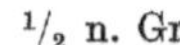

$^{1}/_{2}$ n. Gr

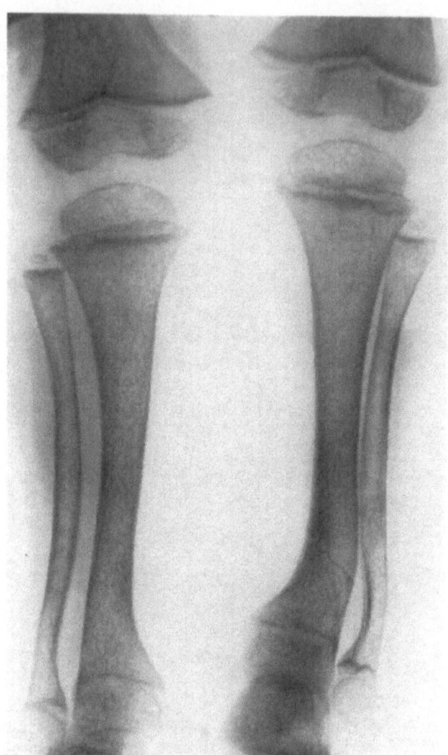

Im 4. Lebensjahr: Unterschenkelverkrümmung — Crura vara — besonders rechts.

In the fourth year. Crooked lower legs — Crura vara — especially the right.

Serie 102.

2.

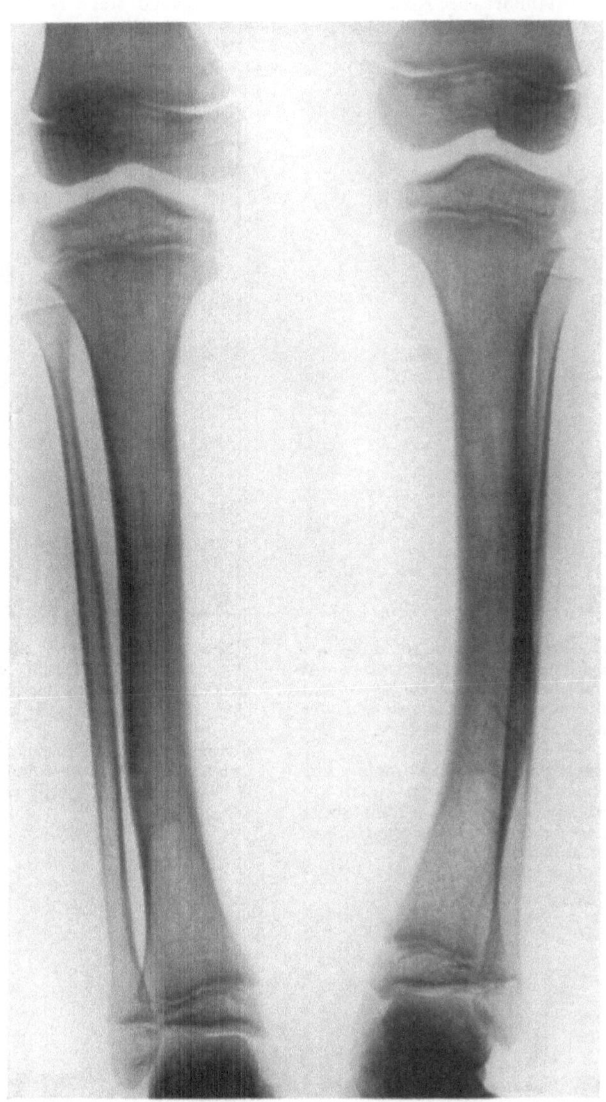

Im 9. Lebensjahr sind Tibia und Fibula wesentlich gerader.
In the ninth year the tibia and fibula are considerably straightened.

Serie 103.

MÖLLER-BARLOWsche Krankheit.

Das 8 Monate alte, verwahrloste Kind litt an schwerster Avitaminose, die außer den rachitischen Symptomen auch die des „infantilen Skorbutes" zeigte. Unter gemischter vitaminreicher Kost heilte das floride Stadium rasch ab; die hochgradigen Veränderungen am Knochen erfuhren eine fast vollständige Rückbildung und formale Angleichung.

$^6/_{10}$ n. Gr.   1.

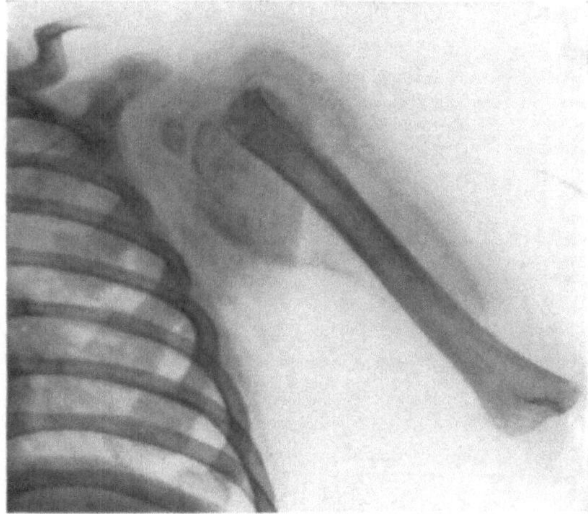

Periostschlauch und mit ihm im Zusammenhang *das proximale Humerusende* (die Epi- und ein Streifen der Metaphyse) *sind durch einen in Verkalkung begriffenen Bluterguß abgehoben,* die Knorpelknochengrenzen der Rippen aufgetrieben und aufgelockert.

The periosteal tube, together with the proximal end of the humerus (epiphysis and strips of metaphysis) are thrust aside by a blood effusion, which is undergoing calcification. The cartilage bone margins of the ribs are swollen and loosened.

Series 103.

MOELLER-BARLOWs Disease.

A neglected child, eight months of age, suffered from a severe form of avitaminosis. In addition to the symptoms of rickets, infantile scurvy was also present. The flourishing stage healed rapidly under the influence of a mixed diet, rich in vitamines. The seriously affected bones became almost completely normal.

2.

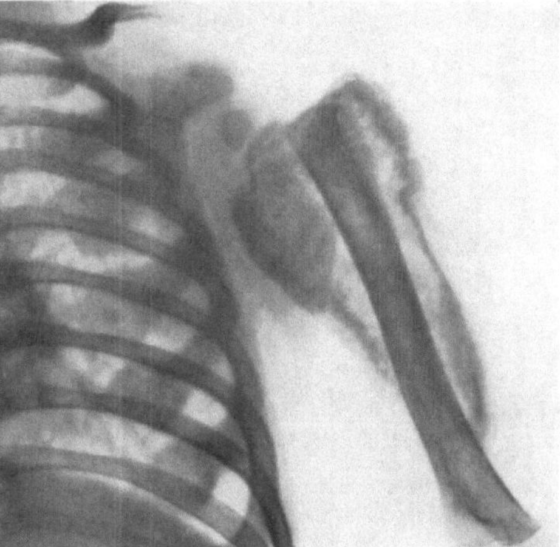

Nach 14 Tagen hat die Verkalkung des subperiostalen Hämatoms unter der Behandlung noch zugenommen; der „rachitische Rosenkranz" ist noch sehr ausgesprochen.

After 2 weeks. The calcification of the subperiosteal haematoma has increased and the „rachitic rosary" is still very pronounced.

Serie 103.

3.

4.

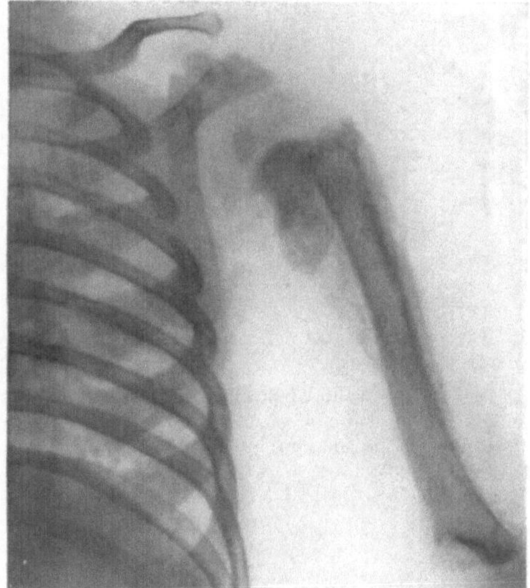

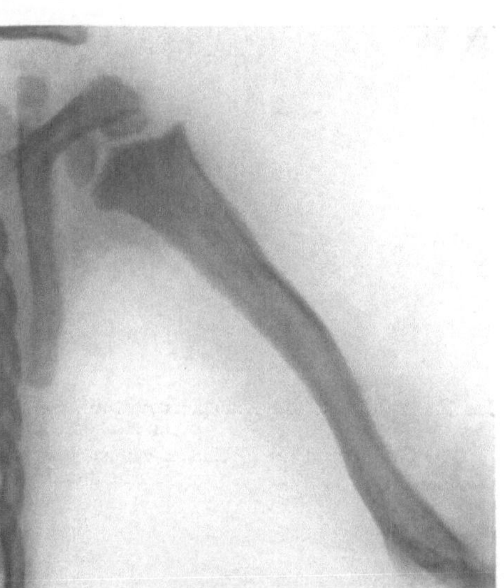

Nach 8 Wochen ist eine erhebliche Verschmälerung der Kalkanlagerung eingetreten, die über-
dies Knochenstruktur anlegt. — Die Auftreibung
der Knorpelknochenzone an den Rippen
ist gleichfalls zurückgebildet.

After 8 weeks. The chalk deposits have become
considerably thinner and bone construction has
commenced. The swelling of the cartilage bone
margins has also decreased.

Nach 1 Jahr ist *ein ausgeglichener Knochenschaft*
vorhanden, der als Folge der schweren Veränderungen lediglich eine Verbreiterung des proximalen
Humerusteiles aufweist.

After one year. The *bone-shaft has become more
regular* and the seriousness of the previous bony
changes is only recognized by the widened proximal
end of the humerus.

Anhang.

Serie 104.

Arthritis urica.

Der 60jährige Mann litt seit Jahren an Gicht mit den charakteristischen Schmerzanfällen, den Uratablagerungen im Gewebe und einem erhöhten Harnsäurespiegel im Blut. Schließlich traten auch Knochentophi auf.

Supplement.

Series 104.

Arthritis Urica.

A man who had reached the age of sixty, had suffered for many years with gout accompanied by the characteristic attacks of pain. Urate deposits in the tissues and the quantity of uric-acid in the blood were above normal. Finally bone-atrophy commenced.

$^2/_3$ n. Gr.

1.

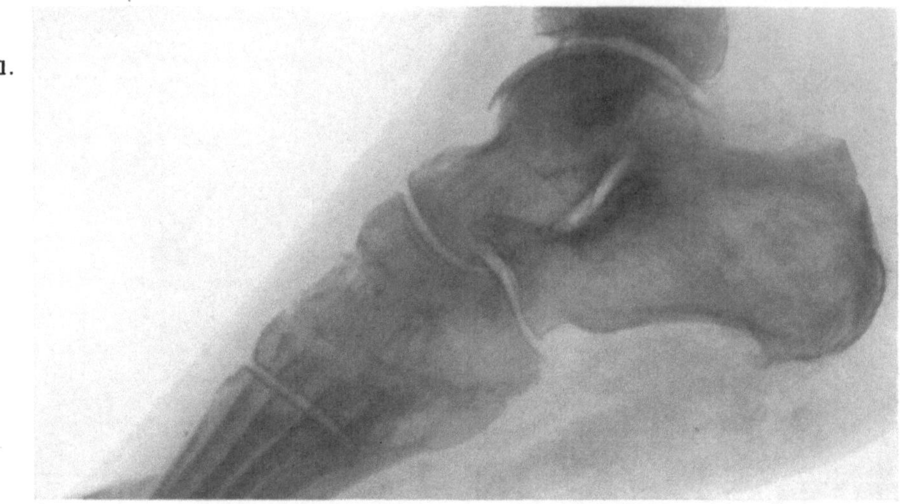

Im Fersenbein ist die Knochenstruktur in einem größeren Bezirk durch Uratablagerungen verwischt; im übrigen ist der Knochen atrophisch.

The bone structure of the calcaneus has been obliterated in a large area by the urate deposit. The bone is atrophied as a whole.

3.

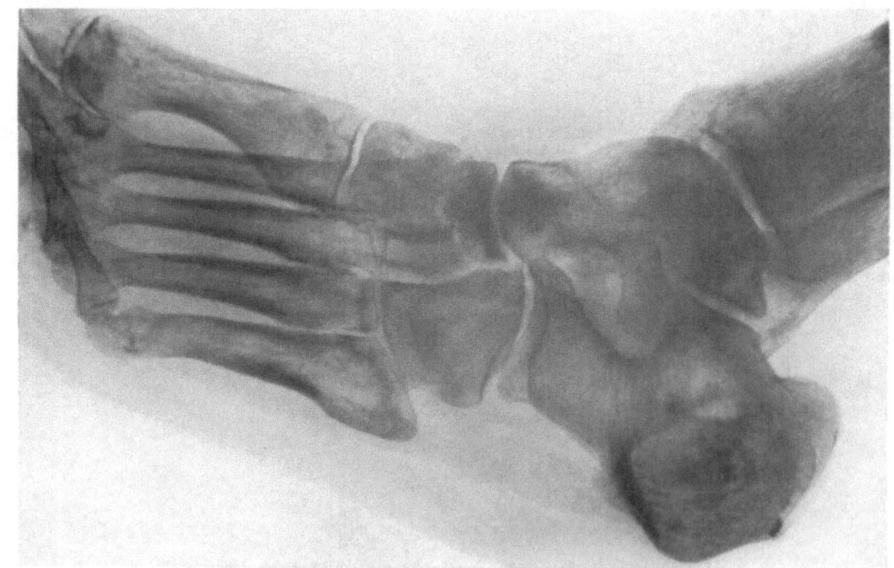

5 Monate später ist der Befund nicht wesentlich verändert.

Five months later. The condition has hardly changed.

Serie 104.

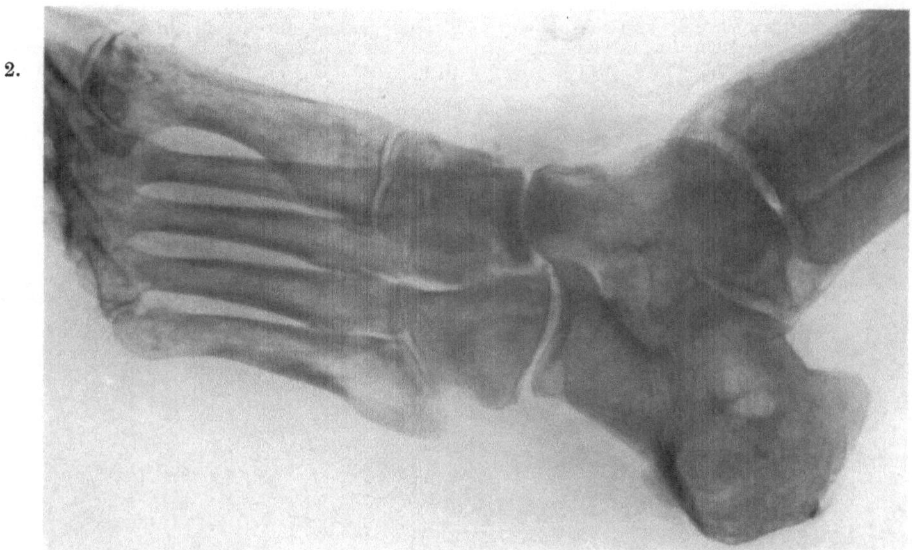

3 Monate später ist der Calcaneusherd kalkreicher; das Kahnbein aber ist usuriert und im Metatarsusköpfchen — am Großzehengelenk findet sich ein „Marktophus".

Three months later the calcaneus is richer in chalk but the os naviculare is eroded and there is a "marrow-tophus" in the metatarsal head in the joint of the big toe.

Anhang.

Serie 105.

Kalkgicht.

Das Leiden begann im 27. Lebensjahr des Mannes mit akuten heftigen Schmerzanfällen zuerst in einem Handgelenk, dann in den Großzehen und später in den meisten anderen Gelenken. Der Harnsäurespiegel im Blut war nicht erhöht. In den ersten 5 Jahren verlief die Krankheit in akuten Schüben und verhältnismäßig langsam, dann aber verschlimmerte sie sich kontinuierlich unaufhaltsam, so daß der Mann im wahrsten Sinn des Wortes versteifte und unbeweglich wurde.

Supplement.

Series 105.

Chalk Gout.

The male patient was in his twenty seventh year when the malady commenced. He had attacks of violent, piercing pain, first in one hand-joint, then in the big toes and later on in most of the other joints. The quantity of uric acid in the blood was not above normal. The disease ran a comparatively slow course in acute stages during the first five years, then it became continually worse and could not be arrested until at last the joints were absolutely stiff and immobile.

$^1/_2$ n. Gr.   1 a.   2 a.

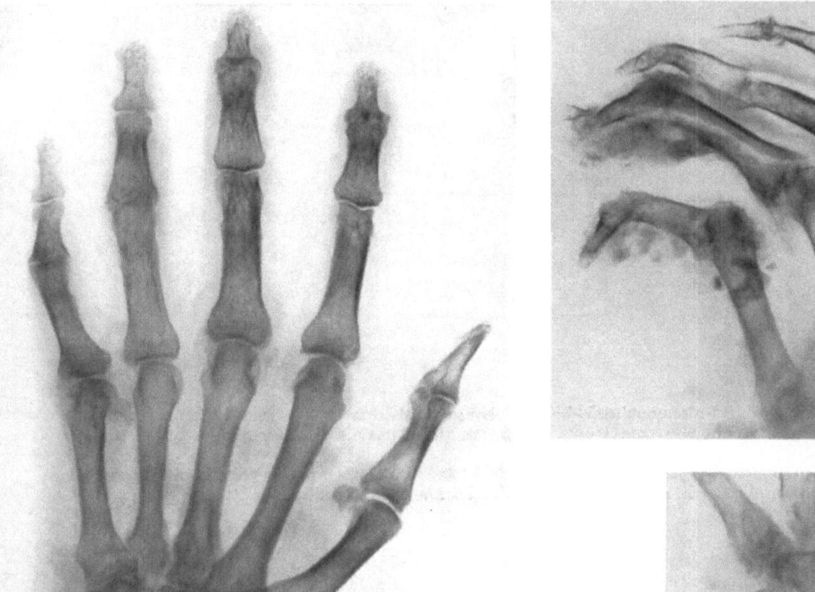

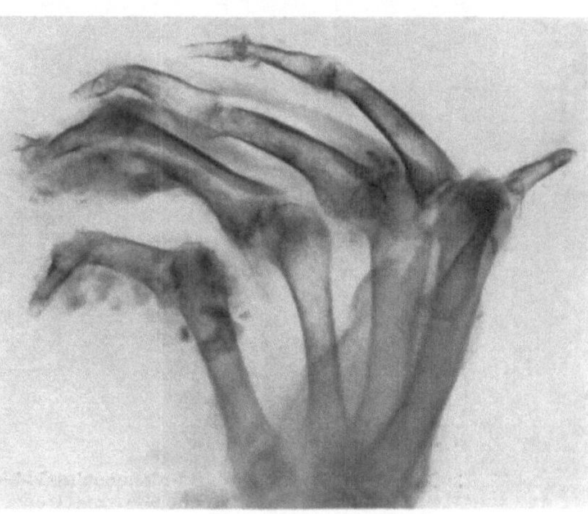

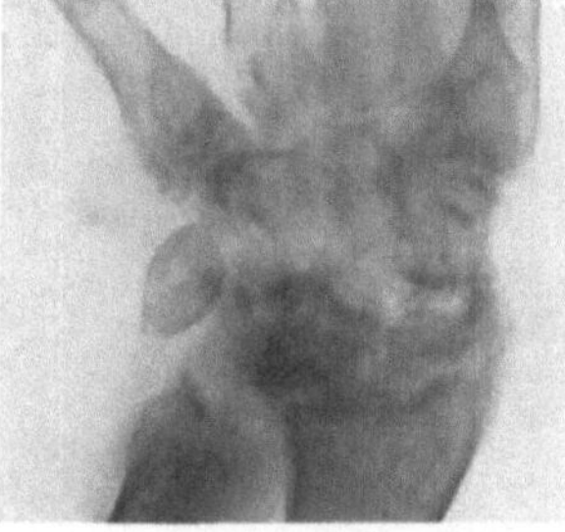

Im 6. Jahr der Krankheit sind einzelne Fingergelenke verödet, an anderen bestehen kleine Randwucherungen.

In the sixth year of the malady. Some of the finger-joints are destroyed and there are small peripheral growths upon others.

$3^1/_2$ Jahre später ist die Hand in Krallenstellung versteift: die Knochen sind hochgradig atrophisch, die Gelenke deformiert und abgeglitten oder ankylosiert. In den Weichteilen aber finden sich ausgedehnte Kalkablagerungen.

Three and a half years later. The hand has stiffened in a claw-like position, the bones are exeedingly atrophious, the joints deformed and disarticulated or stiffened. There are extensive chalk-deposits in the fleshy parts.

Serie 105.

1 b.

2 b.

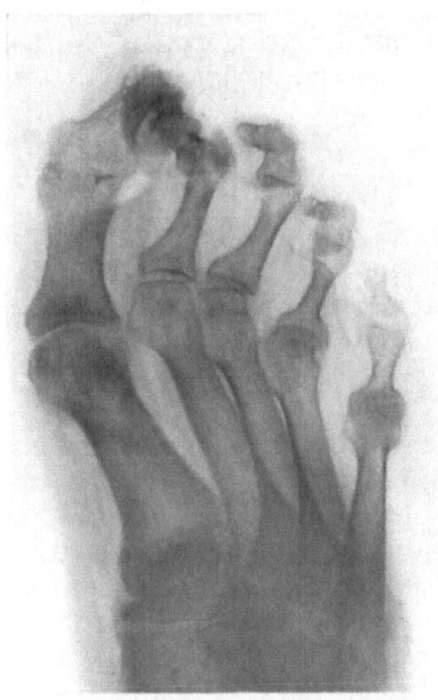 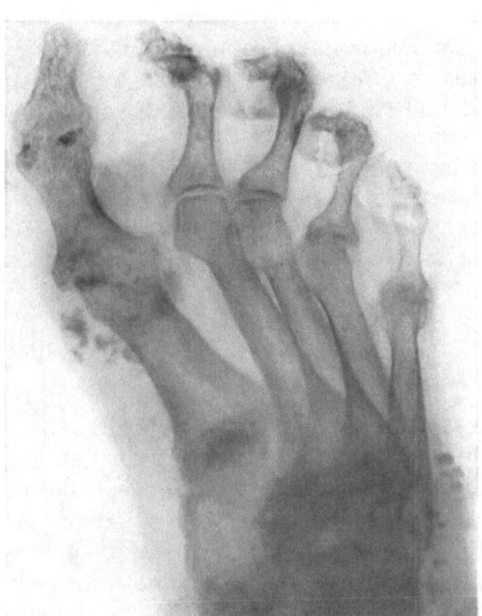

Der Prozeß lief in dem gleichen Zeitraum an den Füßen in der gleichen Richtung ab,
nur nicht ganz so schwer.

The course of the disease in the feet was similar to, but not quite so severe, as that of the hands.
The parts were affected at the same time.

V. Kapitel.

Chronische unspezifische Gelenkleiden.

A. Chronischer Gelenkrheumatismus.

*Die primären Kapselentzündungen des chronischen Gelenkrheumatismus haben
eine schlechte Prognose.* Mögen sie als akuter Gelenkrheumatismus beginnen und
dann in Schüben oder allmählich fortschreiten — der sog. sekundär-chronische Gelenkrheumatismus der Klinik —, oder mögen sie von vornherein schleichend ver-
laufen, der pathologische Prozeß ist unaufhaltsam progredient und *endet erst mit
dem Narbenstadium der Synovialis und oft sehr schweren Knorpel-Knochenverände-
rungen.* Dadurch entstehen Versteifungen der Gelenke in Kontrakturstellungen.
an den Händen und an den Füßen groteske Verunstaltungen (Serien 106 u. 108).
Die Ankylose kann rein bindegewebig-kapsulär (Serie 107 u. 109) sein, sie kann aber
auch auf einer breiten Verwachsung der Knorpel-Knochenflächen beruhen, wenn
diese sekundär geschwürig erkranken (Arthritis ulcerosa der Serie 110). In allen
Fällen war eine energische medikamentöse Behandlung verschiedenster Richtung
ebenso wie physikalische und Bädertherapie ohne Einfluß auf das Fortschreiten des
Prozesses. Seine hartnäckige Progredienz und die schweren Folgen läßt der histologische Befund der blanden Entzündung (Serie 107) nicht ohne weiteres vermuten.

Chapter V.

Chronic Unspecific Joint Diseases.

A. Chronic Joint Rheumatism.

The prognosis of primary inflammation of the capsule in chronic joint rheumatism
is unfavourable. Whether it begins as acute joint rheumatism, continuing spasmodi-
cally or progressing slowly (the so-called secondary chronic joint rheumatism of the
clinic), or whether it commences and proceeds gradually, it is impossible to arrest
the pathological process before the synovial membrane is scarred and before serious
cartilage-bone changes have taken place. These changes cause stiffness of the joints
in unnatural positions and sometimes grotesque deformities result (Series 106 and 108).
The ankylosis may be due to the capsular fibrous tissue (Series 107 and 109) but it
may also be caused by the cartilage-bone surfaces growing together after ulceration.
(Ulcerative arthritis — Series 110.) Energetic medicinal, physical and bath treatment
failed in all cases to influence the progress of the disease. The histological examination of the mild inflammation (Series 107) would not lead us to suspect such an
obstinate course nor such serious results.

Serie 106.

Progressiver Gelenkrheumatismus.

„Primär chronisch" begann das Leiden — ein Gelenkkapsel-
prozeß — schleichend bei der bis dahin gesunden Frau im
40. Lebensjahr, ergriff Hände, Füße sowie die meisten
großen Gelenke und war weder durch medikamentöse noch
Bäderbehandlung aufzuhalten.

$^6/_{10}$ n. Gr.   1.

Series 106.

Progressive Joint Rheumatism.

A forty year old woman, who had always been healthy,
became ill with a joint capsule affection which was "primarily chronic". It began slowly, almost imperceptibly
and attacked hands, feet and most of the large joints,
and could not be arrested either by medicine or baths.

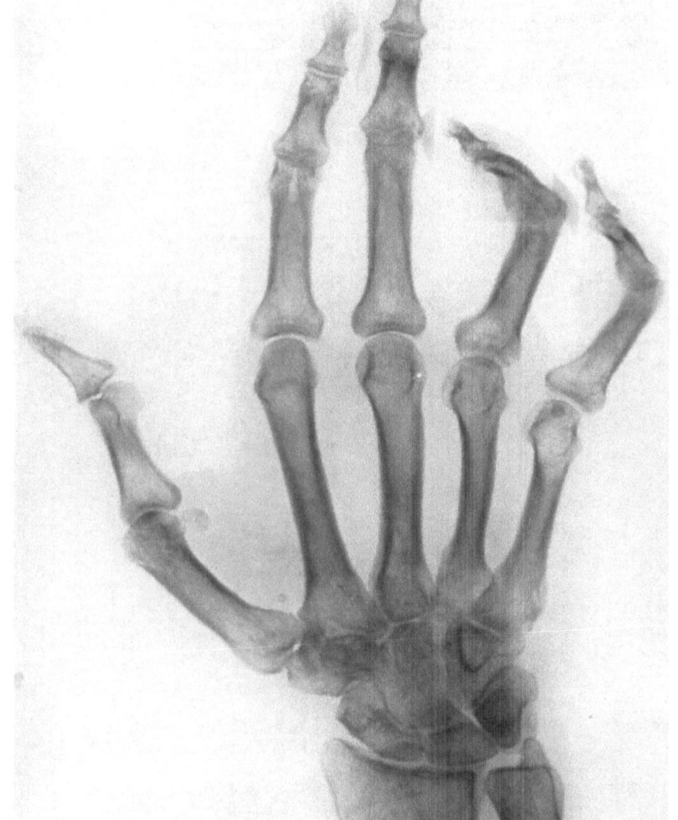

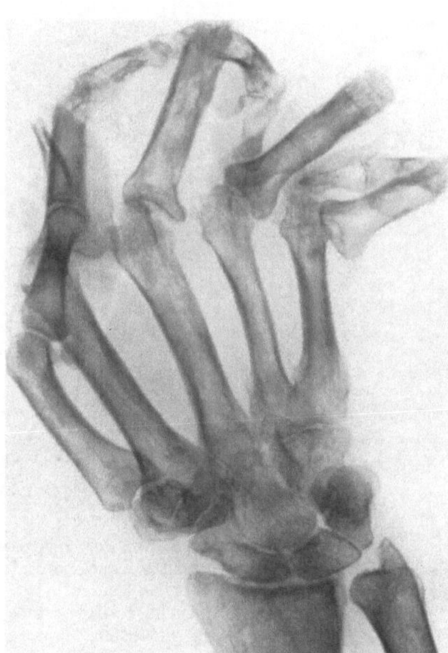

2.

3 Jahre nach Beginn des Leidens zeigen erst der 4. und 5. Finger
die charakteristischen Deviationen der „Spinnenhand".

Three years after commencement of disease, only the fourth and fifth
fingers show the deviation of the "spider-hand".

Nach 6 Jahren sind die Finger in sämtlichen
Gelenken subluxiert, der Knochen hochgradig
kalkverarmt und die Gelenkflächen deformiert.

After six years, all the finger joints are subluxated, the bones extremely decalcified and the
joint surfaces deformed.

Serie 107.

Progressiver Gelenkrheumatismus.

Die 27jährige Frau erkrankte mit einem Erguß eines Kniegelenkes, der zweimal punktiert wurde; wenige Wochen später begann eine zunehmende Versteifung der Halswirbelsäule und eines Ellenbogens. Trotz der energischen und ausgiebigen Arznei- und Bäderbehandlung verlief das Leiden unaufhaltsam progredient, indem die betreffenden Gelenke mehr und mehr versteiften und neue (z. B. Kiefergelenke) ergriffen wurden. — Die Probeexcision aus der Kniegelenkkapsel ergab eine subakute Entzündung ohne spezifische Kennzeichen (aufgelockert-ödematöse Synovialis mit einem epithelartigen Zellbelag ohne Zottenbildung und starker zelliger Infiltration von einkernigen Elementen sowie Plasmazellen).

Series 107.

Progressive Joint-Rheumatism.

A woman, 27 years of age, had a blood effusion in the knee joint. It was aspirated twice. A few weeks later she complained of an increasing stiffness in the cervical portion of the spine and in one elbow. In spite of vigorous treatment (medicine and baths), the condition ran a progressive course. The stiffness increased and other joints (for example, the jaw) became involved. Trial excision of the knee joint capsule revealed a subacute inflammation without specific symptoms. (Loosened synovial membrane with epithelial like cell covering without tuft formation — marked cellular infiltration of mononuclear elements and in addition, plasma cells.)

$^2/_3$ n. Gr.   1.

2.

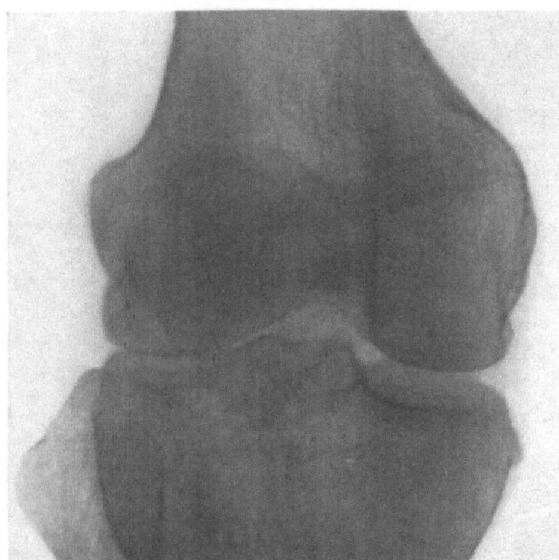

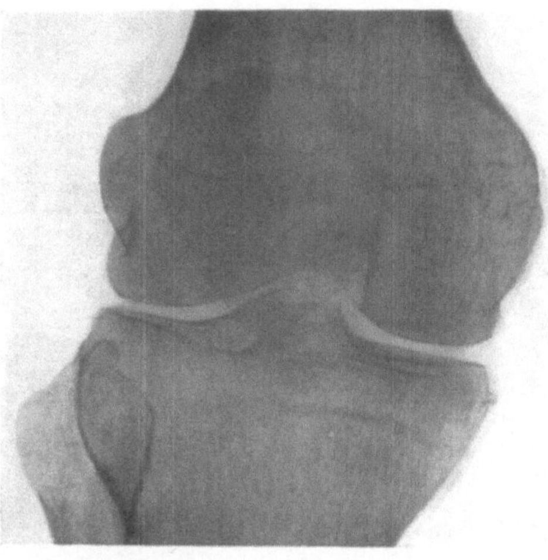

Zu Beginn — im Stadium des Hydrops — besteht kein krankhafter Knochenbefund.

Commencement. At the hydrops stage. Bone not affected.

Nach 1 Jahr sind die Gelenkflächen glatt, der Spalt frei, aber das Gelenk ist kapsulär versteift.

After one year. The joint-surfaces are smooth, the cleft free but the joint capsule is stiffened.

Serie 107.

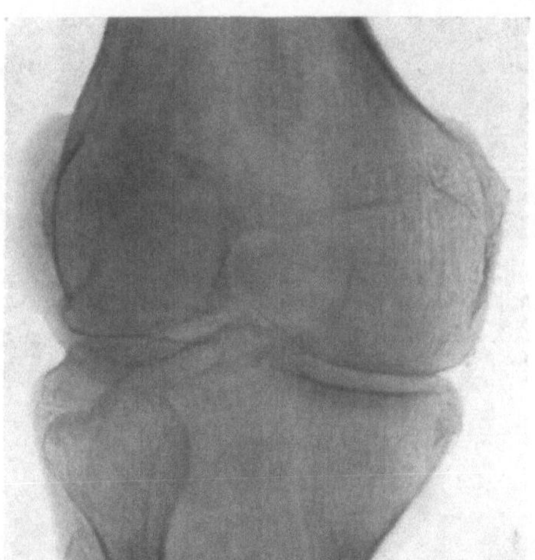

Auch nach $2^1/_2$ Jahren zeigt das in leichter Beugestellung steife Knie, abgesehen von einer Atrophie, keine Veränderungen der knöchernen Gelenkteile.

After two years and a half. The stiffened knee-joint is shown in a slightly bent position. No alteration of the bony parts of the joint has taken place with the exception of atrophy.

<table>
<tr><td>

Serie 108.

Sekundär chronischer Gelenkrheumatismus.

Bei dem nunmehr 62 Jahre alten Mann war der Gelenkrheumatismus *in akuten Schüben* aufgetreten und hatte zuerst die großen, später kleinen Gelenke erfaßt. Ursprünglich ein Kapselprozeß, kam es später zu schweren Veränderungen der knöchernen Gelenkenden.

</td><td>

Series 108.

Secondary Chronic Joint-Rheumatism.

A man sixty two years of age had *acute attacks* of joint-rheumatism. At first the larger joints were attacked; later the smaller joints. It was originally a capsular process but later the bony joint-ends were seriously affected.

</td></tr>
</table>

$^7/_{10}$ n. Gr.   1.

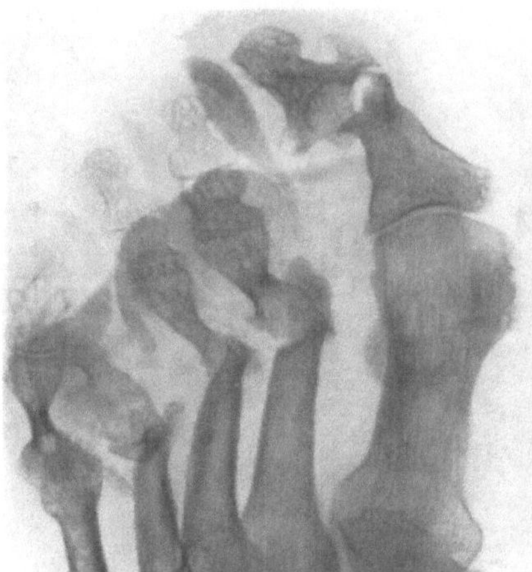 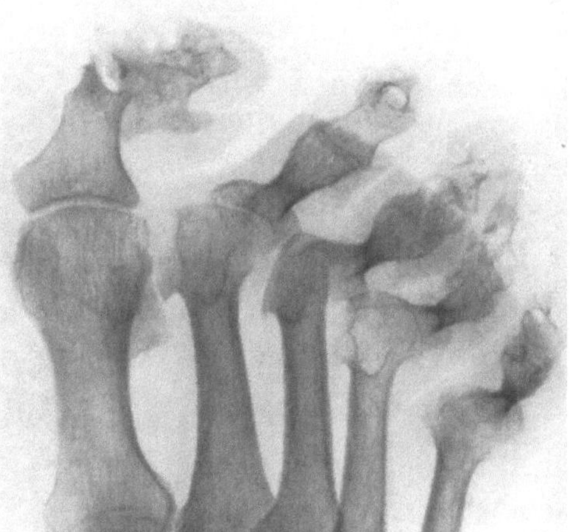

Links (Anfangsstadium) zeigen die *Zehengrundgelenke*, abgesehen von der Knochenatrophie, noch keine Veränderungen; *rechts* (Endzustand) aber sind sie *zerstört und* an den Knochenstümpfen primitiv *neugebildet*.

Commencement. In the *left* foot, with the exception of bone-atrophy, the basal joints of toes show no alteration. *Right* foot (final stage), they are *destroyed* but primitively *newly built* at the bone-stumps.

2.

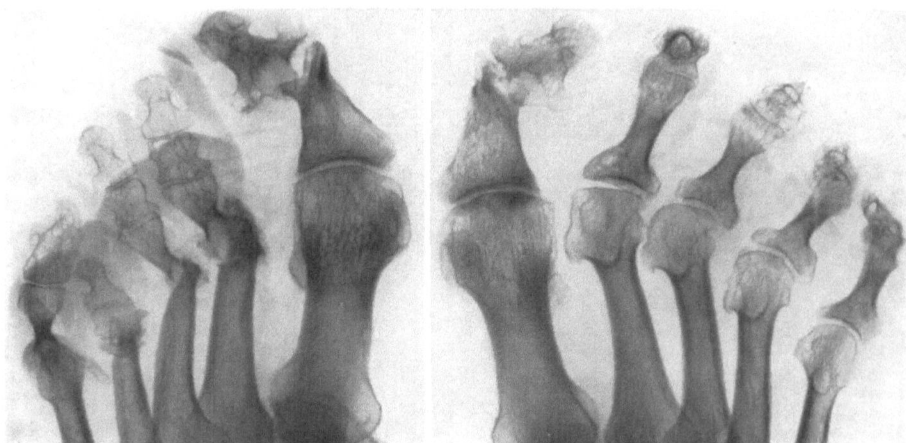

Nach 2 Jahren bestehen links erst Subluxationen, noch keine wesentlichen Knochenveränderungen.

After two years. There are subluxations in the left foot, but so far no great bony change.

Serie 108.

3.

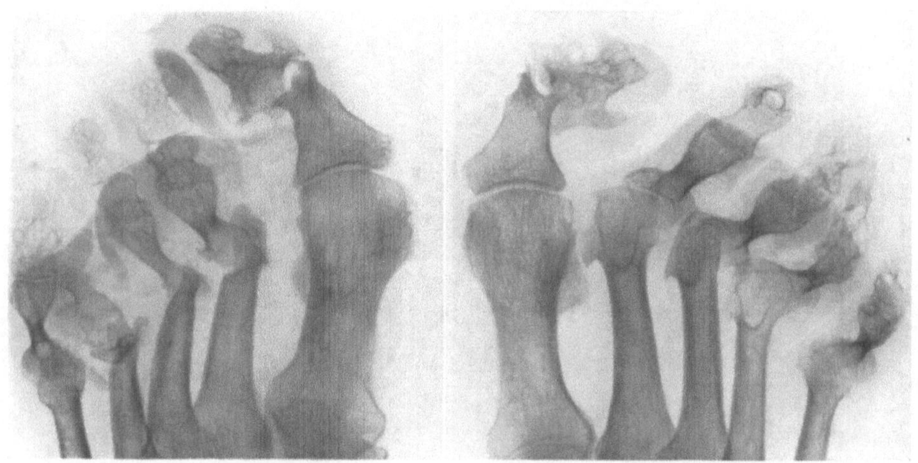

Nach 3¹/₂ Jahren sind die Zehen links weiter abgeglitten und jetzt — sekundär — ist auch die Destruktion der knöchernen Gelenkteile im Gange.

After three years and a half. The left toes have slipped further off and now — secondarily — the destruction of the bony parts of the joints is taking place.

Serie 109.

Primär chronischer Gelenkrheumatismus.

Im 8. Lebensjahr des Knaben begann die Krankheit schleichend mit einer Anschwellung beider Knie- und Hüftgelenke. Die Synovitis führte unaufhaltsam zur völligen Versteifung der Gelenke. — Dabei blieb das Kind in der Entwicklung sehr zurück.

Series 109.

Primary Chronic Joint-Rheumatism.

The patient was a boy in his eighth year and the illness began by a slow, protracted swelling of both knees and hip-joints. The synovitis could not be arrested and led to complete stiffness of the joints. The child's development was greatly retarded.

$^6/_{10}$ n. Gr.   1.

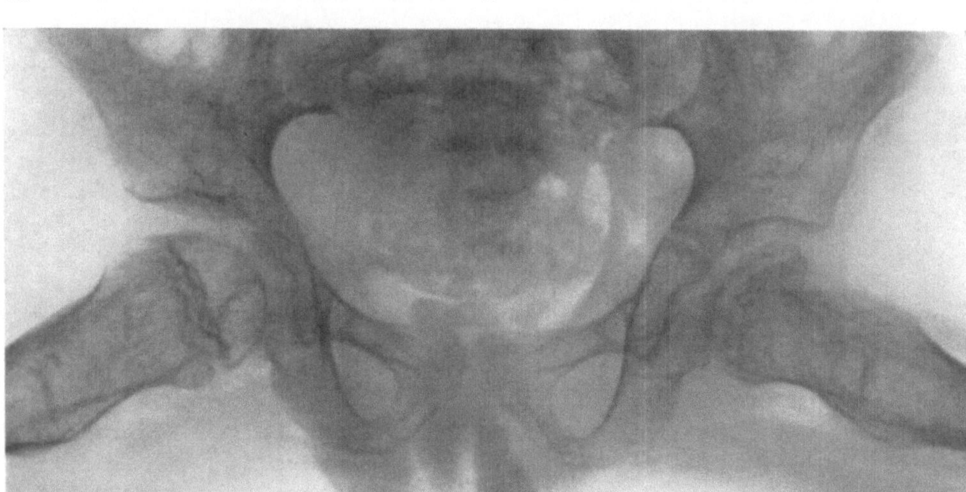

Lebensalter: 8 Jahre. — Das Skelet ist hochgradig atrophisch und die rechte Schenkelkopfepiphyse kümmerlich (Coxa plana!).

Age eight years. The skeleton is extremely atrophied and the epiphysis of the head of right femur is poorly developed (coxa plana).

2.

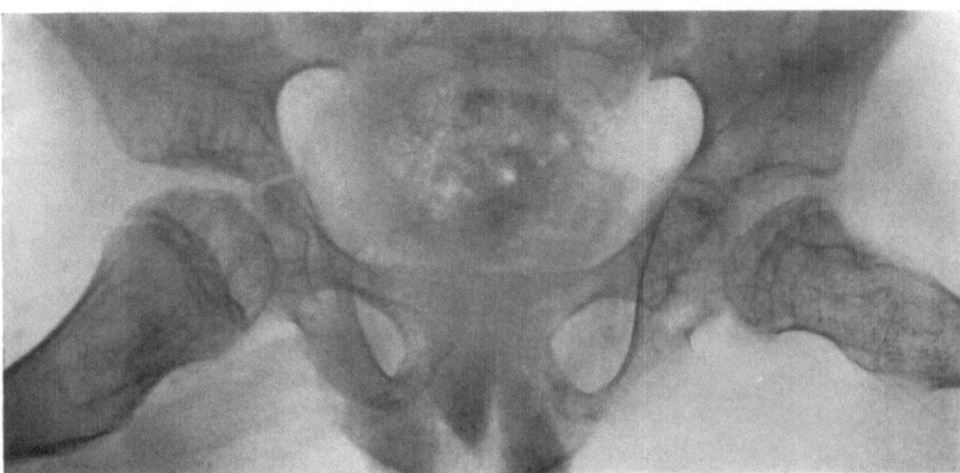

Nach 1 Jahr und
After one and

Serie 109.

3.

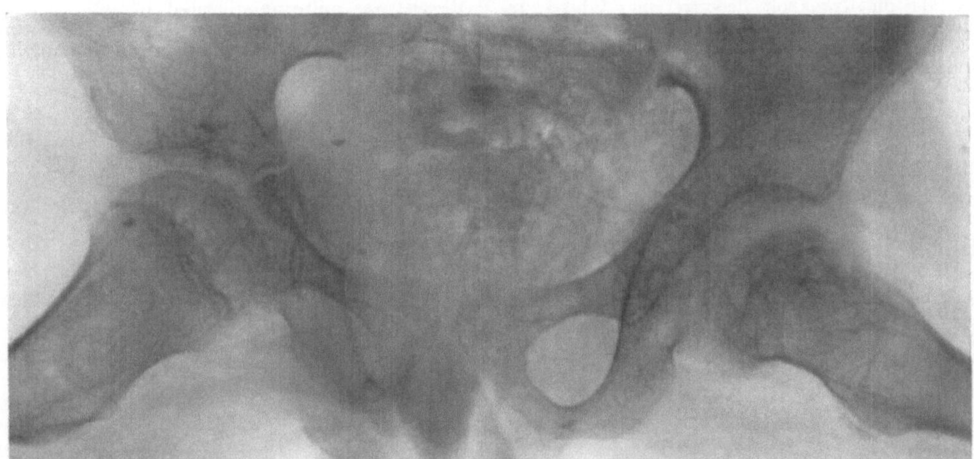

nach 2 Jahren ist ein geringes Wachstum festzustellen, auch der rechte Hüftkopf hat sich
weiterentwickelt (breiter gewordene Kopfkalotte); die Knochenatrophie besteht fort.

after two years. Slight growth is recognizable, the right femoral head has also developed somewhat
(the head-calotte has become wider) and the bone atrophy still exists.

Serie 110.

Primär chronische Polyarthritis.

Bei dem 19 Jahre alten Mann war schleichend und von Schmerzen begleitet in etwa 4 Jahren völlige Versteifung beider Hüftgelenke eingetreten, als dasselbe Leiden auch beide Kniegelenke ergriff. Auch jetzt verlief die Krankheit fieberfrei und führte zur Verödung der Gelenke, therapeutisch unbeeinflußbar. — Der Mann stammte aus einer tuberkulös schwer belasteten Familie, war aber selbst lungengesund.

²/₃ n. Gr.   1.

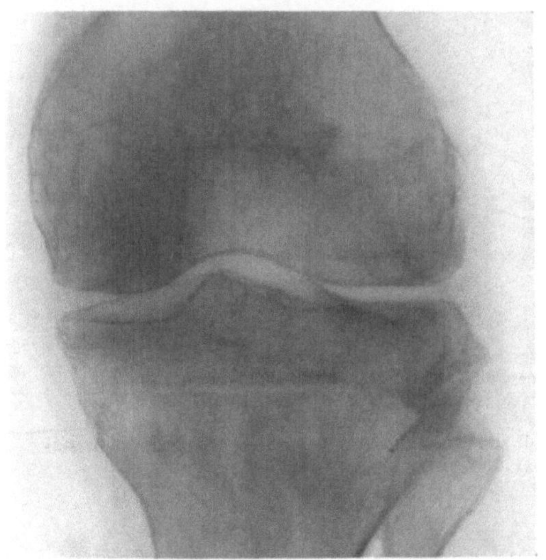

Etwa 1 Jahr nach Beginn sind die Gelenkkonturen scharf, der Gelenkspalt normal, *nur der Knochen atrophisch.*

About one year after commencement. The outlines of joint are distinct and the joint cleft is normal *but the bones are atrophic.*

Series 110.

Primary Chronic Polyarthritis.

A young man of nineteen very slowly developed absolute stiffness in both hip-joints; this took about four years and was accompanied by pain. The knee-joints then also became stiff. No fever was present. The disease was quite uninfluenced by any therapy and at last the joints were destroyed. The patient himself had healthy lungs, though there was a family history of tuberculosis.

2.

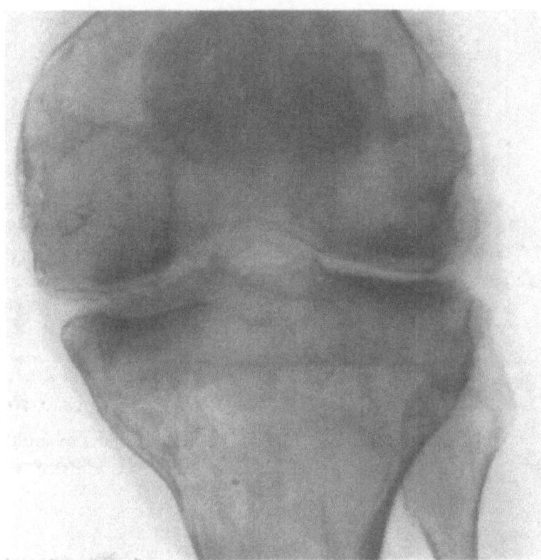

2 Jahre später sind die *Gelenkflächen* aufgelockert, *usuriert* und stellenweise bereits verlötet (Arthritis ulcerosa).

Two years later. The *joint-surfaces* are loosened, *eroded* and in parts already grown together. (Arthritis ulcerosa.)

Serie 110.

3.

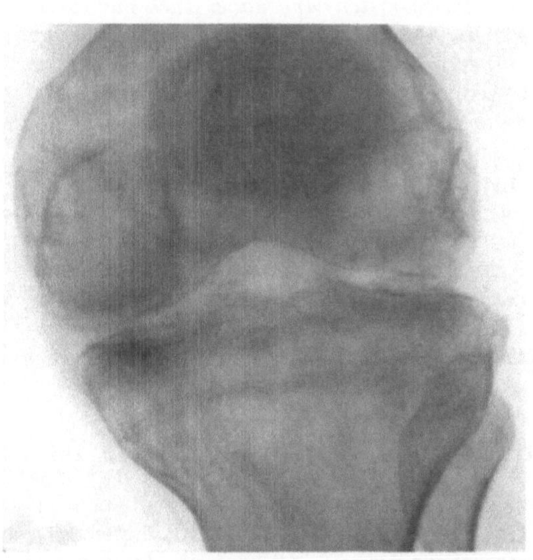

4 Jahre nach Beginn ist der Gelenkspalt ganz aufgehoben, Femur und Tibia sind bereits in ganzer
Ausdehnung — noch etwas locker — *knöchern verwachsen.*

Four years after commencement. There is no joint cleft and tibia and femur are already completely
united by bone, though somewhat loosely.

B. Arthritis deformans — tabische Arthropathie.

Die andere Gruppe der unspezifischen chronischen Gelenkleiden ist prognostisch viel günstiger. Dieser — der Arthritis deformans — liegt primär eine Schädigung des Gelenkknorpels (Elastizitätsverminderung) zugrunde, indem er aufgefasert und bis in den Knochen ausgeschliffen wird, so daß dann reaktiv die charakteristischen osteophytären Randwucherungen entstehen. Die Reihen 111—114 zeigen, daß *der Prozeß langsam fortschreiten und dabei auch zur Bildung eines freien Gelenkkörpers führen kann.* Oft aber erreicht *das Leiden nur einen geringen Grad und bleibt wenigstens für längere Zeit stationär.* Entsprechend der Lokalisation in verschiedenen Gelenken wechseln die Erscheinungsformen. Bei der hypertrophischen Form der Arthritis deformans (Serie 114) führt ein schleichender Umbau, der sich über Jahre erstreckt, zu einer starken Vergrößerung des Gelenkes.

Die neuropathischen Gelenkveränderungen, wie sie am häufigsten bei der Tabes dorsalis vorkommen, stellen anatomisch einen besonders schweren Grad der Arthritis deformans dar. Mögen sie auf einer Erkrankung der trophischen Zentren des Rückenmarkes beruhen, oder auf den rücksichtslosen Gebrauch des analgetischen und porotischen Gelenkes zurückzuführen sein, *es handelt sich dabei um einen Prozeß, der zuerst einen hochgradigen Zerfall bewirkt, dann aber — wie die Serien 117—120 alle zeigen — trotz des fortbestehenden Grundleidens ein Heilbestreben deutlich erkennen läßt.*

B. Arthritis Deformans — Tabetic Arthropathy.

The prognosis of the other group of chronic unspecific joint diseases is much more favourable. Arthritis deformans is primarily caused by a deterioration of the joint cartilage (decrease of elasticity). It becomes frayed and torn away by friction and the reaction causes characteristic peripheral osteophytic outgrowths. Series 111—114 show that the process may advance slowly and lead to the formation of an independent joint body. Frequently the disease reaches a certain degree, which may be only trifling and then it remains stationary for a long time. The aspect varies according to the joint attacked. Hypertrophic arthritis deformans causes joints to become considerably enlarged by a very gradual change which extends over many years.

The neuropathic joint deformities which are most frequent in dorsal tabes, represent anatomically an especially severe degree of arthritis deformans. Whether these deformities are caused by a disease of the trophic centers of the spine, or whether they are due to regardless use of the analgetic and porotic joint, this process always causes first severe decomposition but it will show later on a distinct tendency to heal, despite the continuation of the main affection. (Series 117—120.)

Serie 111.

Arthritis deformans.

Der schleichende Gelenkprozeß des 54 jährigen
Mannes hatte schon längere Zeit dumpfe Schmerzen
verursacht, als die erste Röntgenaufnahme des
Knies gemacht wurde. In den folgenden 5 Jahren
erfuhr er noch gewisse Veränderungen: Proliferation
und Resorption, beides aber nur in geringem
Ausmaß.

Series 111.

Arthritis Deformans.

The fifty-four year old man had had dull pain
for a long time, caused by a protracted joint-
process, when the first X-ray photo of the knee
was taken. It went through various alterations
in the subsequent five years, but there was only
a slight amount of proliferation and resorption.

$^6/_{10}$ n. Gr.   1.

2.

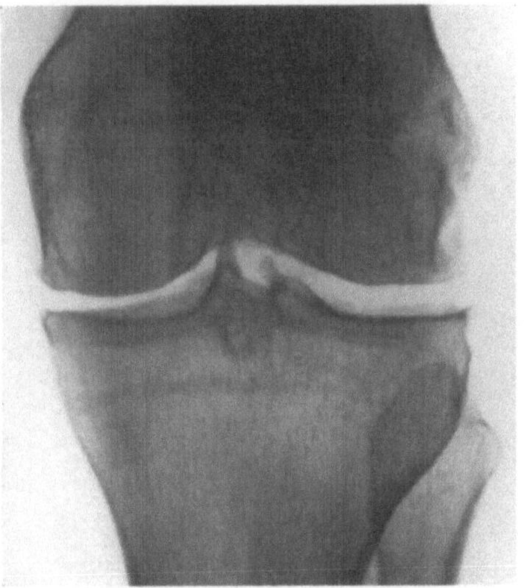

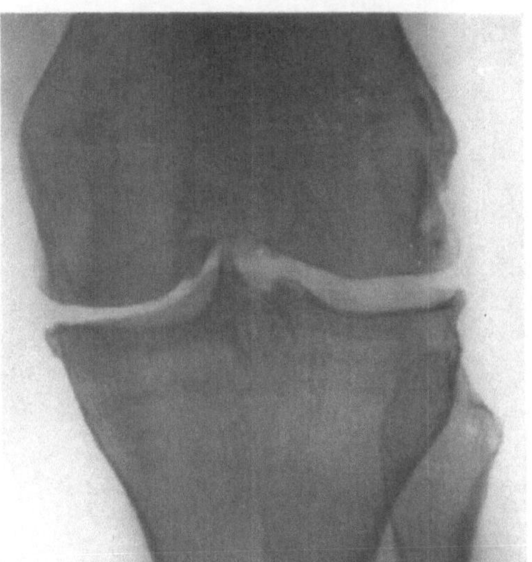

Verknöcherung der Kreuzbänder und geringe
osteophytäre Randwucherungen.

Ossification of crucial ligaments and mild
osteophytic growth at the periphery.

5 Jahre später sind die Wucherungen an den Gelenk-
rändern und in Fossa intercondyloidea etwas größer;
das eine Kreuzband aber tritt nicht mehr in
Erscheinung.

Five years later, the growth proliferation at the
edges of the joint and the fossa intercondyloidea
has somewhat increased, but one crucial ligament
is now invisible.

13*

Serie 112.

Arthritis deformans.

Der eigenartige Knorpel-Knochenprozeß verlief bei
der 44jährigen Frau langsam progredient.
Wa.R. negativ.

Series 112.

Arthritis Deformans.

This curious cartilage-bone process ran a slow
progressive course. W.R. negative. The patient
was a woman forty four years of age.

$^2/_3$ n. Gr.   1.

2.

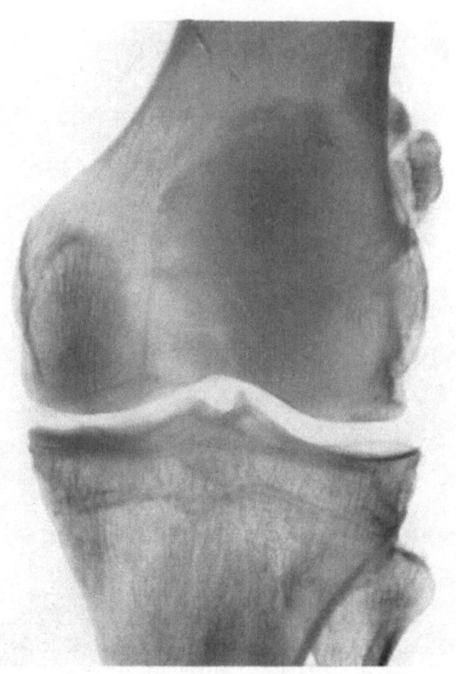

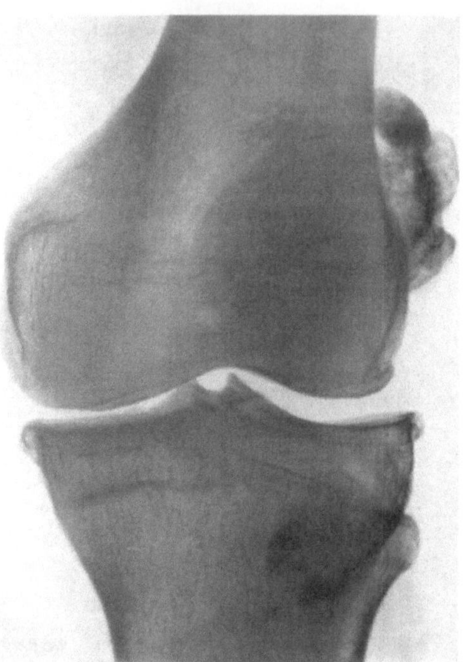

An der Außenseite der Patella finden sich plumpe,
breite Randwülste, während das Kniegelenk im
übrigen von dem Prozeß nicht betroffen ist.

There are coarse wide thickened edges on the outer
side of the patella, while the knee-joint is not
involved.

2 Jahre später sind auch die charakteristischen
osteophytären Randwucherungen der Tibia
vorhanden.

Two years later. The characteristic osteophytic
peripheral growths of the tibia are also present.

Serie 113.

Arthritis deformans.

Der schleichend entstandene Prozeß war in den beiden Jahren progredient und führte zur Lösung eines freien Gelenkkörpers.

Series 113.

Arthritis Deformans.

The slowly advancing process led, in two years, to the formation of a loose joint-body.

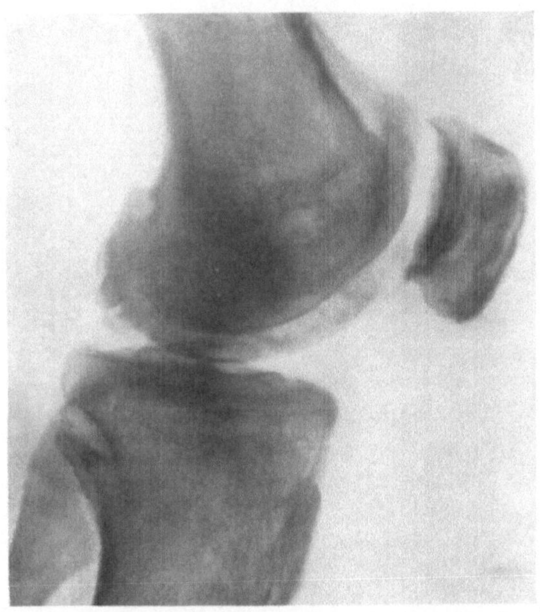

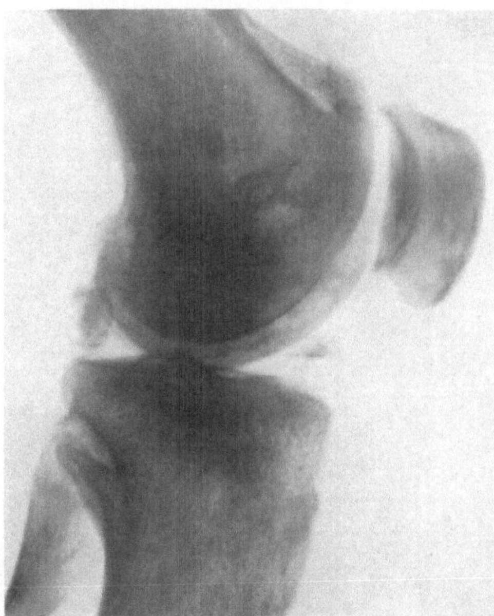

Am Femur und an der Patella sind arthritische Wucherungen erkennbar (42 jährige Frau).

Arthritic changes in the femur and patella are recognizable. (Woman of 42.)

2 Jahre später haben die Veränderungen zugenommen und eine *Gelenkmaus* hat sich gebildet.

Two years later. The condition has advanced and a "joint-mouse" has formed.

Serie 114.

Arthritis deformans coxae.

Bei dem 55 Jahre alten Kutscher machte sich ein Hüftleiden allmählich bemerkbar und führte — von Schmerzen begleitet — nach Jahren zu völliger Versteifung des Gelenkes. Keine Lues.

Series 114.

Arthritis Deformans of the Hip.

A coachman 55 years of age became gradually affected with hip-disease which led, after years of pain, to absolute stiffness of the joint.

$^1/_2$ n. Gr.   1.   2.

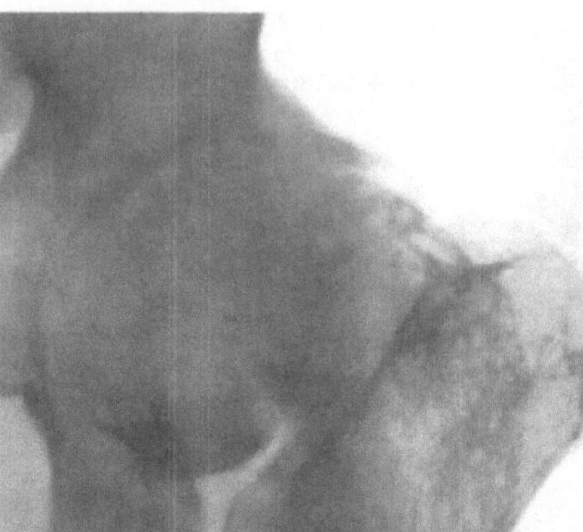

Im 3. Jahr der Krankheit ist die *„Hypertrophie"* *des Gelenkes* bereits sehr deutlich.

After three years the joint shows very distinct hypertrophy.

Nach $5^1/_2$ Jahren sind der Gelenkkopf und Pfannenrand weiter gewuchert.

After $5^1/_2$ years the head and side of the joint have grown exuberantly.

3.

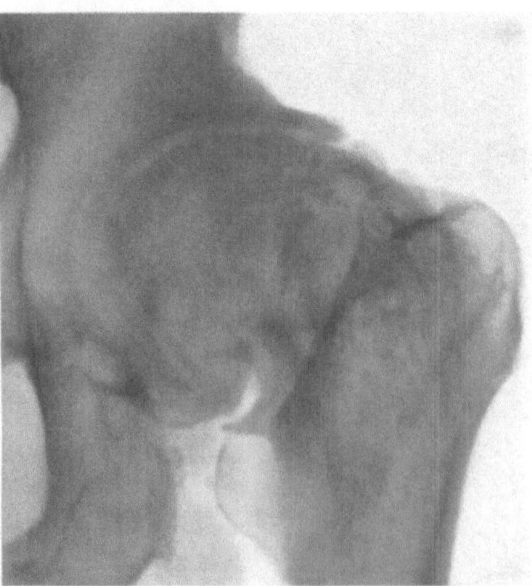

Nach 8 Jahren ist der Krankheitsprozeß noch mehr fortgeschritten: der Schenkelkopf ist unförmlich, der Hals in ihm aufgegangen und das Pfannendach entsprechend verlängert.

After 8 years. The deformity has progressed; the head of the femur is distorted, the neck ingrown and the roof of the acetabulum is correspondingly deepened.

Serie 115.

Spondylitis deformans.

Der 50 jährige Arbeiter klagte seit einem Jahr über ziehende Schmerzen und Steifheit im Rücken. Damals bestanden bereits erhebliche deformierende Veränderungen an der Wirbelsäule; im Laufe der nächsten Jahre aber blieb das Leiden — unbehandelt — auf dieser Stufe stehen und verschlimmerte sich nicht.

$^2/_3$ n. Gr.   1.

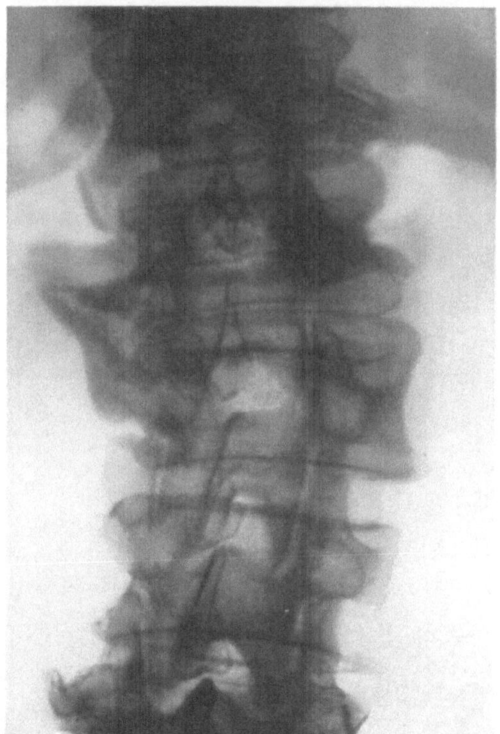

Skoliose mit Spangenbildung und Randwülsten auf der konkaven Seite.

Scoliosis with bridge formation and puffed edges on the concave side.

Series 115.

Spondylitis Deformans.

For about one year, a workman fifty years of age complained of contracting pains and stiffness in the back. At that time extensive deformities in the spine were already present. No treatment was given during the subsequent years and there was no alteration in the condition — neither improvement nor otherwise.

2.

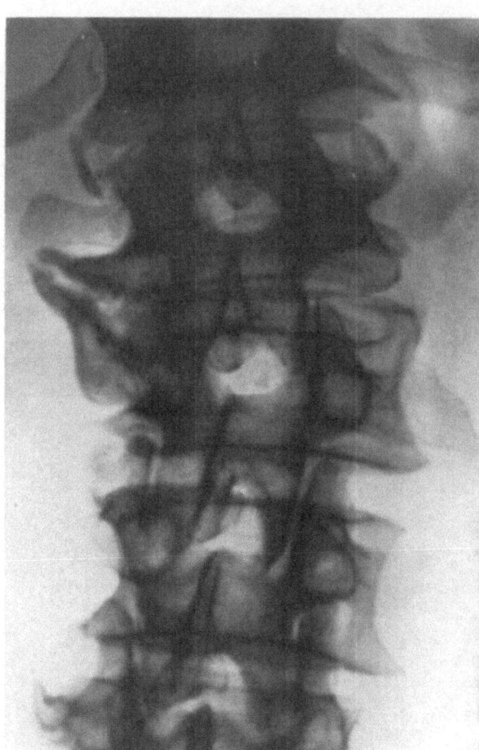

Nach 5 Jahren ist der Befund genau der gleiche.

After five years. Condition quite unchanged.

Serie 116.

Arthritis deformans.

Als Folge des Senkfußes — sinnfällig sekundär — entstand bei dem jungen Mann die Arthritis deformans mit ausgeprägten Randwülsten im Sprunggelenk und in allen Fußwurzelgelenken; sie blieb nach Ausbildung der Deformität stationär.

$^2/_3$ n. Gr.   1.

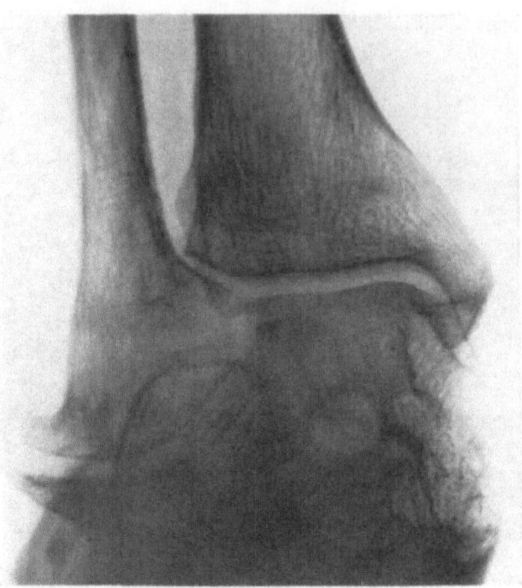

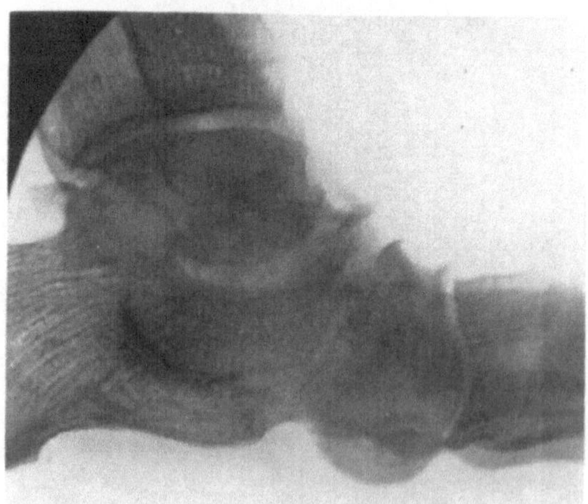

Schwerer Plattfuß mit Deformierung der Fußwurzelknochen und osteophytären Randwucherungen an allen Gelenken. (Keine Tabes dorsalis.)

A severe form of flat foot. The bones at the base of the foot are deformed and there is a peripheral osteophytic growth in all joints. (No tabes dorsalis.)

Series 116.

Arthritis Deformans.

A young man developed arthritis deformans, caused by sinking of the foot-bones. There was marked thickness of the edge of the ankle and in all the joints of the base of the foot. The condition remained stationary.

2.

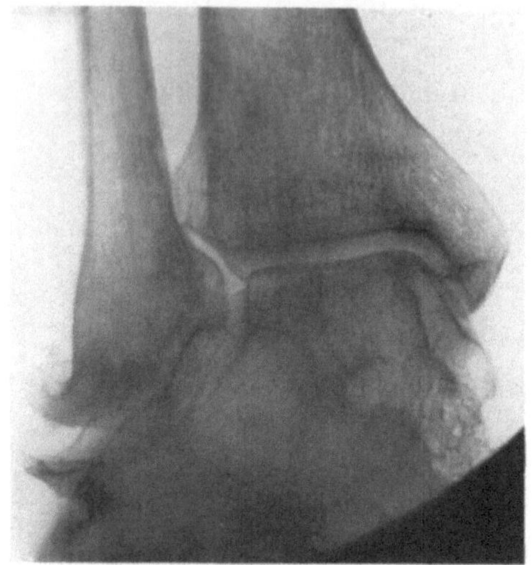

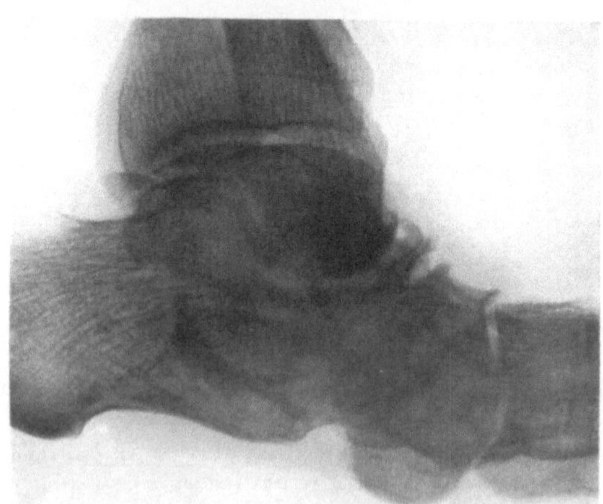

Nach 4 Jahren ist der Zustand unverändert.

After four years. The condition is unaltered.

Serie 117.
Arthropathia tabica.

Die neuropathische Gelenkzerstörung zeigt trotz des
fortbestehenden Grundleidens Heilbestreben:
Reparation und sinnvolle statische Abstützung.

Series 117.
Tabetic Arthropathy.

Despite the continuation of the main affection, the
neuropathic destruction of joint shows a tendency
to heal. Reparation and efficient statical support.

$^1/_2$ n. Gr.　　　　　　1.　　　　　　　　　　　2.

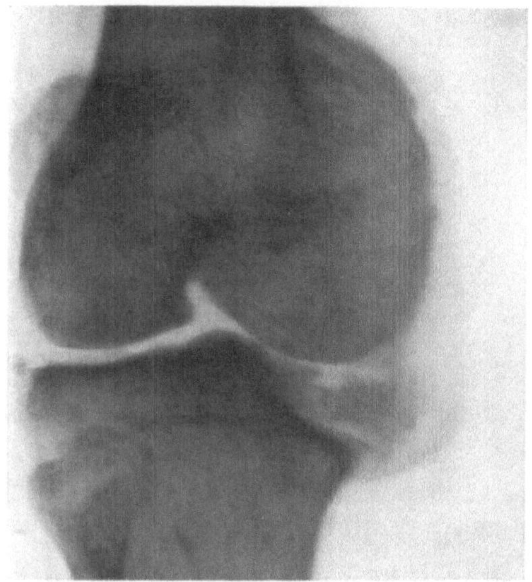
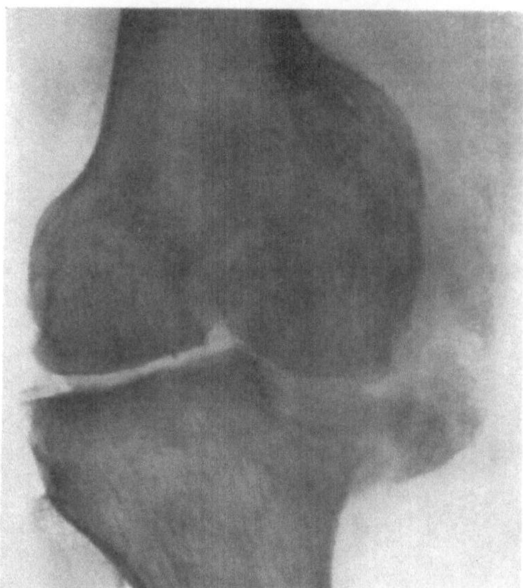

Neben paraartikulären Kalkablagerungen ist vor allem
ein ausgedehnter Zerfall des medialen Tibiacondylus
erkennbar.

Besides peri-articular calcification, an extensive
destruction of tibial condyle is recognizable.

Nach $^1/_2$ Jahr ist der *Defekt knöchern geflickt* und
die mediale Seite des Gelenkes *durch breite para-
artikuläre Verkalkungen statisch abgestützt.*

After one year and a half the *defect has healed by
ossification* and the medial side of joint is *statically
supported by peri-articular calcification.*

3.

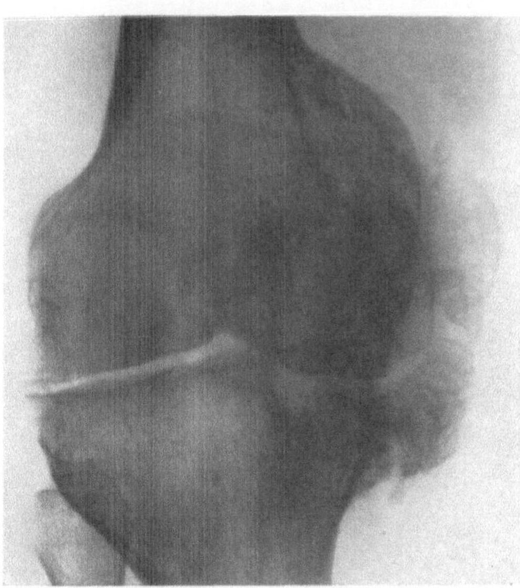

Nach 3 Jahren haben sich die „reparatorischen" appositionellen Prozesse weiter entwickelt:
das Knochengewebe ist dichter.

Three years later. The development of the reparative appositional processes has advanced.
The bone is more compact.

Serie 118.

Arthropathia tabica.

Auch in diesem Fall zeigt der neuropathische
Gelenkprozeß *Reparationen.*

Series 118.

Tabetic Arthropathy.

In this case also, the neuropathic joint-process
shows *restitution.*

$^6/_{10}$ n. Gr.　　　　　1.

2.

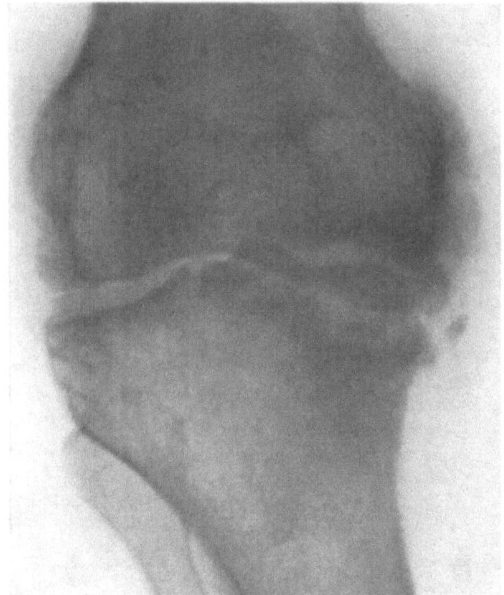

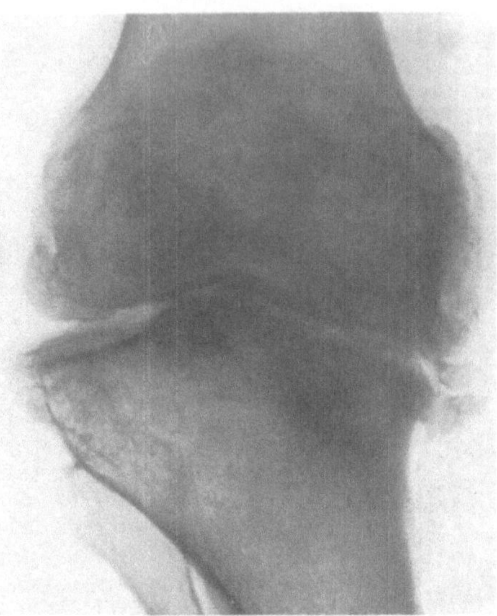

Die medialen Gelenkflächen sowohl des Femur
als besonders der Tibia sind zerstört; ein größeres
Stück der Tibia liegt gelöst in dem Zerfallsgebiet.

The medial joint surfaces of femur and tibia,
particularly the latter, are destroyed. A large
piece of the tibia lies loose in the destroyed area.

8 Jahre später sind *die Gelenkflächen geglättet und
knöchern ausgeflickt*; ein freier Gelenkkörper ist
nicht mehr vorhanden.

Eight years later the *joint-surfaces are smooth
and rebuilt by bone* but there is no freedom in
joint itself.

3.

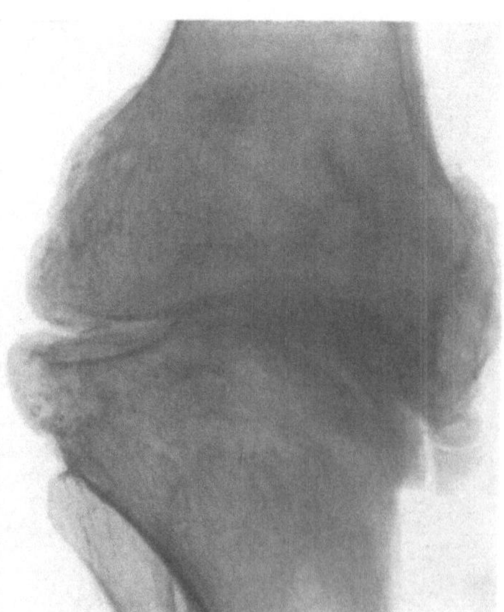

12 Jahre später ist der mediale Tibiacondylus mehr abgeschliffen; im übrigen sind die Gelenkenden
beträchtlich gewuchert und die paraartikulären Verkalkungen haben beträchtlich zugenommen.

Twelve years later the medial tibial condyle has become smoother; the joint-ends have grown
very exuberantly and the peri-articular calcification has increased.

Serie 119.

Malum perforans pedis.

Bei dem 56 Jahre alten Tabiker bestand seit über 1 Jahr ein torpides Druckgeschwür der Fußsohle, das in das schwer zerstörte Großzehengrundgelenk führte. Die Resektion dieses hatte normale Wundheilung im Gefolge; weitere neuropathische Prozesse traten an dem Fuß nicht auf, vielmehr kam es unter der erhöhten Belastung zu ausgleichender Hypertrophie der anderen Mittelfußknochen.

$^6/_{10}$ n. Gr.   1.

Series 119.

Perforating Ulcer of the Foot.

For a year or more, a patient of 56 with tabes, had had a torpid ulcer on the sole of the foot. This had penetrated to the basal joint of the big toe, which was partly destroyed. Resection was followed by normal healing and no further neuropathic trouble ensued. As a reatter of fact, the increased burden caused a compensatory hypertrophy of the other tarsal bones.

2.

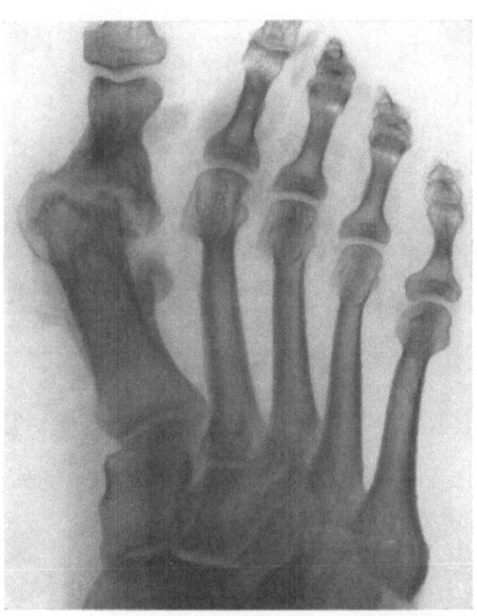

Neuropathischer Prozeß des Großzehengrundgelenkes.

Neuropathic process of the basal joint of the big toe.

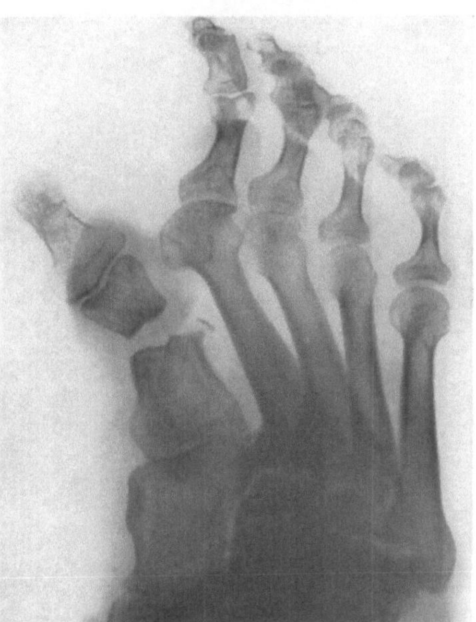

3 Jahre nach der Resektion des Gelenkes sind die Mittelfußknochen infolge der vermehrten statischen Beanspruchung erheblich dicker und stärker geworden.

Three years after resection of the joint, the tarsal bones have become considerably thicker and stronger as a result of the increased statical use.

Serie 120.

Tabische Arthropathie der Wirbelsäule.

Auch an der Wirbelsäule verlief der einer schweren Arthritis deformans entsprechende Prozeß zuerst progredient, dabei stark destruierend, dann aber geschah ein Umschwung: die zerfallenden Wirbelkörper wurden durch neugebildetes Knochengewebe „ausgebessert". Die etwa 50jährige Frau trug von Anfang an ein Stützkorsett und hatte zunehmend gastrische Krisen.

Series 120.

Tabetic Arthropathy of Spine.

This condition, which is analogous to severe arthritis deformans, ran a progressive course at first and caused destruction before improvement could commence. The destroyed vertebrae then "patched" with newly built bone tissue. From the onset, the patient, a woman of fifty, wore a supporting corset and suffered with gastric crises of increasing severity.

$^1/_2$ n. Gr.

1 a.

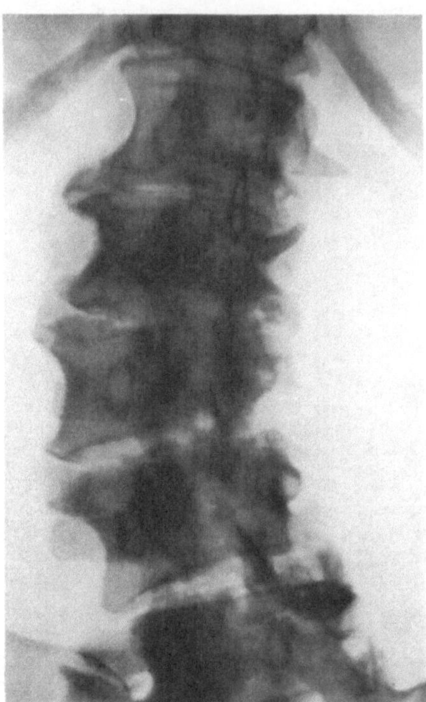

An allen Lendenwirbeln bestehen gewaltige Randusuren und Randwülste, wodurch eine skoliotische Verbiegung der Wirbelsäule entstanden ist.

There is a severe edge-erosion and a thickening of all the lumbar vertebrae. This has caused a scoliotic curvature of the spine.

1 b.

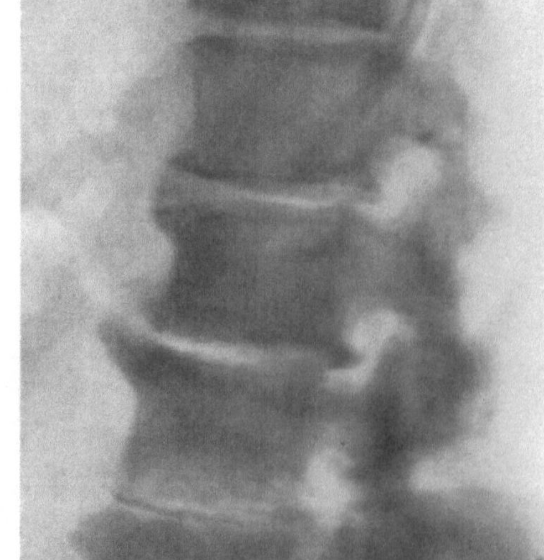

Serie 120.

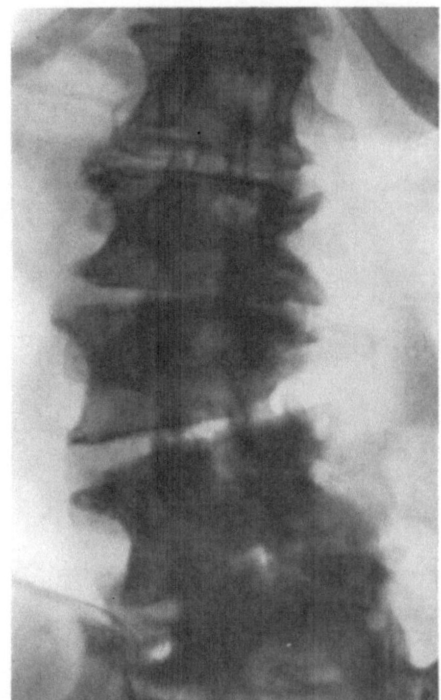

1 Jahr später hat vor allem der Zerfall des III. und IV. Lendenwirbels (Sequester!) sowie die Kalkverarmung der Wirbelsäule zugenommen.

One year later. The destruction of the third and fourth lumbar vertebrae has increased (sequestrum) also chalk impoverishment exists.

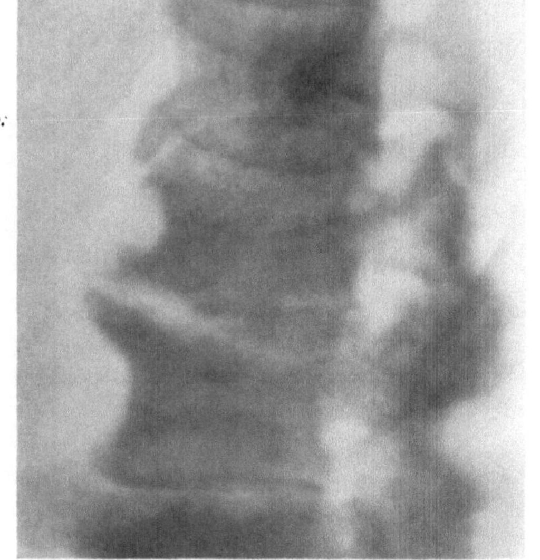

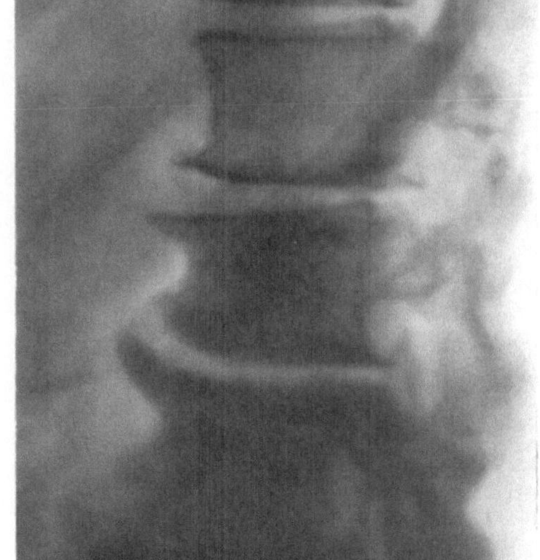

2½ Jahre später bestehen die Wirbelkörper aus festem, zum Teil verdichtetem Knochen und besitzen geglättete Ränder.

Two years and a half later. The vertebral bodies consist of firm, partly compact bone and possess smooth edges.

<table>
<tr><td>

Anhang.

Serie 121.

Blutergelenk (Hämophilie).

Nach einmaliger schwerer Gelenkblutung ent-
wickelte sich bei dem Knaben, der auch andere
hämophile Blutungen durchmachte, eine eigen-
artige Gelenkdeformierung. Im Knochen selbst
traten Blutungsherde nicht auf.

</td><td>

Supplement.

Series 121.

Haemorrhagic Joint (Haemophilia).

A boy who had already had various haemorrhages,
suddenly had a severe haemorrhage into the joint.
This caused an unusual deformation.

</td></tr>
<tr><td>

$^2/_3$ n. Gr.   1.

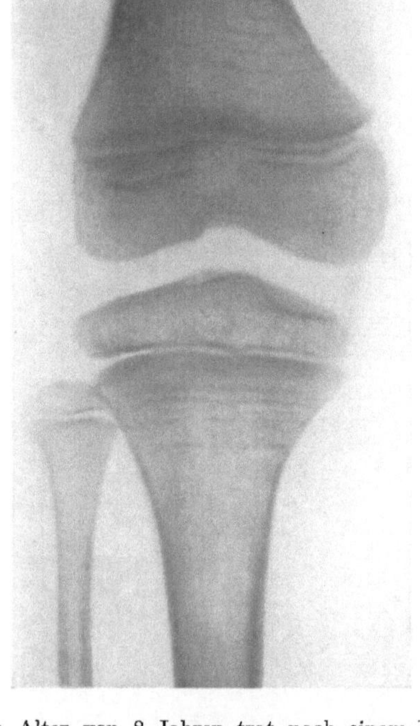

</td><td>

2.

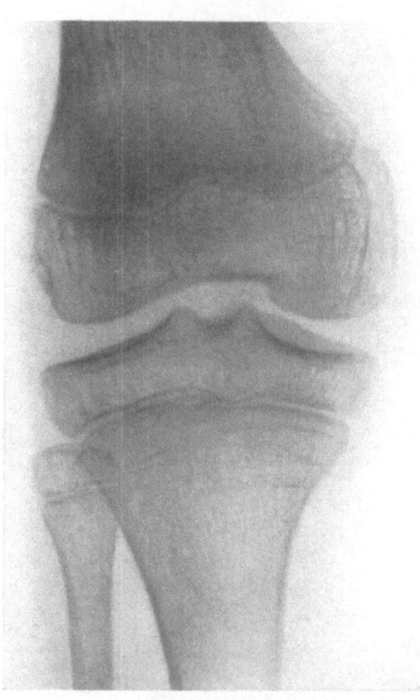

</td></tr>
<tr><td>

Im Alter von 8 Jahren trat nach einem Fall
auf das Knie ein gewaltiger Bluterguß auf.
Noch nach 5 Monaten bestand eine schwammige
Auftreibung des Gelenkes.

8 years of age: After a fall on the knee, a severe
internal blood effusion took place. After 5 months
a spongy swelling of the joint was still present.

</td><td>

Im Alter von 11 Jahren: keine Beschwerden im
Knie, aber eine Abflachung der Gelenkflächen ist
röntgenologisch nachweisbar.

11 years of age: No complaint in knee but a flatness
of the joint surface is shown by X-rays.

</td></tr>
</table>

Serie 121.

3.

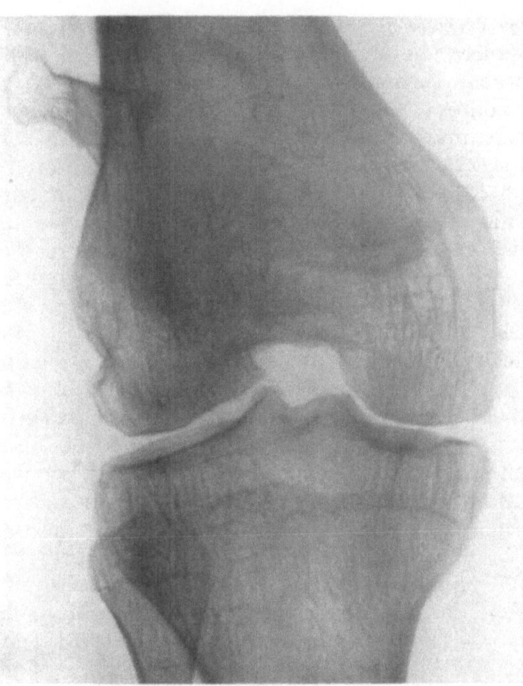

Im 18. Lebensjahr ist die Deformierung der Gelenkflächen noch deutlicher. Außerdem findet sich eine Exostose am Femur. — Subjektiv keine Beschwerden.

18 years of age: The deformity of the joint surfaces is still more distinct, besides which an exostosis of the femur is present. — No subjective complaint.

VI. Kapitel.

Verletzungen.

Heilung des Knochenbruches — Pseudarthrose — Epiphysenverletzung — Gelenkbruch.

Ein Knochenbruch erreicht gewöhnlich eine gewebsvollwertige — knöcherne — Verwachsung. Aus dem durch die Verletzung gereizten Periost und Endost sproßt ein gefäßreiches Keimgewebe, das sich, wie Serie 122 zeigt, über ein osteoides und chondroides Stadium zu echtem Knochen entwickelt, zuerst locker und überschüssig, dann sich verdichtend und abflachend. *Nicht beseitigte Dislokationen werden am Erwachsenen formal geglättet* (Serie 124) und unter bestimmten Bedingungen auch noch verringert (Serie 125). *Beim Kinde aber wird unter günstigen Voraussetzungen* (z. B. Streckung durch die eigene Schwere) *manche Verschiebung noch nachträglich ausgewachsen* (Serie 123 u. 147). Das geschieht nicht nur am Schaft, sondern auch an den Gelenkenden. So erfuhr das Fußgelenk des 16jährigen Mädchens (Serie 136) durch das Wachstum eine Umformung, welche die Absprengung der Knochenecke aufnahm und ausglich.

Eine Störung der Wundheilung am Knochen kann als *einfache Verzögerung* in Erscheinung treten; dann nimmt der Prozeß der Bruchheilung (Serie 128) qualitativ noch den richtigen Weg. Er kann aber auch aus der Richtung der knöchernen Verwachsung abgelenkt werden und zu einer Gewebsformation führen, die nicht mehr Knochen werden kann. So hat in Serie 129 sogar das Knochengewebe der Bruchenden durch die schwere Schädigung eine derartige Umwandlung erfahren und ist somit selbst die Ursache einer *Interpositionspseudarthrose* geworden.

Das Schicksal einer Wachstumsfugenverletzung ist verschieden. Der Oberschenkelbruch in der unteren Epiphysenfuge (Serie 133) heilte nach der exakten Reposition auf dem normalen Wege der Bruchheilung, durch Callusbildung; dadurch aber wurde ein *vorzeitiger Schluß der Wachstumsfuge* herbeigeführt und das Längenwachstum vor der Zeit beendet. In anderen Fällen, in denen die vorzeitige Verknöcherung nicht ausgelöst wird, erfolgt unter dem Einfluß des streckenden Wachstums (Serie 131 u. 132), die Restitutio ad integrum.

Knochenbrüche, welche in das Gelenk hineinführen, heilen gewöhnlich mit einer mehr oder weniger großen Unebenheit der Gelenkflächen, einer sekundären Arthritis deformans (Serie 136). Bei Binnenverletzungen können ausgesprengte Stücke pseudarthrotisch verwachsen oder sehr langsam die feste Knorpel-Knochenverbindung (Serie 139) eingehen.

Chapter VI

Injuries.

Healing of Fractures — Pseudarthrosis — Epiphyseal Injury — Intracapsular Fracture.

Bone fracture is repaired by ossification and usually with complete compensation. Germ tissue, replete with blood vessels, sprouts from the periosteum and endosteum which, owing to the injury, is in a state of irritation (Series 122) and by means of osteoid and chondroid stages, becomes genuine bone. At first it is loose and exuberant, but later it becomes compact and smooth. The displaced bone ends of an adult, if not correctly set, become smooth (Series 124) and under certain conditions become a little smaller (Series 125). By correct treatment (e. g. extension by its own weight), a child may completely outgrow the displacement (Series 123 and 147). This applies not only to the shaft but also to the joint ends. The ankle joint of the 16 year old girl (Series 136) was cured in this way. It was remodelled by growth and levelled.

A disturbance in the healing of the bone wound may only be due to delay, the fracture repair then qualitatively taking the right direction (Series 128). This proceeding however, is sometimes diverted from ossification and results in the formation of tissue which can never become bone. Such a case is seen in series 129. The bone tissue of the joint ends has been so transformed that it has been the cause of an interposition pseudarthrosis.

The course of an epiphyseal injury varies. The femur fracture through the lower epiphyseal line (Series 133) healed in the normal way by means of callus formation, after accurate apposition had been obtained. This led to the closing of the epiphyseal line before the correct time though, and thus further longitudinal growth was prevented. Complete restitution follows under the influence of growth (Series 131 and 132) where there has been no previous ossification.

Bone fractures which involve the joint heal with more or less irregularity of the joint surfaces. (Secondary arthritis def. — Series 136.) In the case of internal injury, the broken off pieces may unite and form a pseudarthrosis or may become a firm cartilage-bone unity.

Serie 122.

Frakturcallus.

Die exakt adaptierten Fragmente heilten mit reichlichem Callus, der in typischer Weise die Bruchstelle umwucherte, sich lamellär schichtete, zunächst an Masse zunahm, sich dann aber verdichtete und mehr und mehr abflachte.

Series 122.

Fracture Callus.

The exactly adapted fragments healed with considerable callus which grew round the broken part. It was deposited in layers in a typical manner; at first increasing in bulk, later thickening and becoming more level.

$^2/_3$ n. Gr.   1.   2.   3.

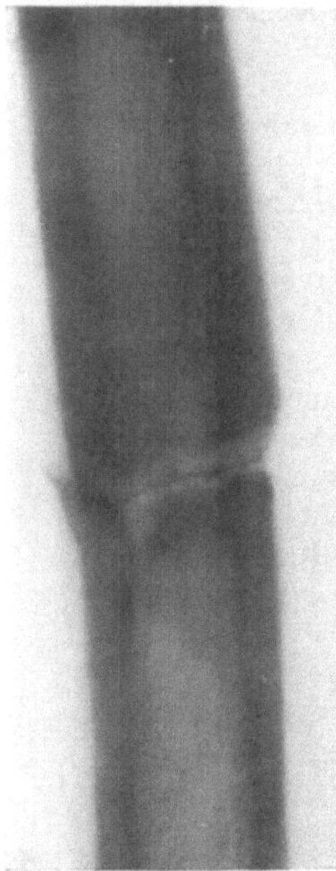 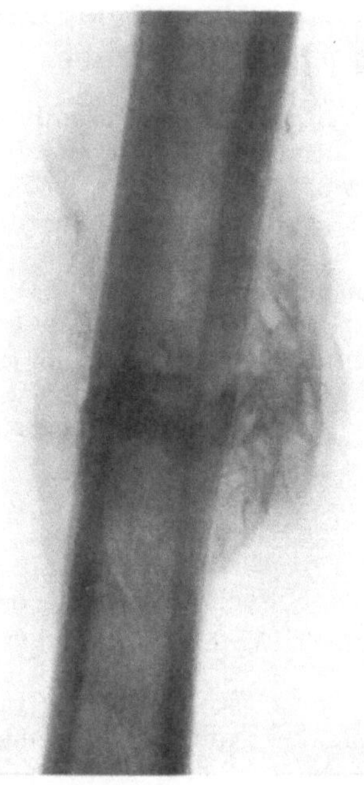 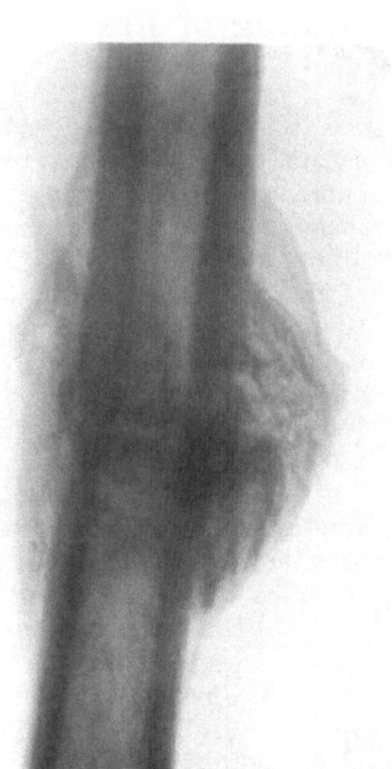

Der exakt reponierte Knochenbruch zeigt 10 Tage nach dem Unfall einen Kalkschwund der Bruchenden.

Ten days after accident the exactly adapted fracture shows a decalcification at the fracture ends.

Nach 8 Wochen besteht reichlicher Callus, der schon lamelläre Schichtung besitzt.

After eight weeks considerable callus is present. Already lamellated.

Nach 11 Wochen hat der Callus an Masse noch zugenommen, ebenso ist die den Bruchspalt überbrückende Bogenstruktur weiter ausgebildet.

After eleven weeks the callus has increased in bulk and the bow-structure, bridging the cleft has further developed.

Serie 122.

4.

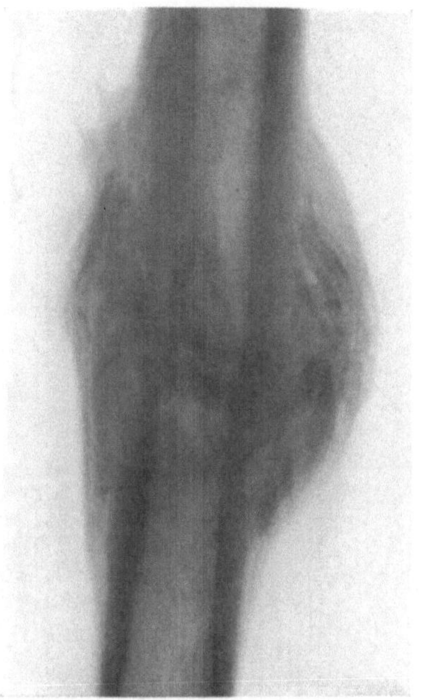

5.

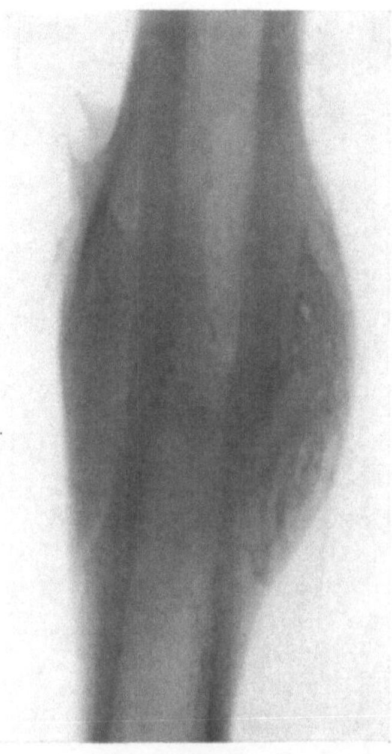

6.

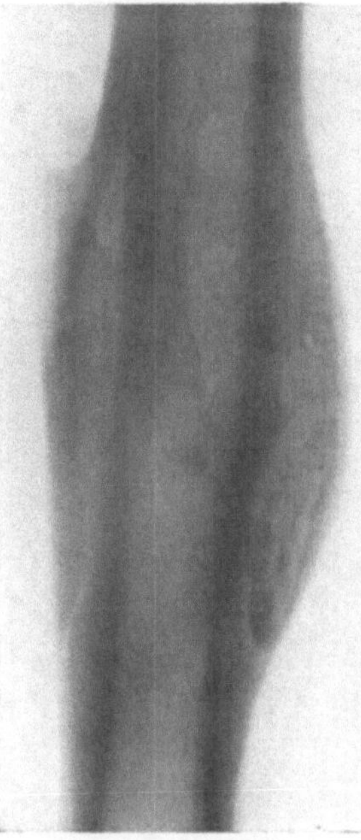

Nach 17 Wochen ist das Stadium der Proliferation auf dem Höhepunkt angelangt.

After seventeen weeks the stage of proliferation has reached its height.

Nach 7 Monaten ist die periostale Knochenschale zwar noch etwas dichter, aber schon flacher.

After seven months the periosteal bone covering is somewhat thicker and also flatter.

Nach 1¹/₄ Jahr ist eine weitere Rückbildung des Callus erfolgt. Eine Bruchlinie ist nicht mehr erkennbar, die Compacta zieht durch die angeglichene Callusschale.

After one year and a quarter a further decrease of callus has taken place. The fracture line is no longer recognizable, the compacta passes through the assimilated callus-covering.

Serie 123.

Oberarmbruch (Kind).

Bei dem 4 jähr. Mädchen wurde die fehlerhafte Stellung des Oberarmes lediglich durch das Wachstum und die Schwere des herabhängenden Armes in wenigen Monaten nahezu ganz ausgeglichen. Ein korrigierender Eingriff geschah nicht.

Series 123.

Fracture of Upper Arm (Child).

Within a few months, the faulty position of the upper arm of a four year old girl was almost entirely corrected by growth and the weight of the dependent arm. A correcting operation was not performed.

⁴/₅ n. Gr.   1.   2.   3.

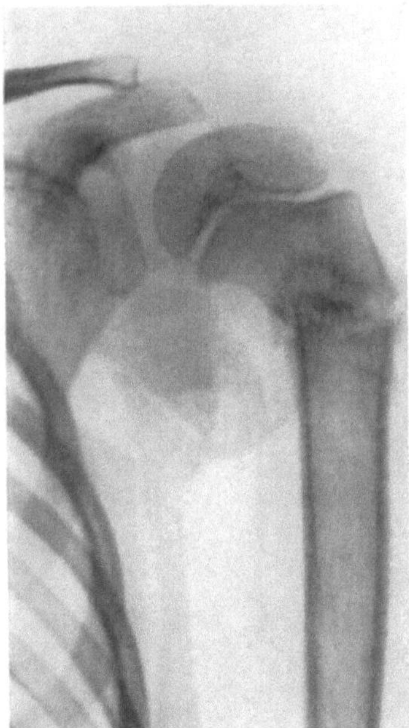 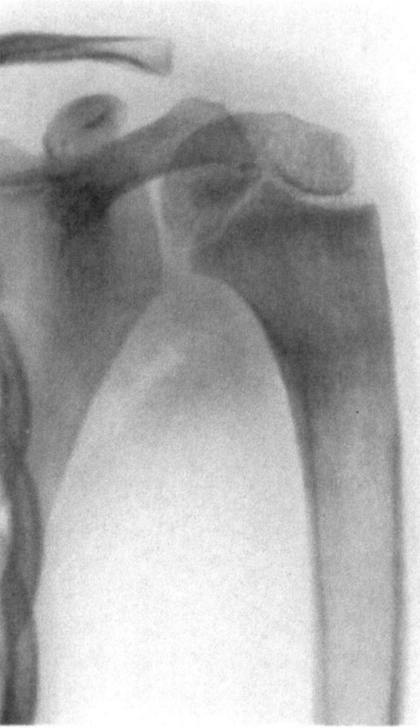 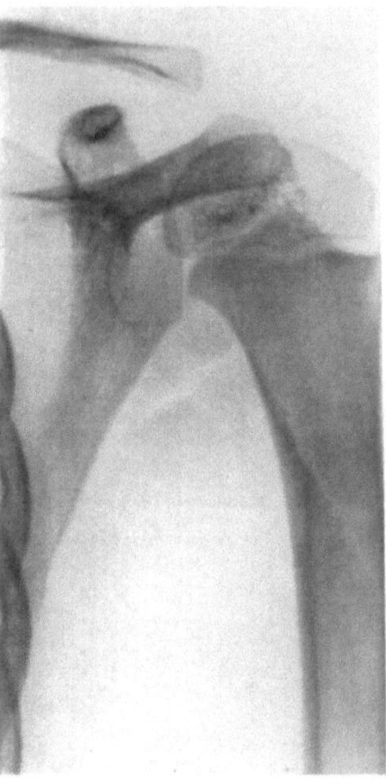

20 Tage nach dem Unfall ist der Knochenbruch bereits fest, aber es besteht eine deutliche Winkelstellung der Fragmente (Dislocatio ad axim).

Twenty days after accident the fracture is firm but a noticeable divergence of the fragments remains. (Dislocatio ad axim).

Nach 4 Monaten ist der Winkel weitgehend gestreckt und die normale Bälkchenstruktur fast wiederhergestellt; eine ringförmige Verdichtung zeigt die Frakturstelle.

After four months the angle is considerably straightened and the normal beam structure nearly restored. The part which was fractured is shown by an annular compactness.

Nach 9 Monaten ist die Bruchstelle weit von der Wachstumsfuge abgerückt und nur noch medial an der Corticalis erkennbar. Der Schaft ist gerade.

After nine months, the part which was fractured has moved a long way from the growth line and is only recognized at the cortex. The shaft is straight.

Serie 124.

Oberschenkelbruch (Erwachsener).

Bei dem 28 jährigen Mann wurde die seitliche Verschiebung
der Knochenenden zwar formal geglättet, aber nicht
— wie beim Wachsenden — beseitigt.

Series 124.

Fracture of Femur (Adult).

A twenty-eight year old man had a fracture of the femur.
The dislocated bone ends became smooth again but not
normal as would have been the case had he not finished
growing.

$^7/_{10}$ n. Gr.   1.   2.   *Anhang:* $^1/_2$ n. Gr.

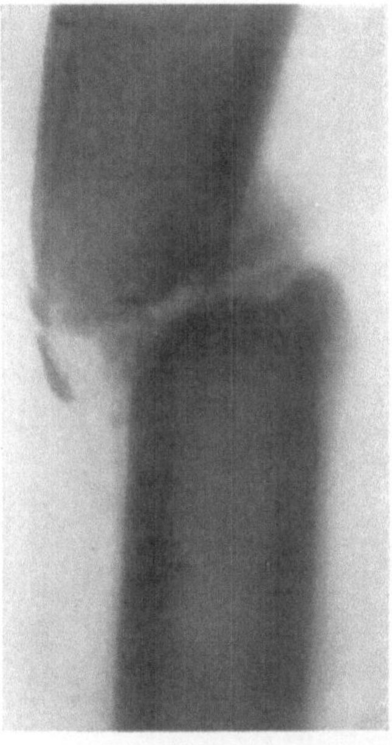 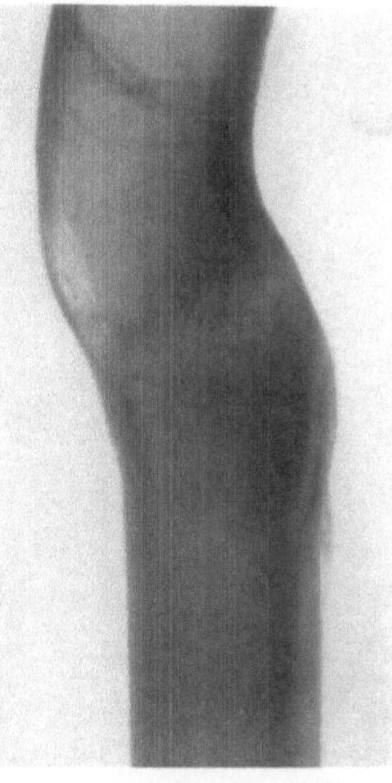 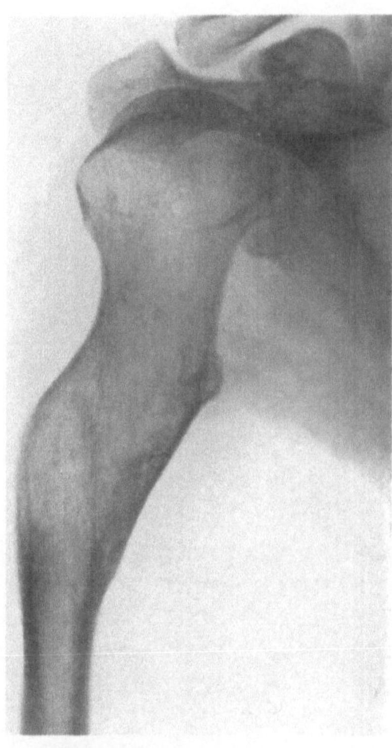

5 Wochen nach dem Unfall sind
die seitlich verschobenen Bruchenden durch Callus verwachsen,
die Kanten der Knochen treten
noch hervor.

Five weeks after the accident the
laterally displaced fractured ends
are joined together by callus. The
edges of the bone are still
prominent.

Nach 4 Jahren ist lediglich die
äußere Form geglättet.

After four years only the outside
shape has been smoothed.

Noch 30 Jahre nach der im 25. Lebensjahr erlittenen Verletzung ist an der er-
haltenen Corticalis die Dislocatio ad latus
erkennbar; nur ein Ausgleich der Form
ist geschehen.

Supplement:

Thirty years after the accident, which
happened when the man was twenty eight.
The dislocatio ad latus is seen at the cortex.
Only the shape has become regular.

Serie 125.

Frakturcallus.

Die stark verschobenen Bruchenden hat ein
„zielstrebiger" Callus auf einem weiten ge-
wundenen Wege vereinigt und im Laufe der
Jahre in geradezu erstaunlichem Maße einander
genähert und der geraden Linie angeglichen.

Series 125.

Fracture Callus.

The widely displaced fracture ends have been
united in a roundabout way by a "purposeful
gravitating" callus. In the course of years they
have drawn together and assumed a straight
line in a truly remarkable manner.

$^6/_{10}$ n. Gr.   1.   2.

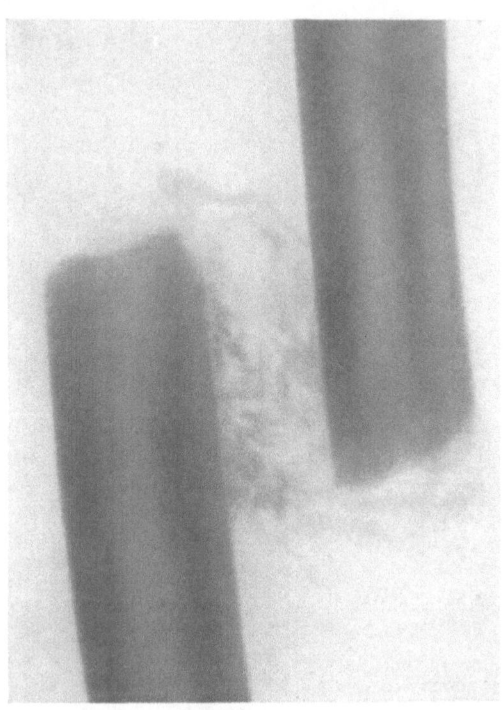

5 Wochen nach dem Unfall sind die Bruchflächen
der weit auseinanderstehenden Fragmente durch eine
Callusstraße verbunden.

Five weeks after accident, the fracture surfaces of the
widely gaping fragments are connected by callus.

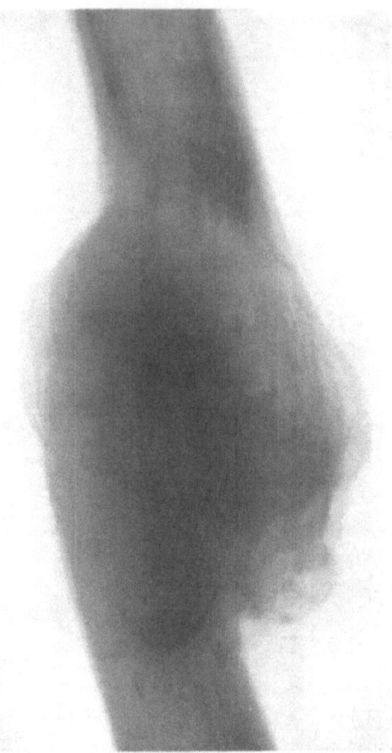

Nach 10 Jahren berühren sich die Fragmente und sind durch ein dichtes wirres
Knochengeflecht fest verwachsen.

After ten years the fragments are grown
together and united by compact
irregular bony tissue.

Serie 126.

Wirbelfraktur.

Der schwere Schaden der beiden Wirbel ist durch
das Wachstum erheblich gebessert worden: aus der
ineinander gepreßten Knochenmasse haben sich
wieder zwei durch eine Zwischenwirbelscheibe
getrennte Wirbelkörper herausdifferenziert.

$^7/_{10}$ n. Gr.   1.

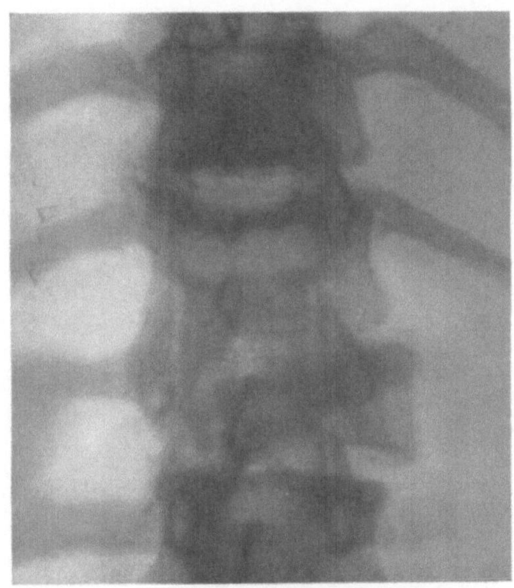

Die frische Kompressionsfraktur des 12. Brust- und
1. Lendenwirbels (15jähriges Mädchen).

The recent compression fracture of the twelfth dorsal
and first lumbar vertebrae. (Girl of fifteen).

Series 126.

Fracture of Vertebrae.

The severe injury to both vertebrae was considerably
improved by growth. Two vertebral bodies, divided
by a disc between the vertebrae, were formed out
of the bone mass which had been crushed together.

2.

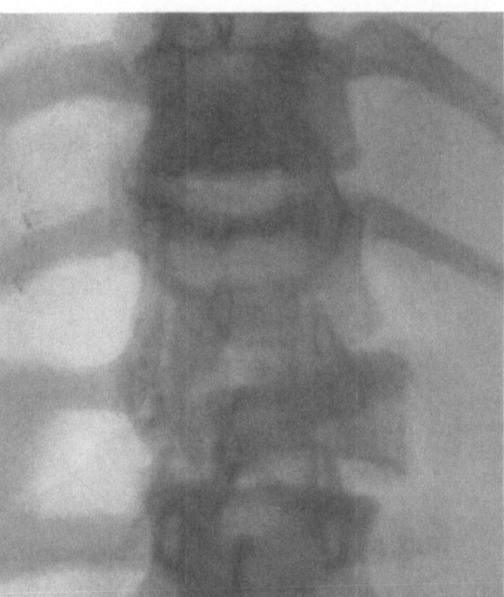

7 Jahre später — im 23. Lebensjahr — sind die
beiden verletzten Wirbelkörper zwar deformiert,
aber *gewachsen* und als zwei feste, abgegrenzte
Knochenblöcke wiederhergestellt; auch die Zwischenwirbelscheibe ist erkennbar.

Seven years later, in the twenty third year. The two
injured vertebral bodies are deformed but have
grown and become two firm distinct bone blocks.
The disc between the vertebrae is also recognizable.

Serie 127.

Komplizierte Unterschenkelfraktur.

Trotz der besonders schweren Verletzung — einem Verkehrsunfall — konnte die Amputation des Unterschenkels vermieden und knöcherne Verwachsung in guter Stellung erreicht werden. Nach der primären Wundversorgung und Ruhigstellung im Gipsverband heilte die blande Entzündung und schließlich setzte auch — als die „Commotio ossium" überwunden war — die knöcherne Verwachsung der später stellungskorrigierten Fragmente ein.

Series 127.

Complicated Fracture of Lower Legs.

In spite of the severe injury, which was due to a traffic injury, amputation was avoided and bony union in a good position was obtained. After primary treatment of the wound and rendering it immobile with plaster of Paris, the inflammation subsided. After the "commotio ossium" had been effectively treated, the bony fragments finally united after their position had been corrected.

1.

$^1/_4$ n. Gr.

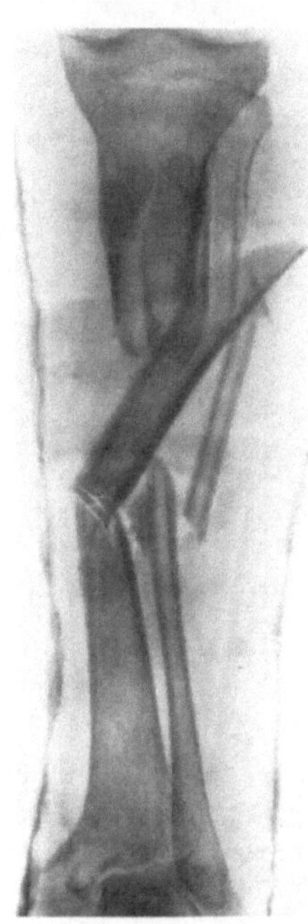

2.

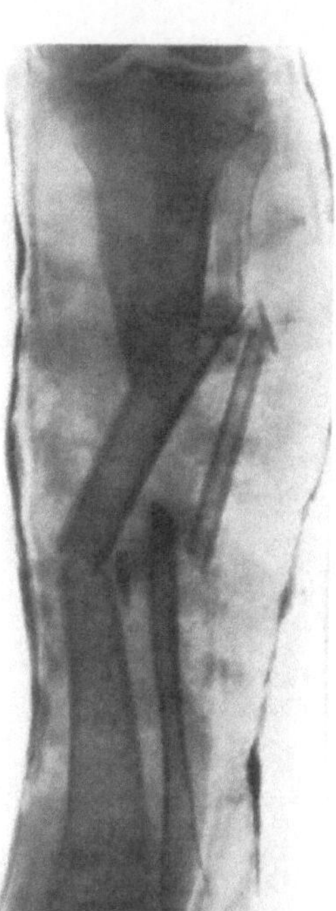

Abgesehen von der großen Weichteilwunde bestehen Splitterung und Stückbrüche beider Unterschenkelknochen.

In addition to the large wound of the soft parts, there is splintering and fragmentation in the lower part of both lower legs.

Nach 8 Wochen ist noch keine Spur Callus gewuchert; das ausgesprengte mittlere Tibiadrittel ist nicht ausgestoßen und wurde jetzt durch Drahtnaht am oberen Ende adaptiert.

After eight weeks there is no trace of callus. The displaced middle third of the tibia has not been expelled and was therefore fixed by a wire suture in its upper end.

Serie 127.

3.

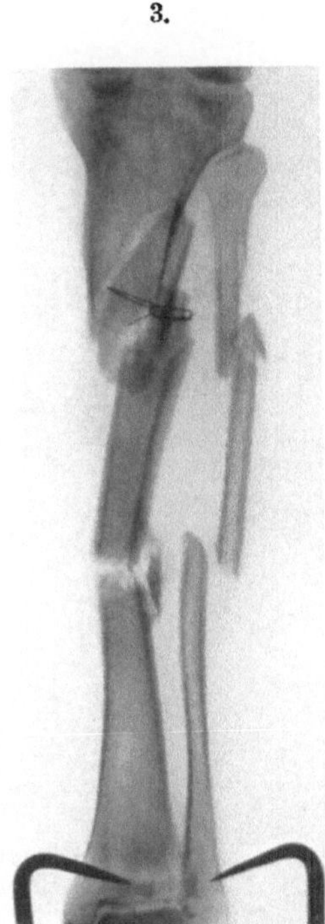

4.

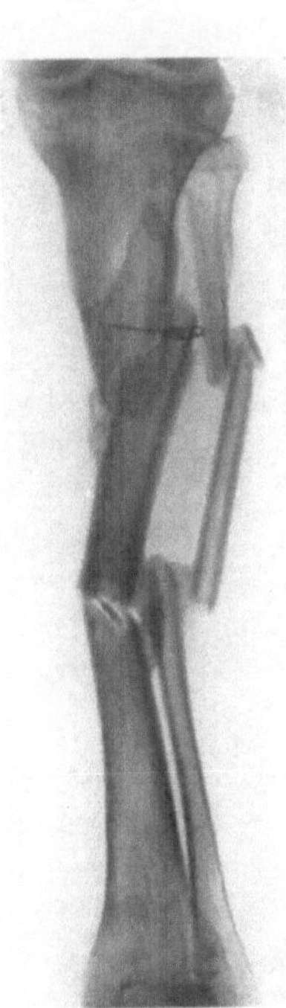

Der noch nicht ausgeglichene distale Knick (Disloc. ad axim.) wurde durch Klammerextension gestreckt.

The distal deformity, which has not yet been reduced (disloc. ad axim), was stretched by clamp extension.

Nach ¹/₂ Jahr ist an allen Bruchstellen mehr oder weniger Callus vorhanden.

After six months, callus is present in all fractured parts.

Serie 128.

Verzögerte Knochenbruchheilung.

Der 15 jährige gesunde Knabe erlitt den Bruch der
Vorderarmknochen durch Fall auf die Hand. Die
knöcherne Verwachsung der sich breit berührenden
Knochenenden vollzog sich außerordentlich langsam
und hatte nach 9 Monaten noch nicht die normale
Festigkeit erreicht, so daß aus geringfügiger Ursache
erneut an derselben Stelle die Fraktur geschah. Auch
diese konsolidierte verzögert. Nur langsam wurde
der eben notwendige Callus aufgebracht, der sich
aber qualitativ normal zu Knochensubstanz entwickelte und nicht aus dieser Richtung in die der
Pseudarthrose abirrte.

Series 128.

Delayed Healing of Fracture.

A healthy boy of fifteen fell on his hand and broke
the bones of his forearm. The bone ends were well
placed but the union took an extraordinarily long
time. It was so weak that the bones broke again in
the same place from quite a slight cause. The union
was further delayed, but very slowly the absolutely
essential callus appeared. Normal bony union and
not pseudarthrosis resulted.

4/5 n. Gr.   1.   2.   3.

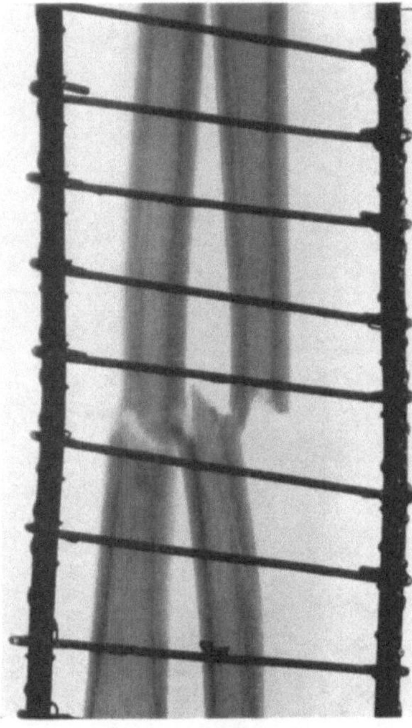 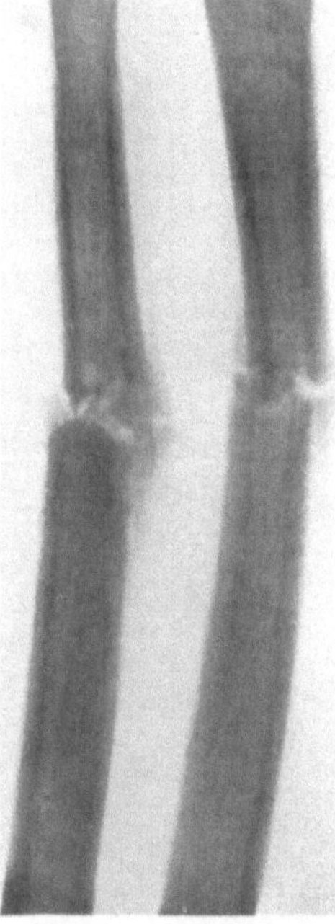 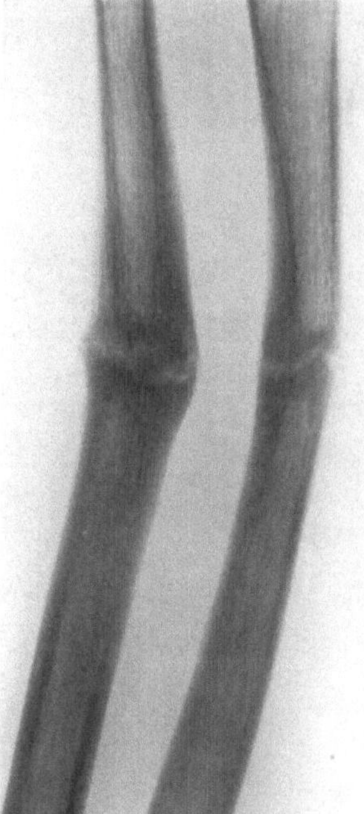

Querbruch beider Unterarmknochen mit
seitlicher Fragmentverschiebung
des einen.

Diagonal fracture of both bones of
forearm. One has slipped aside.

7 Wochen später sind die
Bruchenden gut adaptiert,
aber der Spalt ist noch
offen; *auffallend wenig
Callus* ist gewuchert.

Seven weeks later, the fractured ends are well adapted
but a cleft still remains.
*Remarkably small amount
of callus* has been formed.

Auch nach 1/2 Jahr ist der
Bruchspalt noch deutlich und
nur geringe periostale Knochenwucherung erfolgt.

After six months, the cleft is
still distinct and only very little
periosteal bone-growth has
followed.

Serie 128.

4.

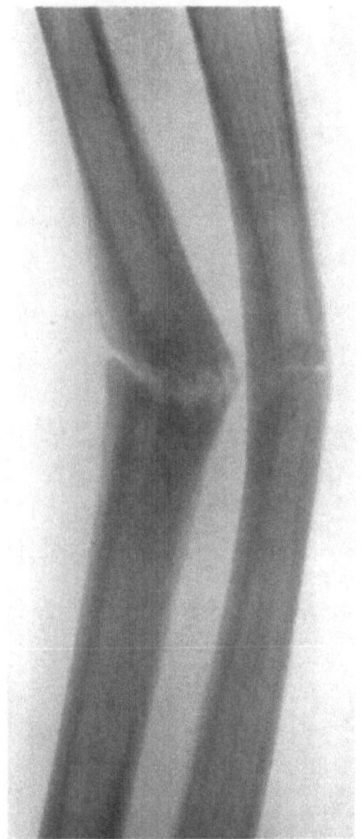

5.

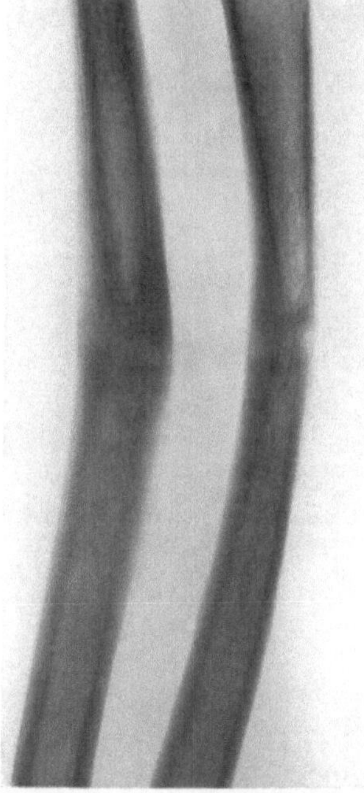

6.

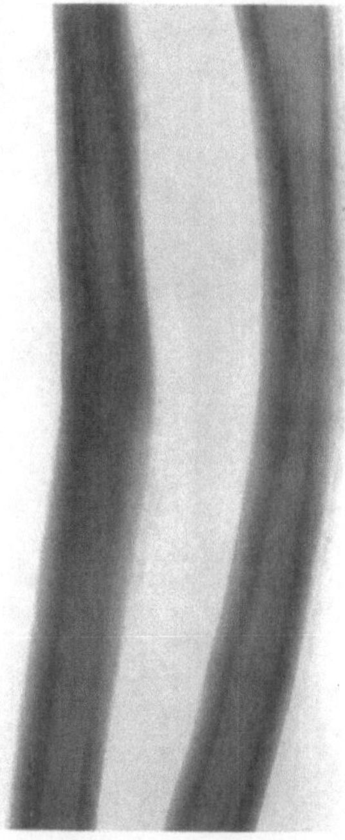

Nach ³/₄ Jahren ist der Unterarm *an denselben Stellen erneut gebrochen.*

After nine months, *the forearm has broken again in the same place.*

Nach 14 Monaten ist der Bruchspalt beiderseits knöchern verwachsen — *ohne jeden Überschuß an Callus.*

After fourteen months. The clefts have closed and union has occurred — *without any superfluity of callus.*

Nach 2 Jahren sind die Bruchstellen nur noch an der geringen Strukturunregelmäßigkeit zu erkennen. — Normales Wachstum.

After two years the fractured part is only recognizable by the slight irregularity in structure.
Normal growth.

Serie 129.

Pseudarthrose des Unterschenkels.

Der kräftige 36 jährige Mann erlitt eine komplizierte Unterschenkelfraktur durch direkte Gewalt-
einwirkung. Die Wunde heilte schnell, doch der
Knochenbruch wurde nicht fest und führte trotz
breiter Berührung der Bruchenden zur Pseudarthrose:
an den schwer geschädigten Knochenenden entstanden Randnekrosen, die durch den Wundprozeß
narbig umgewandelt wurden und als ein dem Knochen
fremdes Gewebe zwischen den Bruchenden liegen. —
So ist durch Knochengewebe selbst eine „Interpositionspseudarthrose" entstanden.

Series 129.

Pseudarthrosis of Lower Leg.

A strong healthy man, 36 years of age, in an accident
received a complicated fracture of the lower leg. The
wound itself healed rapidly, but despite extensive
apposition the fracture did not become firm and led
to pseudarthrosis. The bone ends were considerably
injured and became necrotic at the edges; the necrotic
tissue in the course of cicatrization remaining in the
form of foreign tissue between the fractured ends
and giving rise to "interposition pseudarthrosis".

$^2/_3$ n. Gr.   1.   2.

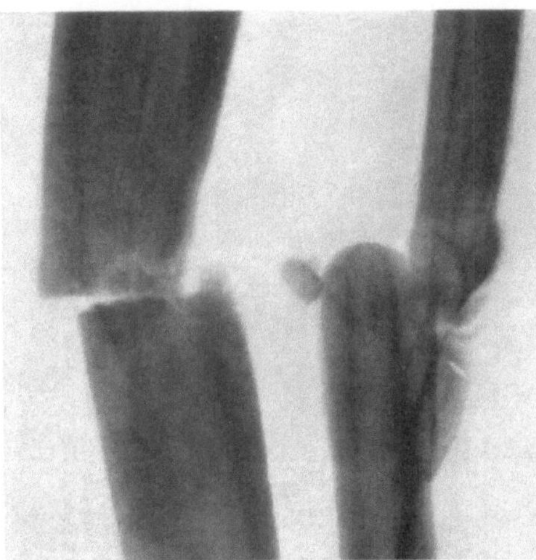

Der frische Knochenbruch zeigt breite Berührung
der Tibiafragmente (in beiden Bildebenen).

The recent fracture shows extensive contact of the
fibrous fragments (in both planes).

6 Wochen später ist eine Ecke der oberen Bruchfläche
demarkiert.

Six weeks later, a corner of the upper surface
of fracture shows demarkation.

5.

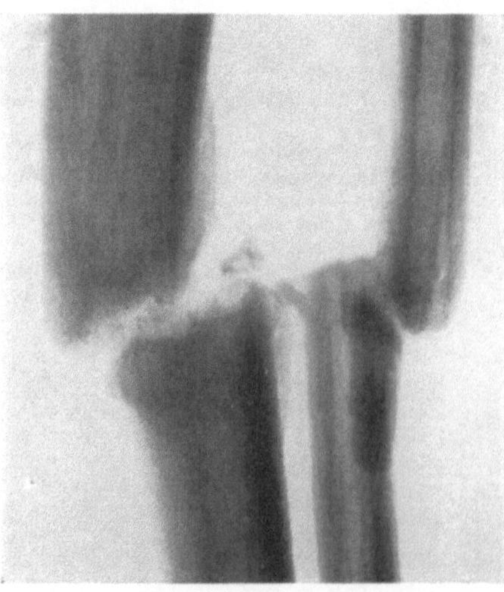

6 Monate nach dem Unfall sind die Knochenenden noch mehr ausgeschliffen und der Spalt noch deutlicher:
das Falschgelenk ist ausgebildet und befand sich nach weiteren 5 Monaten in demselben Zustand.

Six months after the accident the bone ends are further consumed and the cleft more distinct. The false
joint is complete. No alteration after a further five months.

Serie 129.

3.

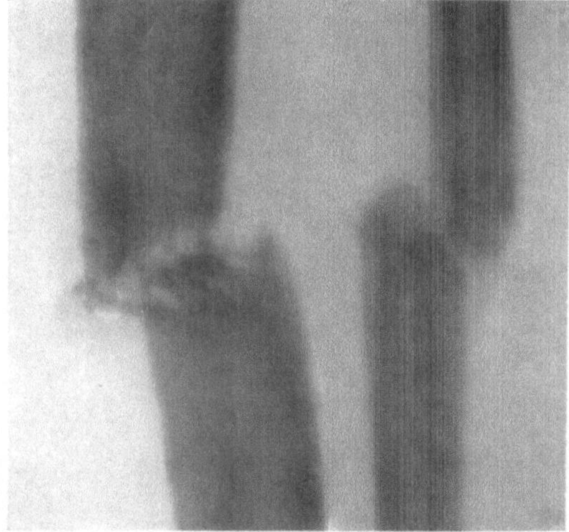

4.

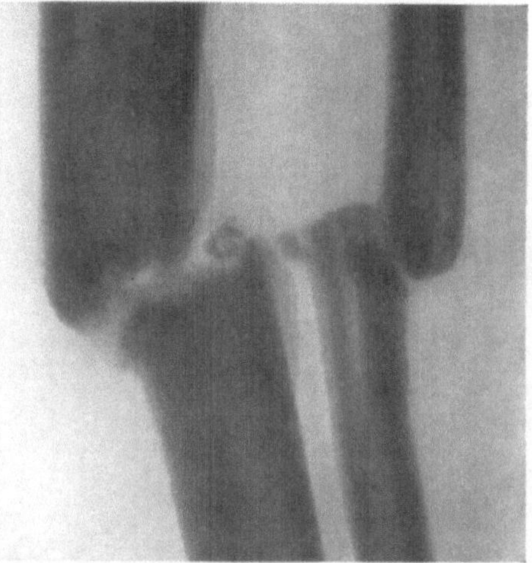

Nach weiteren 3 Wochen ist der kleine Sequester des oberen Fragmentes resorbiert bzw. narbig umgewandelt; inzwischen ist aber auch eine Sequestrierung an der unteren Bruchfläche erfolgt.

Within another three weeks the small sequestrum of the upper fragment has been absorbed in the course of cicatrization. In the meantime, sequestration of the lower fracture surface has taken place.

Nach knapp 5 Monaten sind die Randsequester nicht mehr erkennbar.

After just five months the marginal sequestra are no longer recognizable.

Serie 130.

Pseudarthrose am Unterarm.

Der durch direkte Gewaltwirkung entstandene Splitter-
bruch beider Unterarmknochen zeigte trotz sachgemäßer
Schienenbehandlung noch nach 5 Monaten keinen Callus,
weshalb die Naht der angefrischten Knochenenden ausgeführt wurde. Auch dann heilte nur der Bruch der Ulna
knöchern, am Radius entstand trotz der Drahtfixierung
eine Pseudarthrose, die bei der Pro- und Supination einen
Teil der Funktion des Radiusköpfchengelenkes übernimmt.

Series 130.

Pseudarthrosis.

The two forearm bones had sustained a comminuted fracture caused by direct force. Although correctly treated
and put into splints, no callus had formed: at the end
of five months. The bones were therefore scraped and
joined with wire. Even then only the ulna fracture ossified.
In spite of the wire fixation, pseudarthrosis developed at
the radius, which, during pronation and supination, partly
encroached upon the function of the radius head.

$^6/_{10}$ n. Gr.   1.   2.

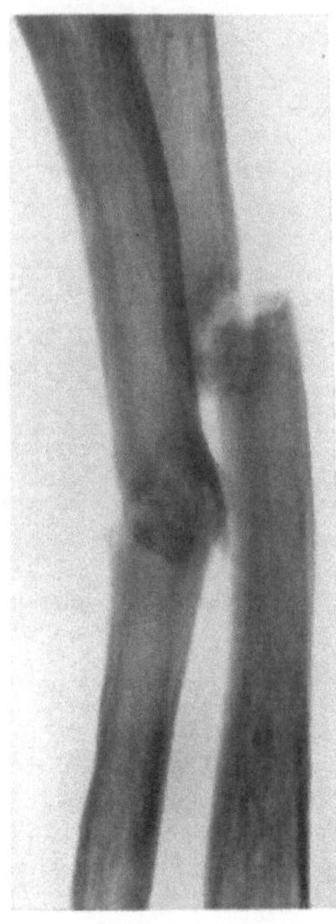
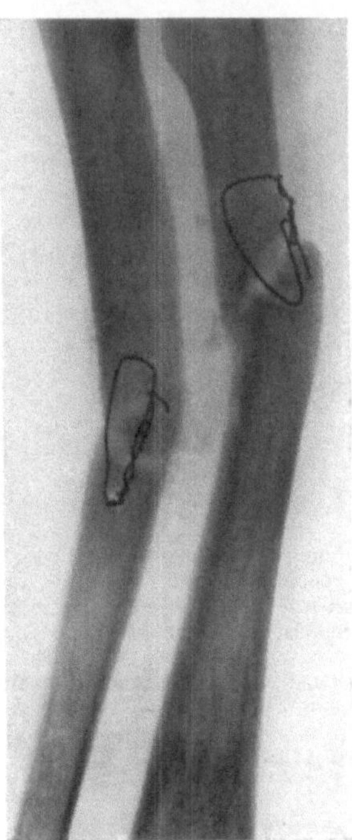

5 Monate nach dem Unfall fehlt jede Calluswucherung.

Five months after accident, there is no callus growth.

8 Monate nach der Verletzung — 3 Monate nach der Knochen
naht — ist der Bruch noch nicht geheilt.

Eight months after accident and three months after the bon
ends had been joined by wire, there was no sign of healing

Serie 130.

3.

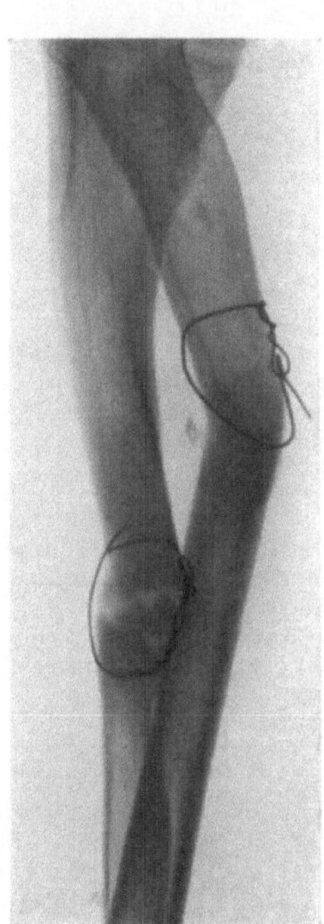

Nach 2 Jahren ist der Bruch der Ulna knöchern verheilt, am Radius aber hat sich eine Pseudarthrose ausgebildet.

After two years, the fracture of the ulna has ossified but pseudarthrosis has developed in the radius.

Serie 131.
Typische Radiusfraktur.

Das 14jährige Mädchen erlitt durch einen Sturz
eine schwere Radiusfraktur. Obwohl eine genaue
Einrichtung nicht gelang und obwohl der Bruch
durch die Wachstumsfuge ging, sind nach Abschluß des Wachstums die Verletzungsfolgen am
distalen Radiusende ausgeglichen: Struktur und
Form sind glatt, eine Wachstumshemmung war
nicht eingetreten.

Series 131.
Typical Fracture of Radius.

A girl of fourteen had a fall which caused a
severe fracture of the radius. Although an exact
setting was not obtained and although the fracture passed through the epiphysis, the effects of
the injury at the distal end of the radius were
counteracted. The structure and shape became
smooth and growth was not hindered.

⁴/₅ n. Gr.   1.   2.

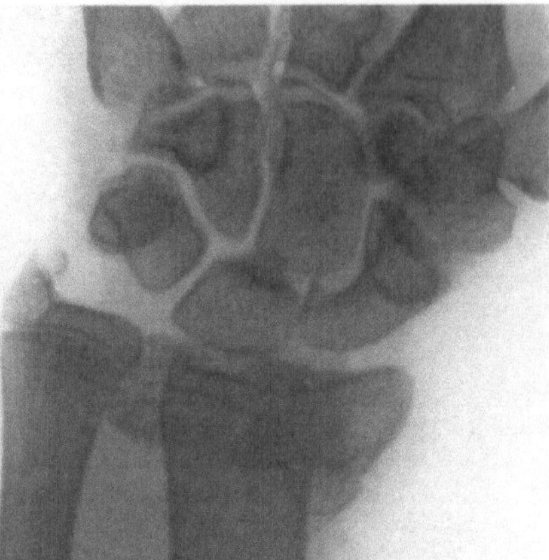
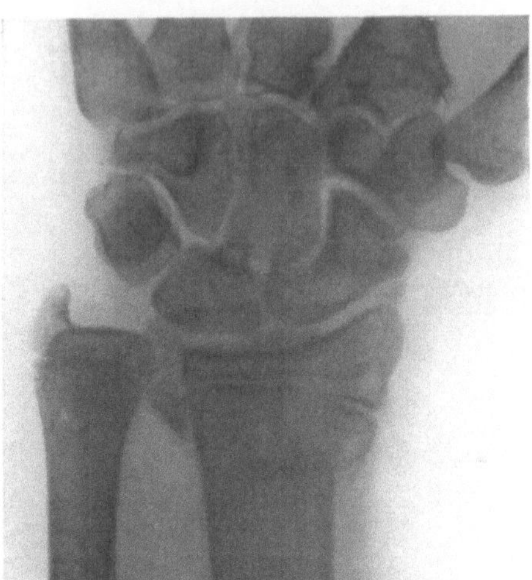

Der frische Knochenbruch: Mehrfache Splitterung und Stauchung der Bruchstücke; Fraktur
der Epiphysenfuge.
The recent fracture. Considerable splintering
and jumbling together of the broken pieces;
fracture of epiphyseal line.

Nach der Einrichtung ist die Stauchung nur
teilweise ausgeglichen.
After setting, the jumbling only partly
counteracted.

3.

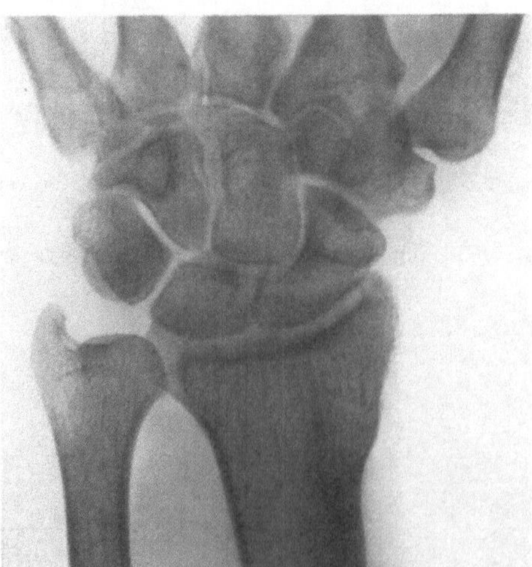

Nach 7 Jahren ist das distale Radiusende wohl geformt, kaum erkennbar verdickt.
After seven years, the ends of the radius are well shaped and very slightly thicker.

Serie 132.

Series 132.

Radiusfraktur.

Fracture of Radius.

In wenigen Wochen glich das Wachstum die Verletzung des peripheren Radiusendes aus, mit Wiederherstellung der geschädigten Wachstumsfuge.

Within a few weeks, the injury of the peripheral ends of the radius was repaired by growth and the injured growth area was restored.

$^3/_4$ n. Gr.   1.   · 2.   3.

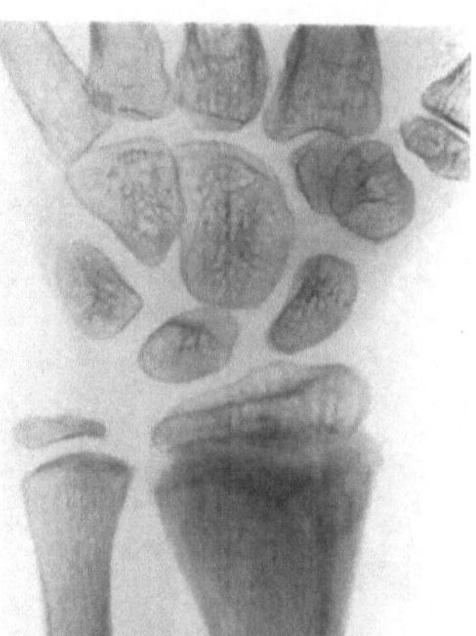

Bruch des distalen Radiusendes mit Stauchung und Splitterung der Wachstumsfuge.

Fracture of the distal radial end with crushed and splintered epiphysis.

3 Wochen später ist der die Epiphysenfuge durchziehende Bruchspalt ausgefüllt.

Three weeks later. The fracture-cleft which passes through the epiphyseal line is filled out.

Nach 8 Wochen ist auch die äußere Form geglättet.

After eight weeks. The outer shape also has become smooth.

4.   5.

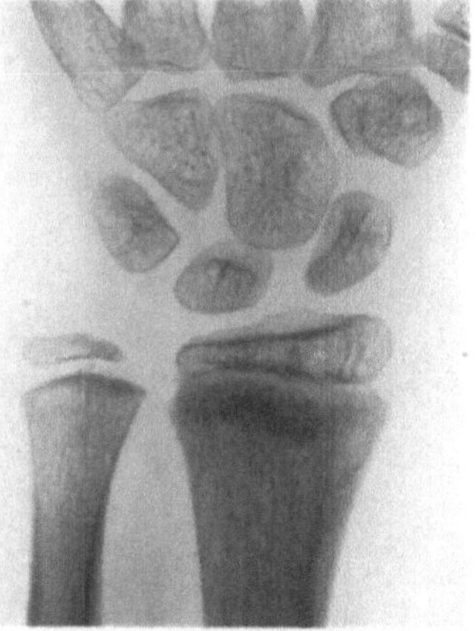

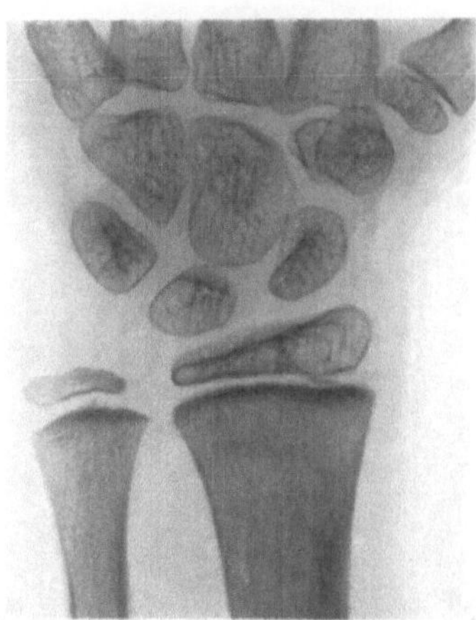

Nach $^1/_4$ Jahr ist ein weiterer Ausgleich durch die Wachstumsstreckung erfolgt.

After three months. Growth has resulted in a further uniformity.

Schon nach $^1/_2$ Jahr lassen Form und Struktur des Knochens die stattgehabte Verletzung nicht mehr erkennen; die Epiphysenfuge ist wiederhergestellt, nur ein verkalkter Strich in ihr deutet die Bruchlinie an.

Six months later. The shape and structure of the bone defy recognition of the late injury. The epiphysis line has been renewed and the fracture is only indicated by a chalk-line.

Serie 133.
Epiphysenfraktur.

Der Oberschenkelbruch in der Wachstumsfuge
wurde, nachdem er genau eingerichtet war, in
normaler Zeit knöchern fest. Aber dadurch verknöcherte der Wachstumsknorpel und verlor seine
proliferierende Fähigkeit, so daß vor der Zeit (im
10. Lebensjahr) das von dieser Stelle ausgehende
Längenwachstum ein Ende fand.

Series 133.
Fracture of the Epiphysis.

The fracture of upper leg through the epiphysis,
after exact correction, became bonily firm within
a normal period. But the growth-cartilage ossified
and lost its capability of proliferation, thus causing
longitudinal growth to be suspended in this
situation. (Patient, aged 10.)

$^{1}/_{2}$ n. Gr.

1.

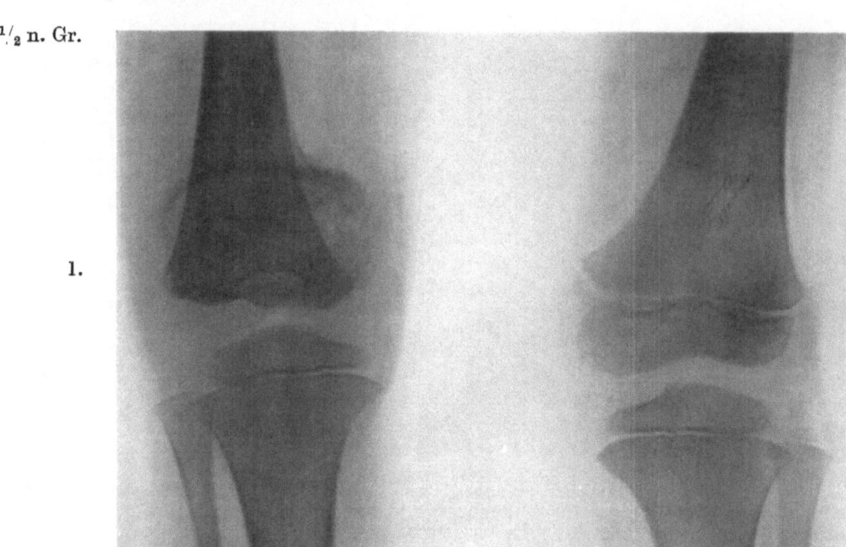

Bruch des linken Oberschenkels in der unteren Wachstumsfuge mit weiter Verschiebung der Fragmente.
Fracture of the left femur through the lower epiphysis with wide displacement of fragments.

2 a.

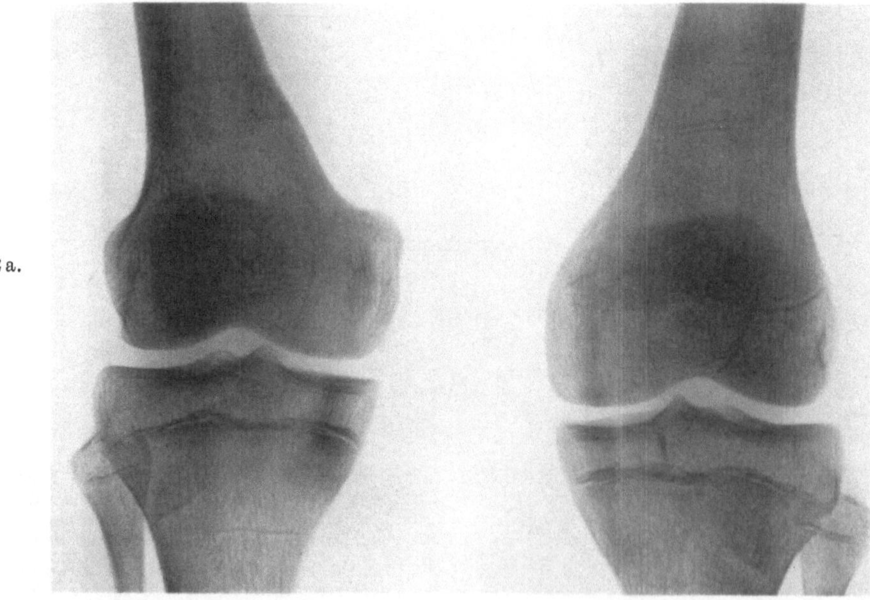

Nach 5 Jahren — im 16. Lebensjahr — ist an dem verletzten Femur keine Spur einer Wachstumsfuge
erkennbar, während sie am anderen Oberschenkel noch angedeutet ist.
After five years, in sixteenth year. No sign of epiphysis in the injured femur is recognizable, while
in the other femur it is just visible.

Serie 133.

4/10 n. Gr.   2 b.

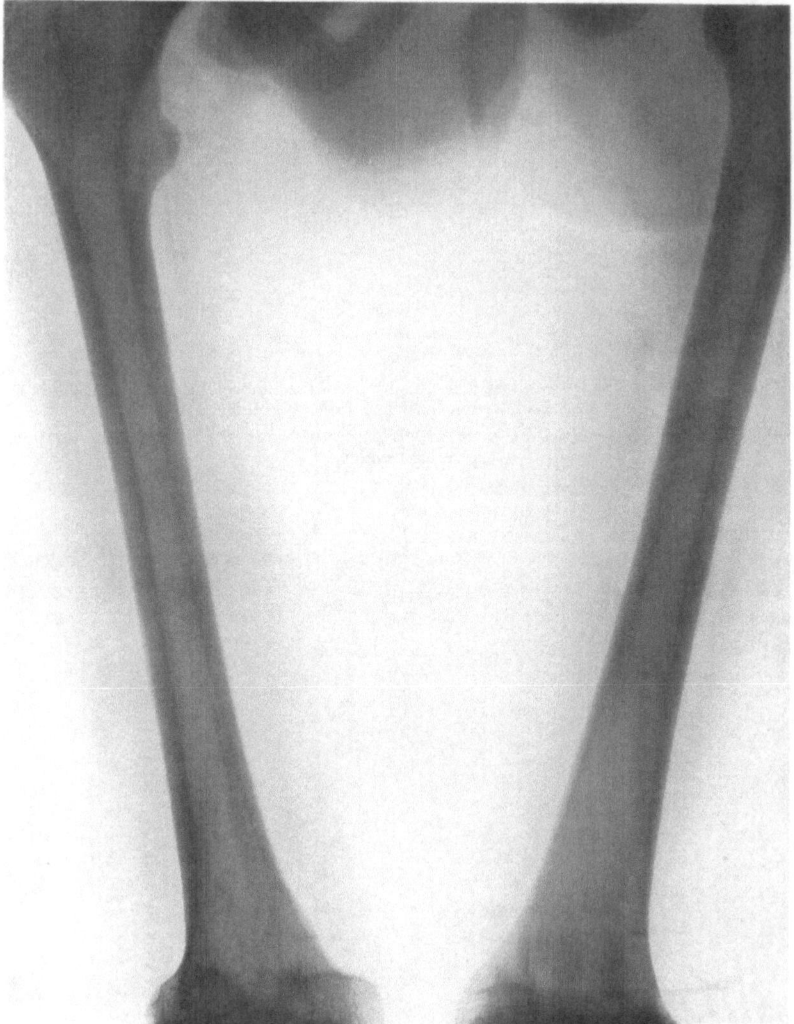

Es besteht eine Verkürzung von 5 cm.
There now remains a shortening of 5 cm.

Serie 134.

Symphysenfraktur.

Der offene Symphysenbruch an der linken Knorpel-
Knochengrenze heilte ohne Eiterung; er hatte eine
frühere Ossification des verletzten Knorpelfugenteiles
zur Folge.

Series 134.

Symphysis-Fracture.

The open symphysis fracture at the left cartilage-
bone boundary healed without pus formation. A premature ossification of the injured part of cartilage
border ensued.

1.

⁶/₁₀ n. Gr.

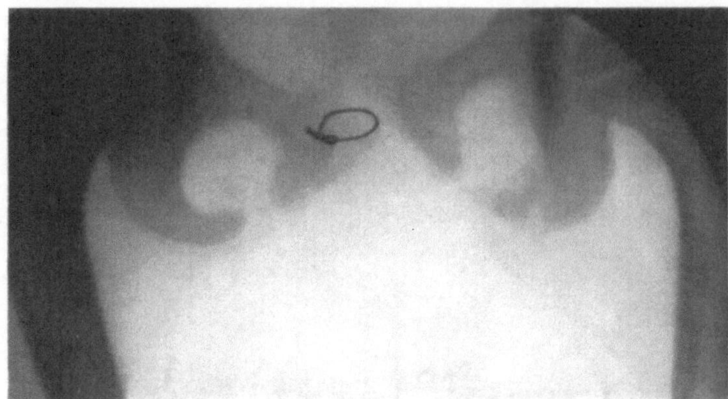

Der durchbrochene Beckenring ist durch eine Drahtnaht, welche links den Knochen
und rechts den Knorpel faßt, vereinigt.

The broken pelvis ring has been united by wire which passes through the bone on the left and the cartilage
on the right.

2.

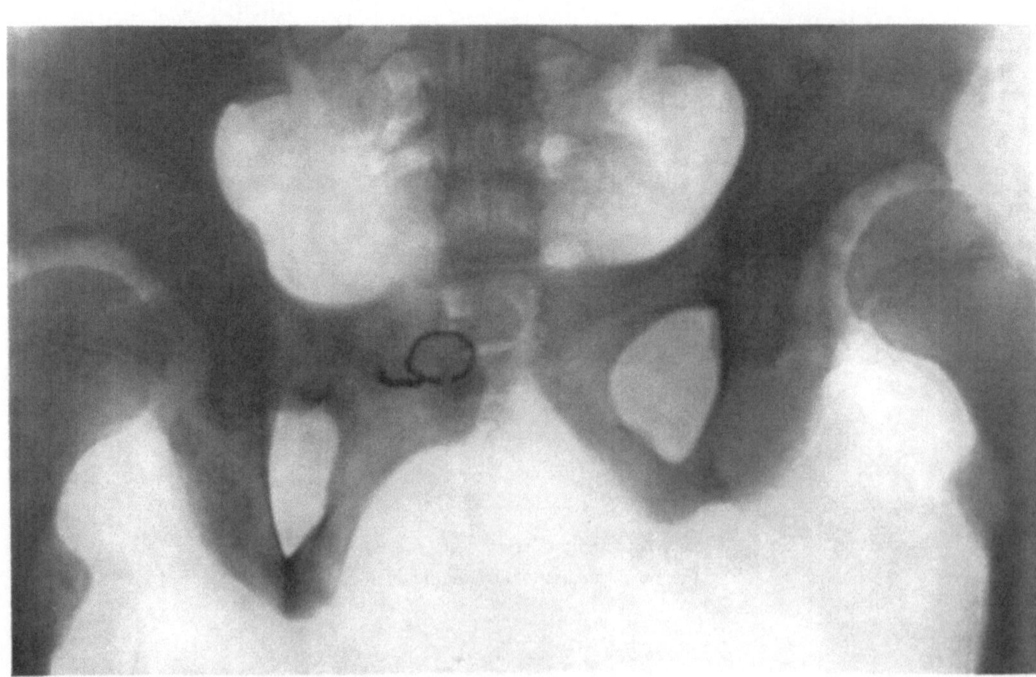

Nach 6 Jahren — im 10. Lebensjahr — ist die Ossification links, d. i. an der Bruchlinie, ausgedehnter erfolgt;
der Drahtring ist gesprengt, das Becken etwas unsymmetrisch.

After six years. (The patient is now ten.) The ossification (viz. at the line of fracture), is more extensive on the left.
The wire ring is broken and the pelvis is somewhat unsymmetrical.

Serie 135.

Patellarfraktur.

Die intraartikuläre Verletzung heilte nach operativer
Knochennaht mit voller Funktion und ohne Schädigung
des Kniegelenkes.

²/₃ n. Gr. 1.

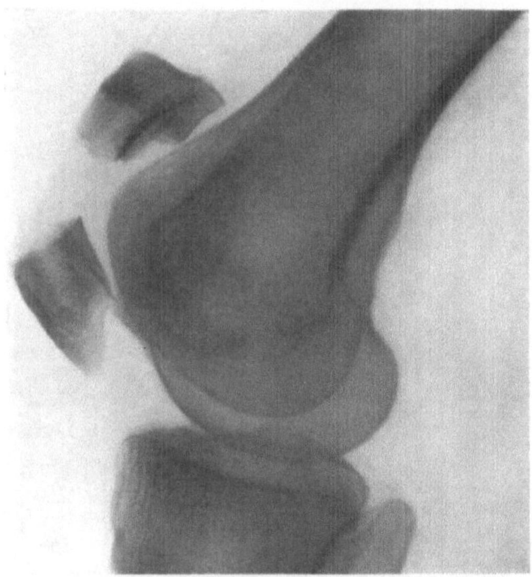

Querbruch der Kniescheibe mit weiter Diastase
der Fragmente.

Diagonal fracture of patella and wide displacement
of fragments.

Series 135.

Fracture of Patella.

After wiring by operation the intra-articular injury
healed with full function and without detriment
to knee-joint.

2.

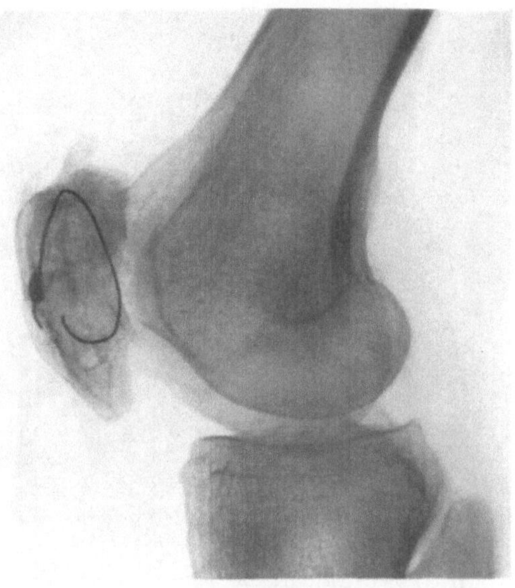

Nach 4 Jahren sind die durch Drahtnaht adaptierten
Bruchstücke fest verwachsen; arthritisch-deformierende
Veränderungen bestehen nicht.

After four years, the fractured parts which were drawn
together by wire, have become firm. Arthritic deformity
does not exist.

Serie 136.

Kniegelenkfraktur.

Der abgebrochene äußere Tibiacondylus heilte (unter Extensionsbehandlung) mit leichter Verschiebung an; dabei wurde in wenigen Monaten volle Funktion und gänzliche Beschwerdefreiheit erreicht.

$^6/_{10}$ n. Gr.   1.

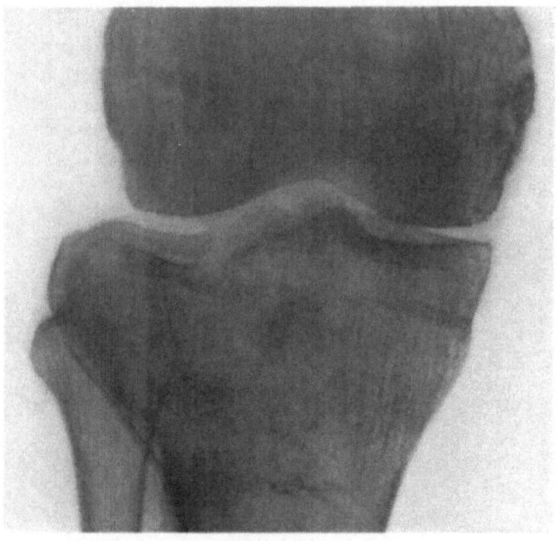

Die frische Gelenkfraktur besteht in einem Abbruch des äußeren Tibiacondylus.

The recent joint fracture consists of the broken — off lateral tibial condyle.

Series 136.

Knee-Joint Fracture.

The broken lateral condyle of the tibia was cured by extension treatment. There was a slight displacement, but within a few months full use was restored and freedom from all complaint attained.

2.

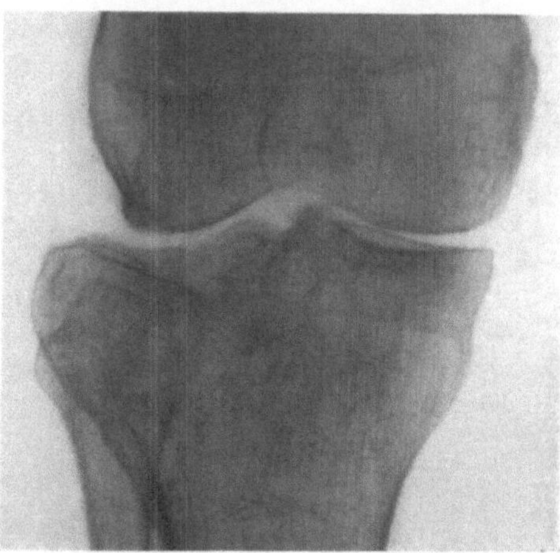

Nach $^1/_4$ Jahr zeigt die verwischte Knochenstruktur die Verwachsung im Bruchspalt an.

After three months. The obliterated bone structure shows the union in the fracture cleft.

Serie 136.

3.

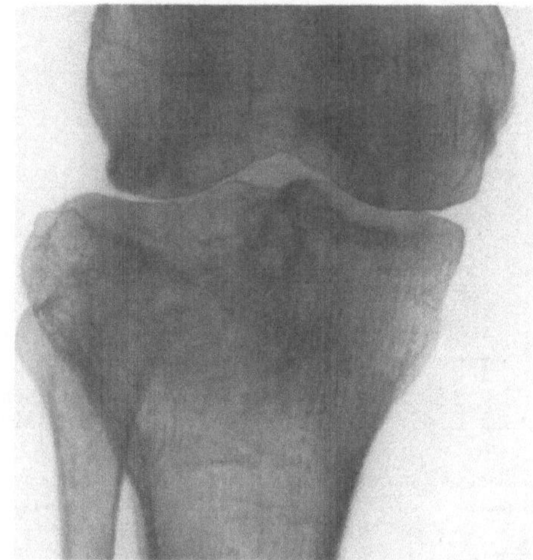

4.

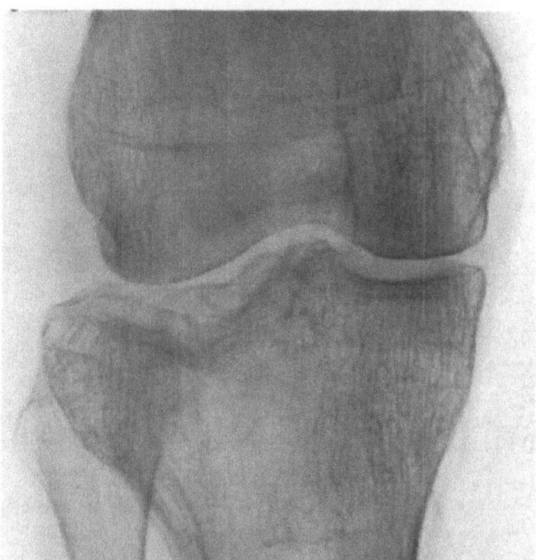

Nach 5 Monaten beginnt die Bälkchenstruktur
wieder hervorzutreten.

After five months. The beam structure becomes
evident again.

Nach 9 Monaten ist der Endzustand erreicht:
der Rand der ein wenig tiefer getretenen
Gelenkfläche ist wieder geschlossen.

After nine months. The final stage is reached.
The rim of the joint surface, which has become
somewhat deeper, is again closed.

Serie 137.

Luxationsfraktur des Sprunggelenkes (Mädchen).

Bei dem 16jährigen Mädchen gelang die exakte Reposition der Luxa ionsfraktur nicht, aber das Wachstum glich die Unebenheit aus, indem es die Gelenkenden entsprechend umformte. Geringe Beschwerden blieben bestehen.

Series 137.

Luxation-Fracture of Ankle-Joint (Girl).

A girl sixteen years of age had a luxation-fracture of ankle-joint. The exact reposition was not attained but growth equalized the unevenness by reforming the joint-ends. A slight functional disorder remained.

$^2/_3$ n. Gr.   1.   2.

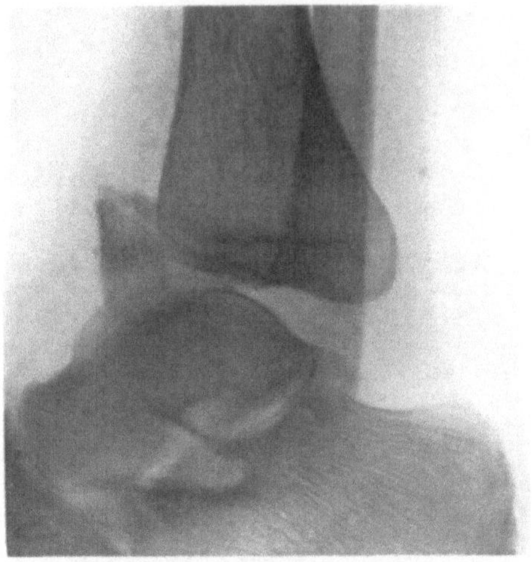 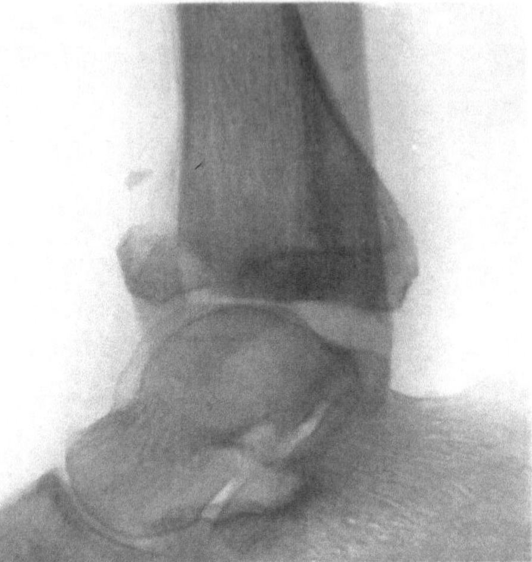

Außer dem Bruch der Knöchel ist die vordere Tibiakante ausgesprengt und das Sprunggelenk subluxiert.

Besides the ankle-fracture, the front tibial edge has sprung off and the ankle-joint is luxated.

Nach 2 Monaten ist das abgebrochene Knochenstück in der verschobenen Lage durch periostalen Callus angewachsen.

After two months, the piece of bone which was broken off has grown in the misplaced position by periosteal callus.

3.

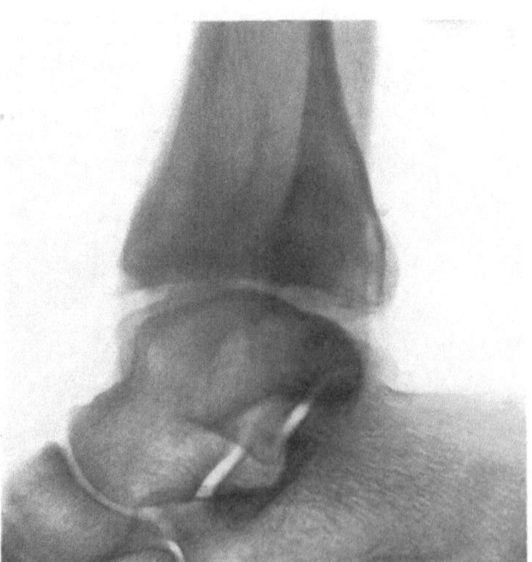

Nach 3 Jahren ist das *Sprunggelenk umgeformt:* das ausgesprengte Knochenstück ist organisch in dem verbreiterten Tibiaende aufgenommen und die Talusrolle entsprechend der veränderten Gelenkfläche der Tibia abgeflacht.

After three years, *the ankle-joint is reformed.* The broken piece of bone has been organically absorbed into the widened tibial end and the talus-roll levelled to correspond to the altered joint surface.

Serie 138.

Luxationsfraktur des Sprunggelenkes (Frau).

Die gleiche Verletzung heilte bei der 38 Jahre alten Frau mit guter Funktion, war aber später immer noch im Röntgenbild genau zu analysieren, da das modellierende Wachstum fehlte.

³/₄ n. Gr.   1.

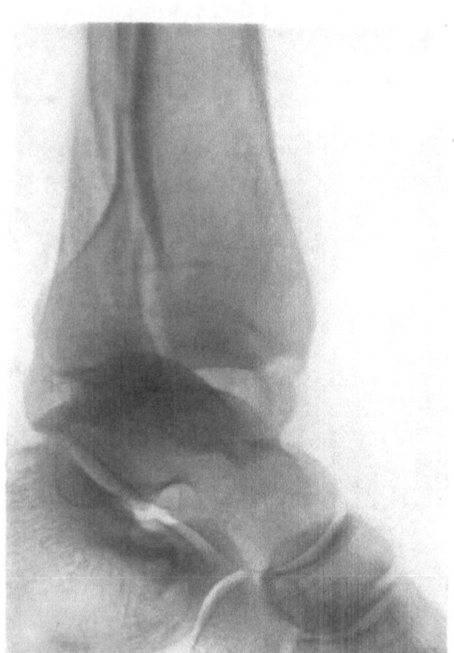

Fraktur beider Knöchel und Abbruch eines kleinen Stückes der vorderen Tibiakante.

Fracture of both ankle bones and a small piece broken off from the anterior tibial edge.

Series 138.

Luxation-Fracture of Ankle-Joint (Woman).

The same injury to a woman of thirty-eight healed with good function. Later, in X-ray-photo it could be distinctly recognized, owing to the absence of modelling growth.

2.

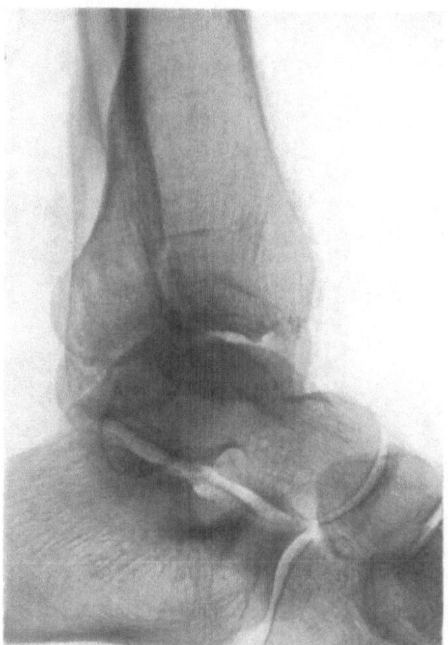

Nach 4 Jahren sind die abgebrochenen Knochenenden in derselben — leicht verschobenen — Stellung knöchern verwachsen; eine Modellierung ist nicht erfolgt.

After four years, the broken bone ends have grown together in a slightly misplaced position. Remodelling has not taken place.

Serie 139.

Binnenverletzung des Knie-
gelenkes.

Durch einen Sturz auf das Knie kam es zu einem
Abriß der Kreuzbänder samt ihrem Ansatz. Nach
Punktion des Blutergusses und vorübergehender
Ruhigstellung war in 5 Wochen volle Beweglichkeit
des Gelenkes erreicht, die anatomische Heilung aber
— das Anwachsen der Eminentia intercondyloidea —
war nach 1 Jahr noch nicht beendet.

Series 139.

Internal Injury of the
Knee Joint.

The patient fell on his knee and the crucial ligaments with their attachements were torn off. The
blood effusion was aspirated and the knee kept
temporarily at rest. Within five weeks, the entire
function was restored. The anatomical healing —
the reattachment of the eminentia intercondyloidea
— was not complete, even after one year.

$^{7}/_{10}$ n. Gr.   1.

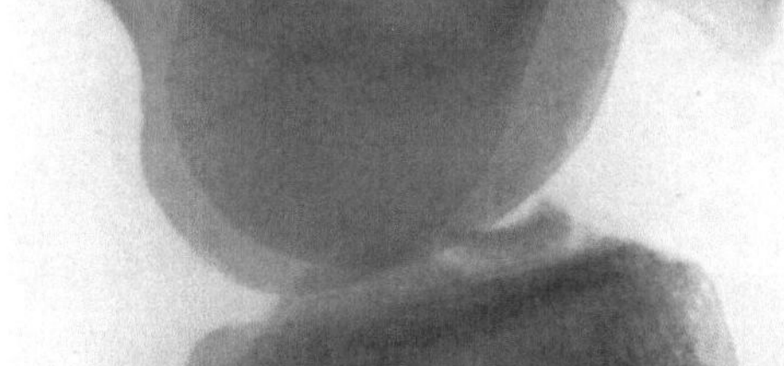

Der Ansatz der Kreuzbänder ist ausgerissen.

The attachments of the crucial ligaments have been
torn off.

2.

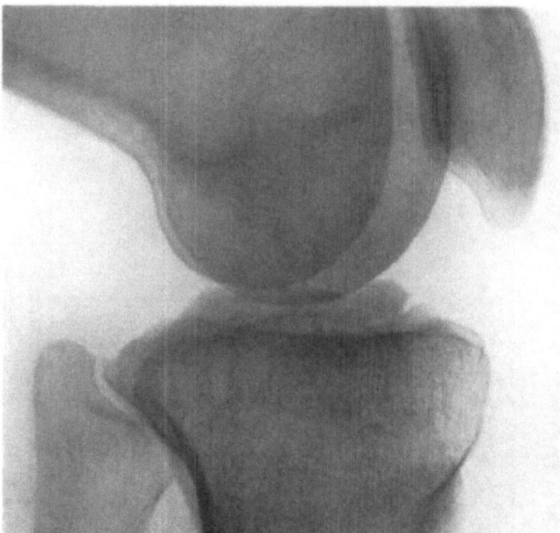

Nach 9 Wochen ist dieses Knorpel-Knochenstück
erst in der Mitte wieder angewachsen.

After nine weeks this cartilage-bone piece is only
reattached in the centre.

Serie 139.

3.

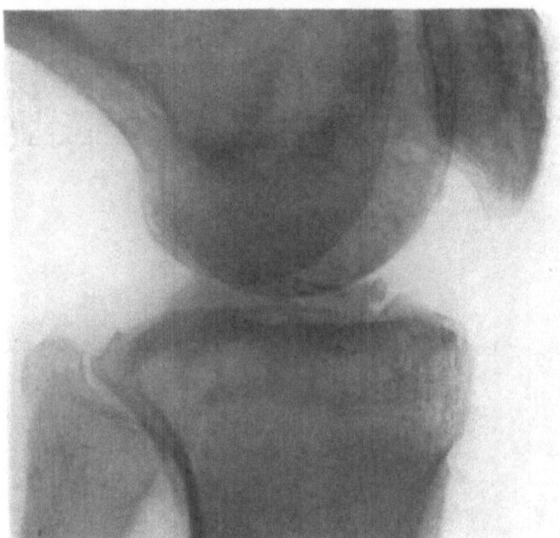

4.

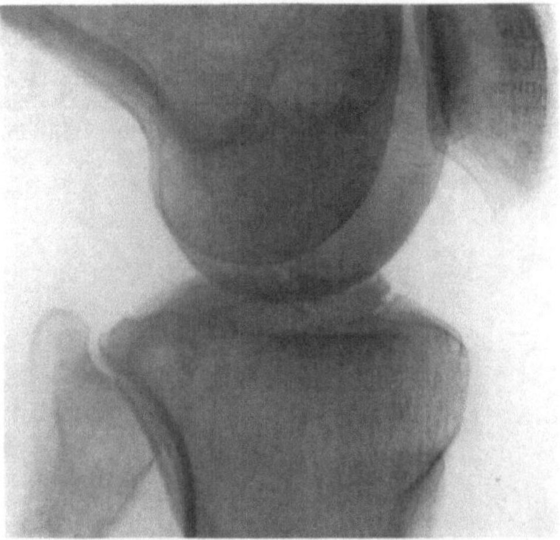

Nach 11 Monaten ist nur eine schmale Knochenspange mehr gewachsen.

After eleven months only a narrow bridge of bone
has grown.

Nach 1¼ Jahr ist seitlich noch ein Spalt vorhanden.

After fifteen months there is still a cleft on the side.

$^6/_{10}$ n. Gr.

5.

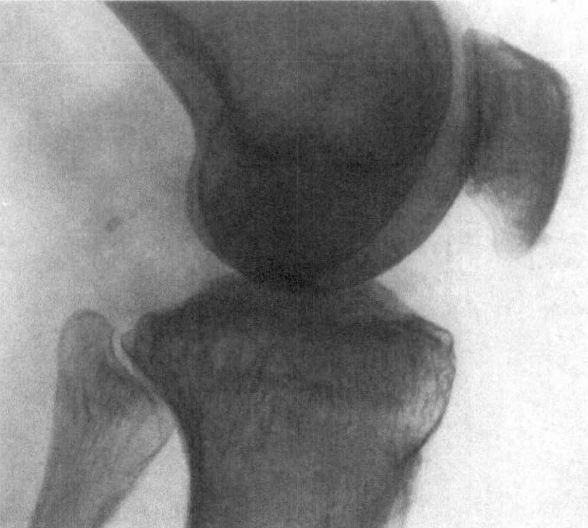

Nach 2 Jahren ist auch diese Lücke ausgefüllt und jetzt erst ist die Ansatzplatte der Kreuzbänder
ganz angewachsen.

After two years this gap has also filled out and the crucial ligaments fully united.

Anhang.

Serie 140.

Fractura colli femoris.

Bei dem 72jährigen Mann heilte die subcapitale (mediale) Schenkelhalsfraktur in charakteristischer Weise: unter zunehmendem Schwund des Schenkelhalses trat eine bindegewebige — pseudarthrotische — Verwachsung des Kopfes mit dem hochgetretenen Knochenschaft ein.

¹/₂ n. Gr.   1.

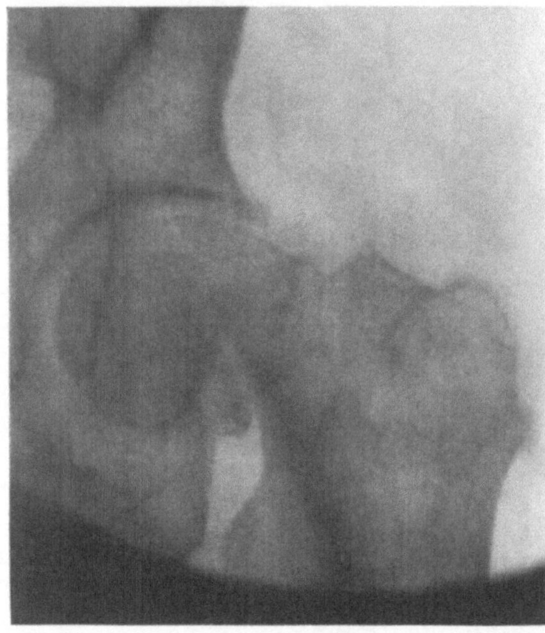

Der frische Knochenbruch zeigt schon einen gewissen Trochanterhochstand.

The recent fracture already shows the displacement of trochanter.

Supplement.

Series 140.

Fracture of Neck of Femur.

In a seventy two year old man the subcapital (medial) fracture of neck of femur healed in a characteristic manner. With increasing resorption of the neck of femur, the head and the updrawn bone shaft are grown together by means of binding texture pseudarthrotically.

2.

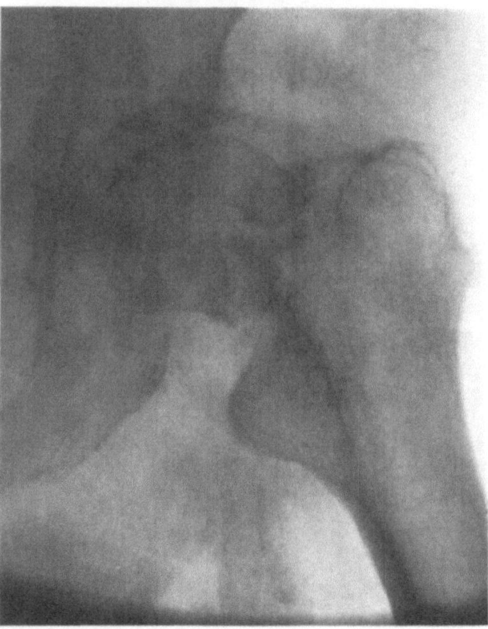

Nach 6 Wochen — Behandlung im Streckverband — ist ein Teil des Schenkelhalses bereits resorbiert.

After six weeks treatment in extension, a part of neck of femur has been resorbed.

Serie 140.

3.

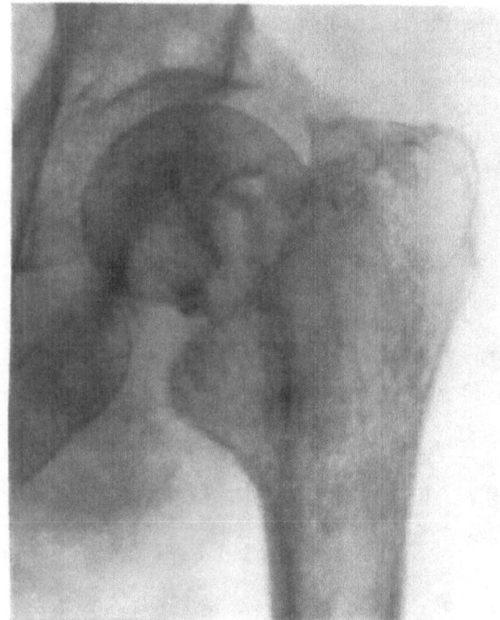

4.

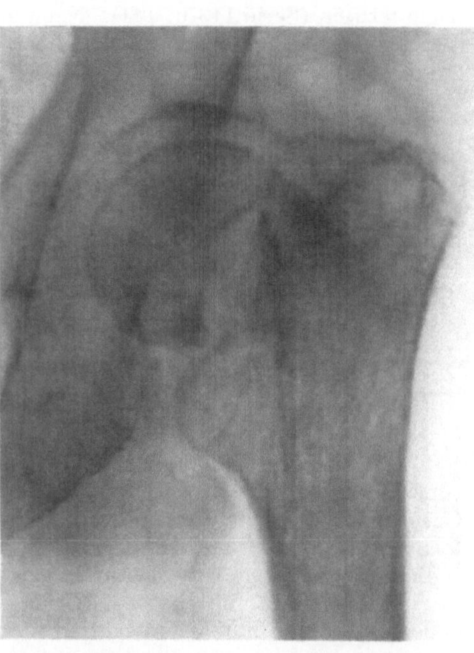

Nach 10 Wochen ist der Schenkelhals ganz ge-
schwunden und der Trochanter noch höher getreten.

After ten weeks, the neck of femur has entirely
disappeared and the trochanter is drawn up still
higher.

Nach 15 Wochen ist die — bindegewebige — Verwachsung so fest, daß der Kranke am Stock gehen kann.

After fifteen weeks the malformation of fibrous tissue
is so firm that the patient is able to walk with the
aid of a stick.

Myositis ossificans — traumatische Knochenatrophie — ischämische Muskelkontraktur.

Leichtere Verletzungen, welche die Gelenke treffen — *Quetschungen und Verstauchungen* —, können *von einer vorübergehenden Kalkverarmung der Knochenenden* begleitet sein (Serie 143 u. 144). Nach einer Verrenkung (besonders des Ellenbogens) kommt es gelegentlich zur Kalkablagerung und Knochenbildung in den paraartikulären Weichteilen. Die bei der Luxation zerrissene Kapsel erfährt leicht degenerative Veränderungen, die in Serie 145 bis zur Verknöcherung führten.

Zirkulationsstörungen an wachsenden Gliedmaßen, wie die sog. ischämische Muskelkontraktur (Serie 147), haben nicht nur eine Degeneration der Weichteile, sondern auch eine Schädigung der Wachstumsfugen zur Folge, die vor der Zeit verknöchern. — Beim Erwachsenen trat im Falle der Serie 146 nach Zerreißung der Hauptschlagader eine Knochenatrophie ein.

Supplement.

Myositis Ossificans — Traumatic Bone Atrophy — Ischaemic Muscle-Contraction.

Slight injuries which affect the joints, such as contusions and sprains are sometimes accompanied by temporary decalcification of the bone ends. (Series 143—144.) Occasionally after a dislocation (particularly of the elbow), calcification and bone formation occur in the peri-articular fleshy parts. If the capsule has been torn, it is liable to undergo a degenerative change which, in series 145, led to ossification.

The results of circulatory disturbances in the growing limbs, such as the so-called ischaemic muscle-contraction (Series 147), led to a degeneration of the fleshy parts and injury to the epiphyseal line with subsequent premature ossification. In the case of an adult (Series 146), bone atrophy resulted from the tearing of one of the main arteries.

Serie 141.

Myositis ossificans circumscripta.

Nach einfacher Verrenkung des Ellenbogens, die sogleich eingerichtet wurde, bildete sich die für diese Verletzung charakteristische Verknöcherung im M. biceps: das retikuläre Bindegewebe des Muskelinterstitiums entwickelte sich weiter zu echtem Knochen.

Series 141.

Circumscribed Myositis Ossificans.

After a simple elbow sprain which was immediately set, the characteristic ossification, which is not uncommon after this injury, formed in the biceps muscle and the reticular connective tissue of the muscle interstitium developed into real bone.

$^2/_3$ n. Gr.   1.   2.

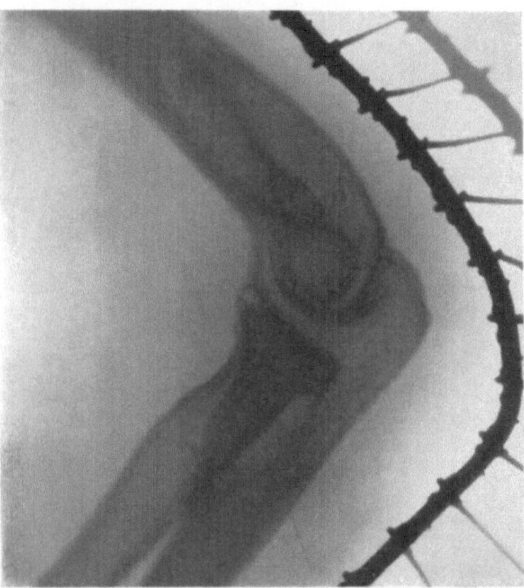

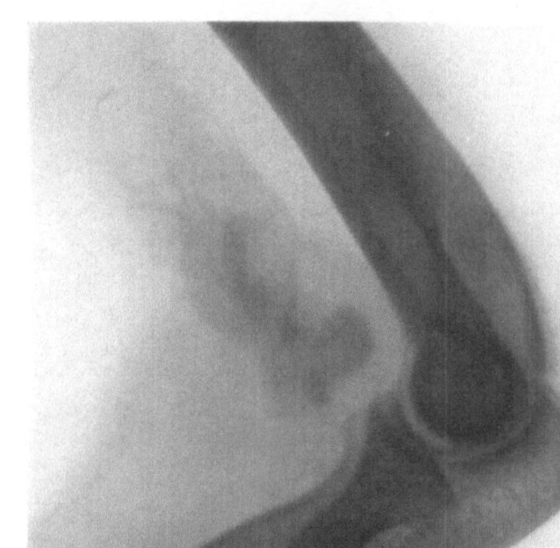

Der frisch eingerichtete Ellenbogen zeigt keine Knochenabsprengung.
The recently set elbow shows no splinters.

4 Wochen nach der Verletzung ist eine ausgedehnte Kalkablagerung in der Muskulatur nachweisbar.
Four weeks after accident, an extensive chalk deposit can be seen in the muscle.

3.

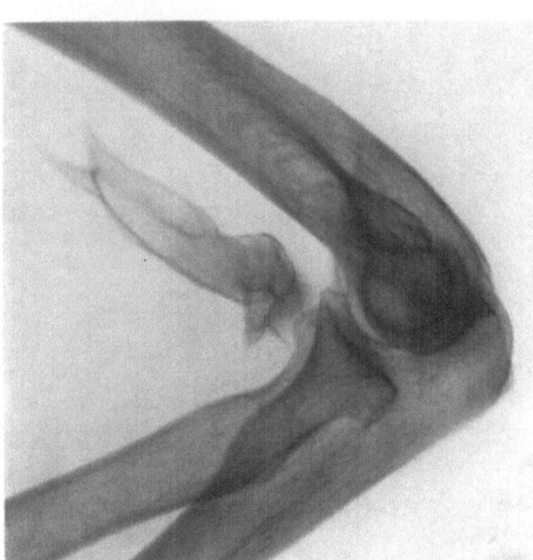

7 Jahre später findet sich an dieser Stelle ein langer, strukturierter Muskelknochen.
Seven years later at the same place there is a long constructed portion of ossified muscle.

Serie 142.

Myositis ossificans circumscripta.

Die Distorsion des Ellenbogengelenkes war mit einer kleinen Knochenabsprengung und einem erheblichen Bluterguß der Weichteile verbunden, der zu Kalkablagerung und Knochenbildung im M. biceps führte.

$^7/_{10}$ n. Gr.

Series 142.

Circumscribed Myositis Ossificans.

Besides the distortion of the elbow-joint, a small piece of bone had splintered and there was a considerable blood-effusion in the fleshy parts which led to chalk-deposit and bone building in m. biceps.

1.

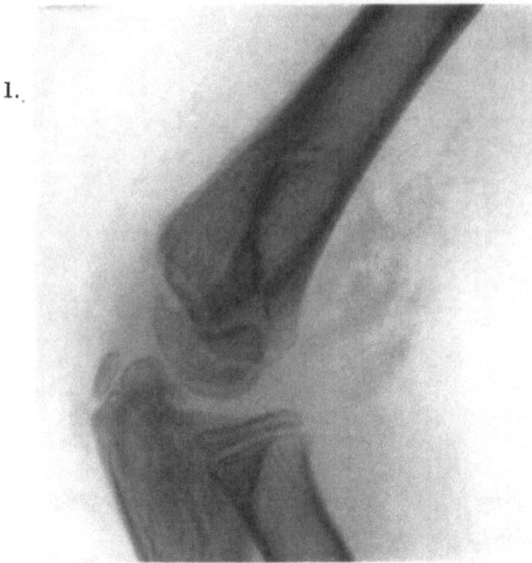

6 Wochen nach dem Unfall ist eine ausgedehnte Kalkablagerung in der Beugemuskulatur des Oberarmes nachweisbar.

Six weeks after accident, an extensive chalk-deposit is visible in the flexor muscles of forearm.

2.

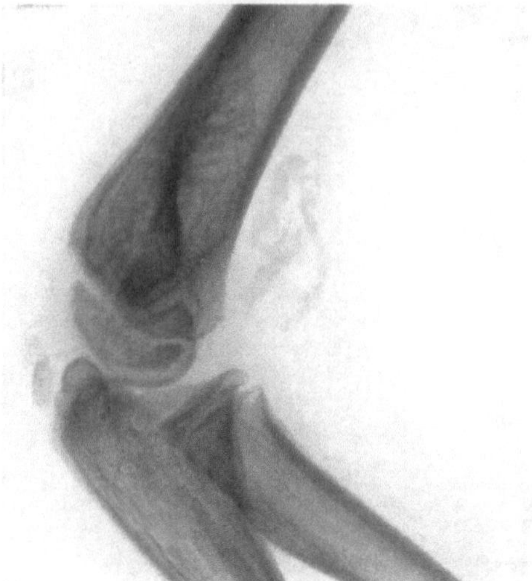

Nach 9 Wochen ist *ein Teil des niedergeschlagenen Kalkes resorbiert.*

After nine weeks, the chalk deposit is partly resorbed.

3.

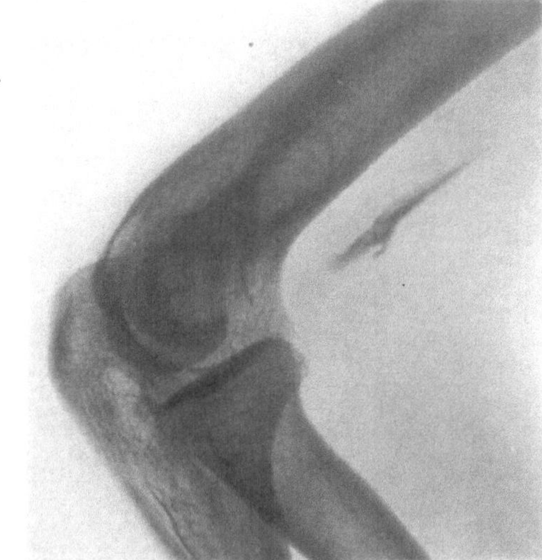

Nach 7 Jahren besteht an dieser Stelle ein schmaler *Knochen*span.
After seven years, there is a small bone-splinter at this place.

Serie 143.

Gelenkverstauchung.

Die Band- und Kapselzerreißung ging mit einem Bluterguß in das Gelenk einher. Ohne daß strenge Bettruhe innegehalten wurde, stellte sich eine *Kalkverarmung* der knöchernen Gelenkanteile (besonders des Femur und der Patella) ein, die in wenigen Wochen mit der Heilung der anderen Verletzungsfolgen gleichfalls ausgeglichen war.

Series 143.

Joint-Sprain.

Besides the torn tendon and capsule there was a blood effusion in the joint. Though the patient was not entirely confined to bed, a decrease of chalk in the joint parts set in, (particularly in the femur and patella), which however, became normal when the sprain healed after a few weeks.

$^6/_{10}$ n. Gr.   1.

2.

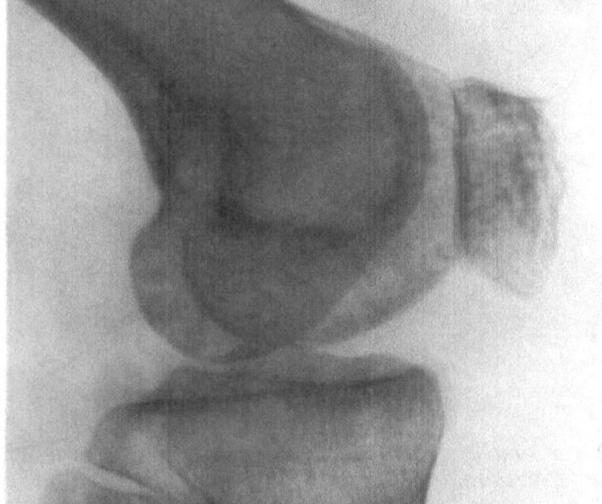

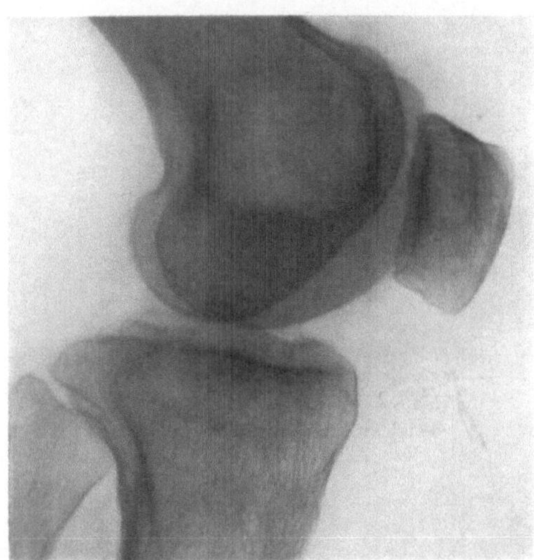

3 Wochen nach dem Unfall ist eine „fleckige Atrophie" (Halisterese) deutlich.

Three weeks after accident. "Speckled atrophy" (Halisteresis) is distinct.

Nach 8 Wochen besteht wieder ein völlig normaler Knochenzustand.

After eight weeks, completely normal condition of bones.

<table>
<tr><td>

Serie 144.

Gelenkkontusion.

Die Knochenatrophie war nach einem Schlag gegen das Knie entstanden, ohne daß ein nennenswerter Erguß vorhanden war. Bettruhe wurde nicht gehalten, aber die Kalkverarmung nahm einen beträchtlichen Grad an und war erst nach Monaten ausgeglichen.

</td><td>

Series 144.

Contusion of the Joint.

The bony atrophy originated from a hit against the knee, but no effusion into the joint worth mentioning, was present. Rest in bed was not considered necessary, but considerable decalcification occurred and was only counteracted after several months.

</td></tr>
</table>

$^6/_{10}$ n. Gr.   1.    2.

<table>
<tr><td>

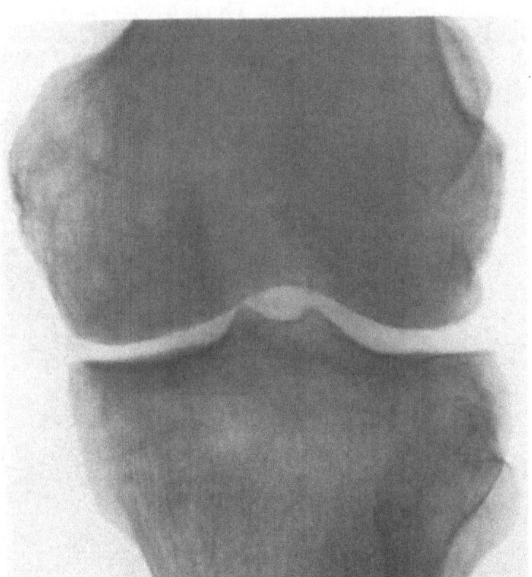

10 Tage nach dem Unfall ist eine unregelmäßig verteilte Kalkverarmung erkennbar.

Ten days after the accident. An irregular decalcification area can be seen.

</td><td>

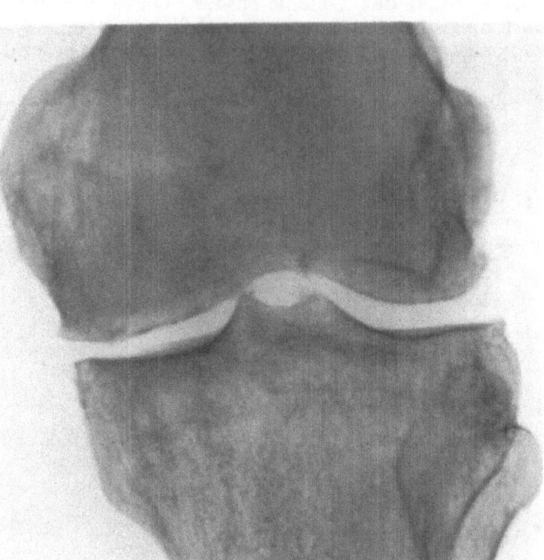

Nach 2 Monaten hat die Halisterese erheblich zugenommen und ist auch in subchondralen Bezirken deutlich.

After two months the halisteresis has increased considerably and is also distinct in the subchondral areas.

</td></tr>
</table>

3.

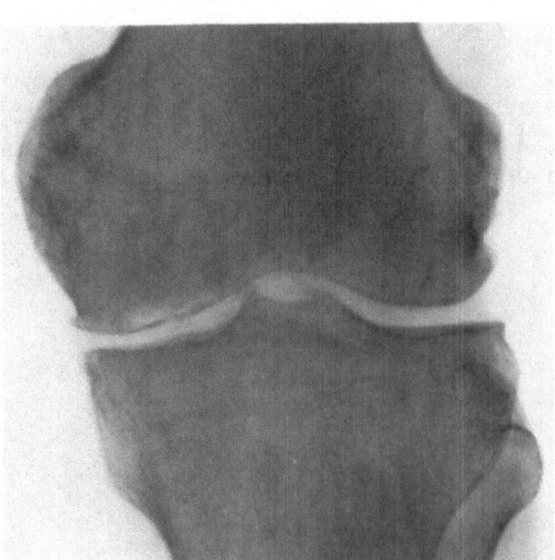

Nach 5 Monaten ist die Atrophie im wesentlichen behoben

After five months the atrophy has practically disappeared.

Serie 145.
Traumatische Arthritis.

Infolge traumatischer Schulterverrenkung, die sofort eingerichtet wurde, entwickelte sich in der verletzten Gelenkkapsel ein Degenerationsprozeß — narbige Umwandlung mit Verkalkungen. Daher klagte der Mann seit dem Unfall über Schmerzen und knackende Geräusche im Gelenk bei Bewegungen des Armes. Im Röntgenbild war ein Hinweis auf die traumatische Synovitis erst nach vielen Monaten in der Verknöcherung des Kapselansatzes ablesbar.

$^2/_3$ n. Gr. 1.

Series 145.
Traumatic Arthritis.

Following upon an accidental dislocation of shoulder, which was immediately set, a degeneration of the joint capsule — scarry change with calcification — developed. The patient complained of pain and crackling sounds in the shoulder-joint whenever he moved his arm. Only after many months could the suggested traumatic synovitis be seen in the X-ray photo, by the ossification of the capsule.

2.

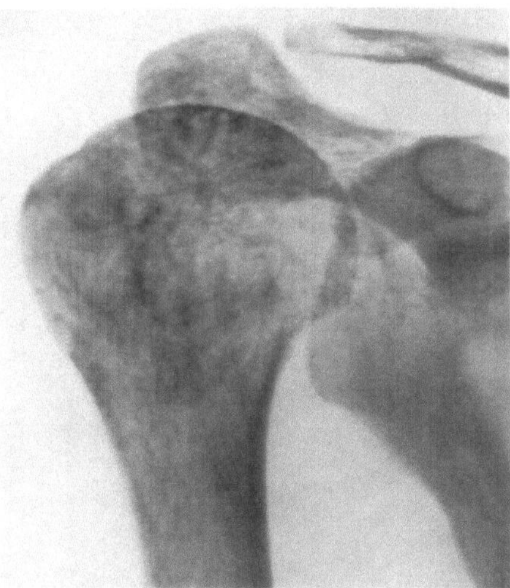

4 Wochen nach der Verletzung besteht eine erhebliche Kalkverarmung („fleckige Atrophie") des Gelenkes.

Four weeks after accident, considerable decalcification at the joint has taken place (Speckled atrophy).

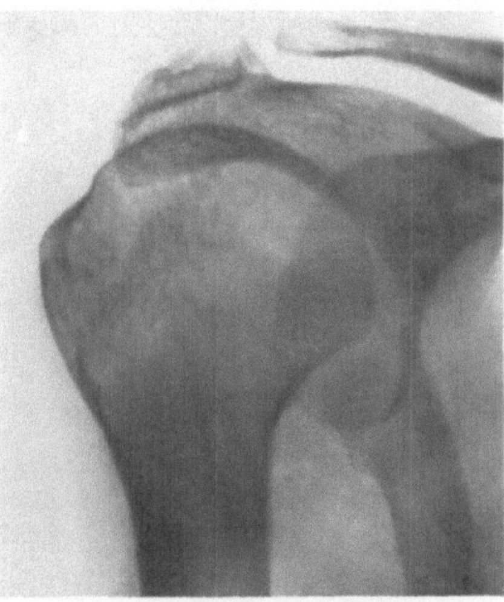

Nach $^1/_2$ Jahr zeigt das Röntgenbild normalen Befund; die Atrophie ist behoben.

After six months, the X-ray photo shows normal condition.

3.

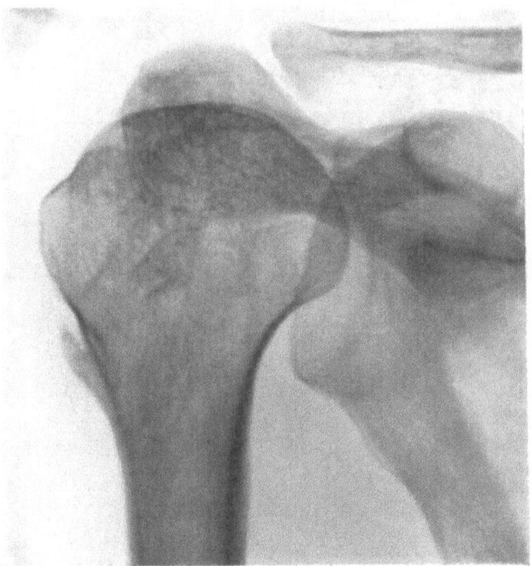

Nach 2 Jahren ist die degenerative Kapselveränderung röntgenologisch an der *Verknöcherung ihres Ansatzes* erkennbar.

After two years, the degenerative change in the capsule is recognized in the Röntgenphoto by the ossification of its attachment.

<table>
<tr><td>

Serie 146.

Knochenatrophie.

Infolge Zerreißung der Art. poplitea kam es zu ausgedehnten Nekrosen der Haut und Unterschenkelmuskulatur, die unter Eiterung in großen Sequestern ausgestoßen wurden. Während des langen Krankenlagers entwickelte sich eine hochgradige Knochenatrophie, die jedoch in einigen Wochen funktioneller Beanspruchung des Beines nahezu ganz behoben war.

</td><td>

Series 146.

Atrophy of Bone.

The tearing of the popliteal artery caused an extensive necrosis of the skin and muscles of the lower leg, which were cast off as sloughs. Considerable bone atrophy developed during the long illness but it almost entirely disappeared after a few weeks functional use of the leg.

</td></tr>
</table>

$^2/_3$ n. Gr. 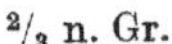    1.

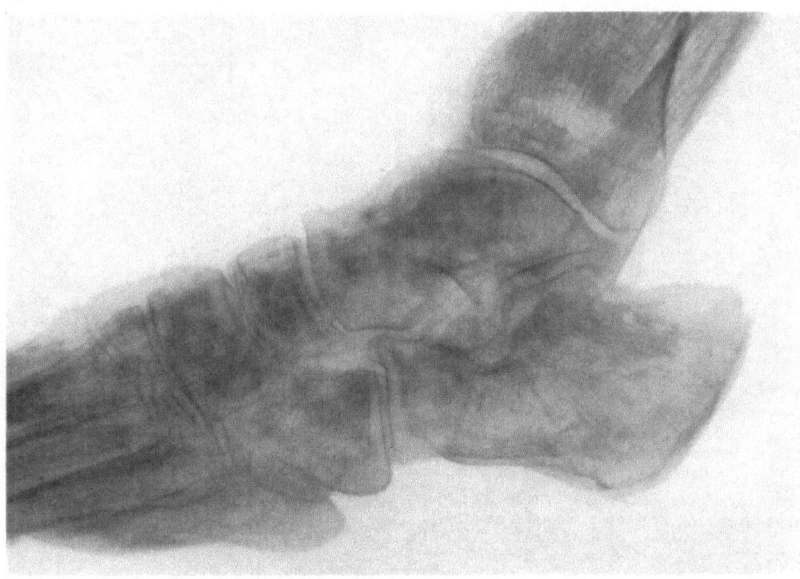

6 Monate nach dem Unfall hat der Kalkschwund des Knochens („fleckige Atrophie") den Höhepunkt erreicht.

Six months after the accident, the chalk consumption of the bone — speckled atrophy — had reached its climax.

Serie 146.

2.

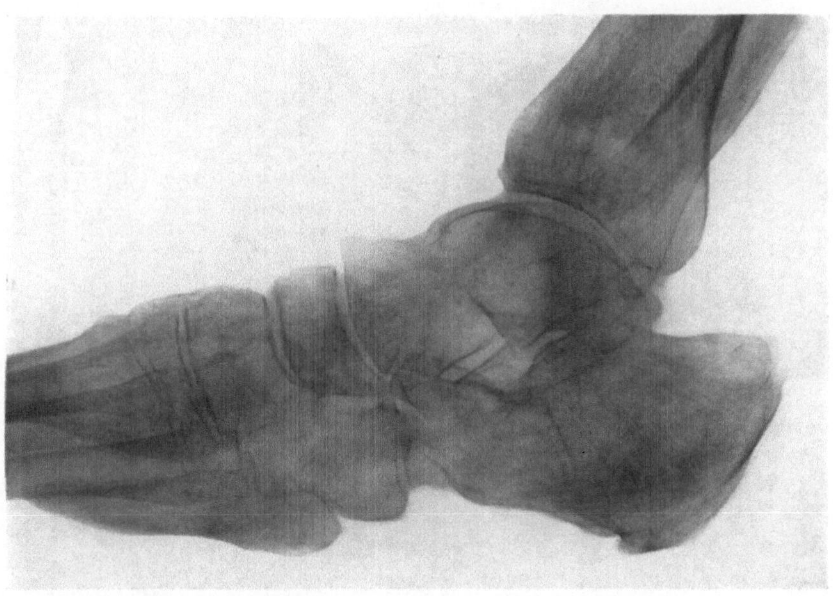

Nach weiteren 3 Monaten regelmäßiger statischer Belastung hat der Knochen fast die normale
Struktur und Kalkdichte wieder erlangt.

Later, after three months constant use, the bone had nearly recovered its normal structure and chalk
compactness.

Serie 147.
Ischämische Muskelkontraktur.

Im Verlauf der Behandlung, welche der 6jährige Knabe wegen der Unterarmverletzung erfuhr, trat der Zustand der ischämischen Muskelkontraktur ein. Die Blutsperre setzte aber auch eine schwere *Schädigung der Wachstumsfugen* des Knochens am Ellenbogen, so daß es zu ihrer frühzeitigen Verknöcherung und infolgedessen zu einer Wachstumshemmung des Unterarmes kam, der im übrigen durch Sehnenverlängerung nahezu voll gebrauchsfähig wurde.

Series 147.
Ischaemie Muscle Contraction.

During the treatment of a six year old boy for an injury to the forearm, an ischaemie muscle contraction set in. The arrested circulation caused considerable disturbance to the growth area in the region of the elbow. Growth of the forearm was prevented by premature ossification. Practically the full use of the arm was obtained by tendon stretching.

$^6/_{10}$ n. Gr.

1 a.

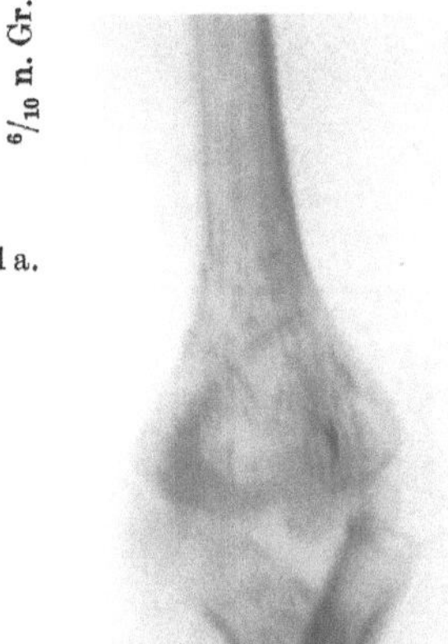

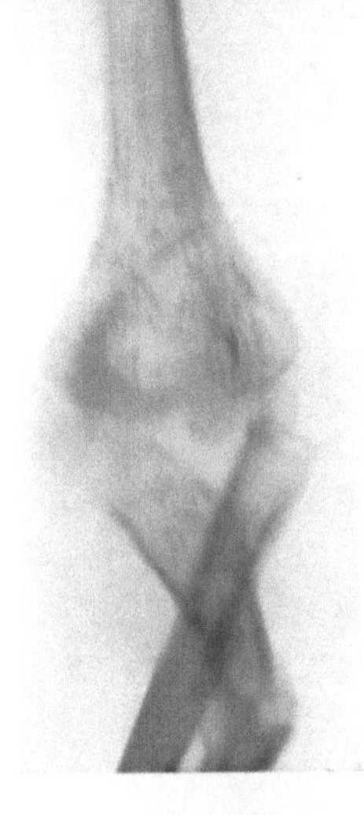

1 b.

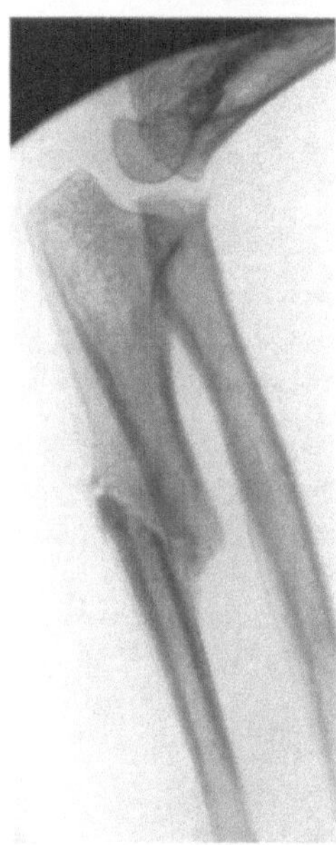

2.

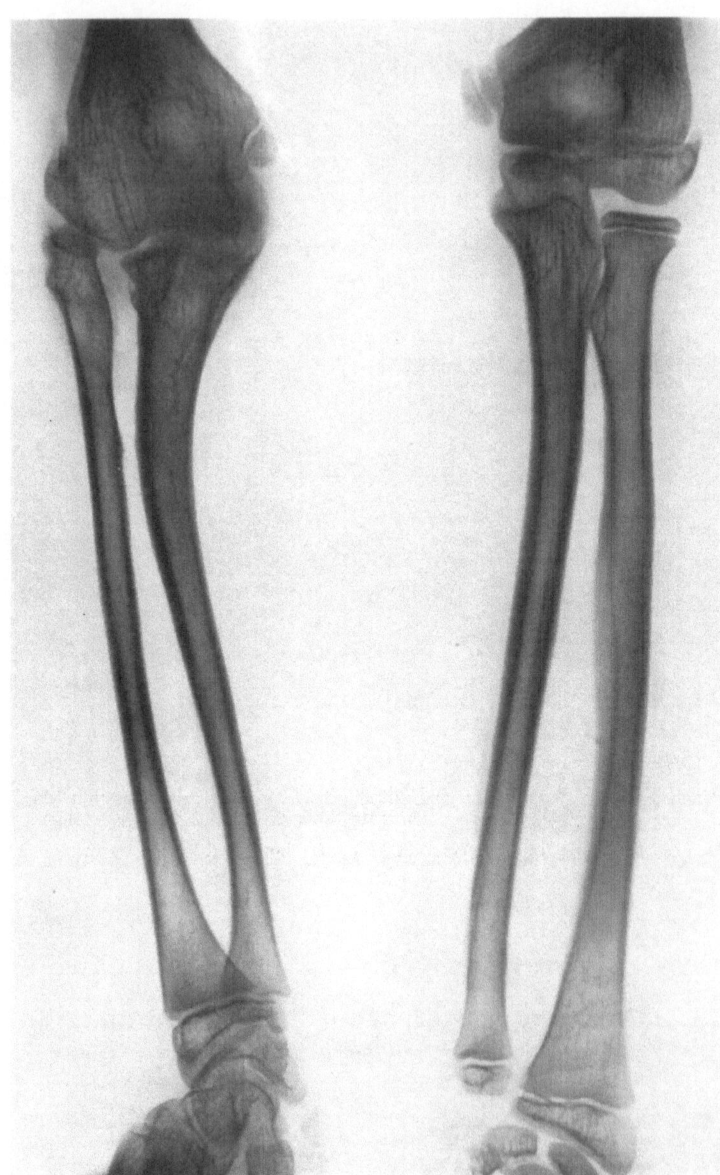

Fraktur der Ulna mit Luxation des Radiusköpfchens.

Fracture of the ulna with luxation of the head of the radius.

7 Jahre später — im 13. Lebensjahr — sind die Hauptwachstumsfugen am Ellenbogen verknöchert und die Verkürzung des Unterarmes beträgt bereits 2 cm. — Die Bruchstelle selbst ist nicht mehr erkennbar.

Seven years later, in the thirteenth year, the main growth areas were ossified and the length of the lower-arm was shortened by two centimetres. The part which was broken is no longer noticeable.

VII. Kapitel (Anhang).

Knochentransplantation und Gelenkbildung.

A. Freie Auto- und Heterotransplantation.

Das Knochengewebe des menschlichen Körpers besitzt einerseits große Lebenszähigkeit bei Zirkulationsunterbrechungen, andererseits eine ideale Regenerationskraft, die größte der feiner differenzierten Gewebe. Infolgedessen läßt sich Knochen frei verpflanzen und wird nach Zerstörung vollwertig erneuert. *Auch nach Beendigung des Wachstums werden große Defekte knöchern ergänzt und es wird*, wie Serie 148 zeigt, *die Wiederherstellung der alten Form angestrebt: eine aufgemeißelte Knochenröhre wird wieder geschlossen.*

In demselben Organismus frei verpflanzt, heilt Knochen ein und wird umgebaut: sein Periost bleibt am Leben, die Corticalis dagegen stirbt ab und wird von der Nachbarschaft (Periost und Wundbett) erneuert. Dieser Vorgang ist auch im Röntgenbild erkennbar. Die aktive Knochenbildung des Transplantatperiostes sehen wir in Serie 149 und 150, den Umbau der Knochensubstanz — ihre Auflösung und Erneuerung — in den Bildern der Serie 149. Unter dem Einfluß der Funktion kann *beträchtliches Dickenwachstum* erfolgen (Serien 148 u. 150), eine interstitielle Streckung in die Länge aber geschieht nicht. — *Artfremder Knochen* (Serie 151) *bleibt ein Fremdkörper und heilt nicht ein.*

Chapter VII (Supplement).

Bone Transplantation and Joint Formation.

A. Independant Auto and Hetero Transplantation.

The bone tissue of the human body has great vitality in cases where there is a disturbance of the circulation and it also possesses an ideal power of regeneration. It has the greatest regenerative power of all the finer differential tissues. Because of this, bone can be independantly transplanted and after the initial destruction will become completely reformed. Even when the growing stage is passed, considerable defects may be repaired and an endeavour is always made to recover the original form, as in series 148, where a chiselled open bone tube closes again.

When bone is independantly transplanted into the same organism, it heals in and becomes renewed. The periosteum continues to live, but the cortex decays and becomes renewed from its surroundings. (Periosteum wound bed.) This proceeding is illustrated, where we see the active bone building of the periosteum in series 149 to 150 and the changing of the bone substance where it is disintegrating and rebuilding in series 149. Functional use influences the thickness of the growth considerably (Series 148—150), but an interstitial longitudinal growth is not obtained. Bone from another species (Series 151) remains a foreign body and does not unite.

Serie 148.

Knochenregeneration und freie Autotransplantation.

Die *Regenerationskraft* der Tibia nach Abschluß des Wachstums ergänzte den großen Meißeldefekt so weitgehend, daß wieder ein geschlossener dicker Röhrenknochen entstand. — Die autoplastisch *frei verpflanzten Knochenspäne* heilten ein und bewiesen ihre knochenbildende Kraft, indem sie untereinander sowie mit dem Lager verwuchsen und ein erhebliches Dickenwachstum entfalteten.

$^6/_{10}$ n. Gr.   1.

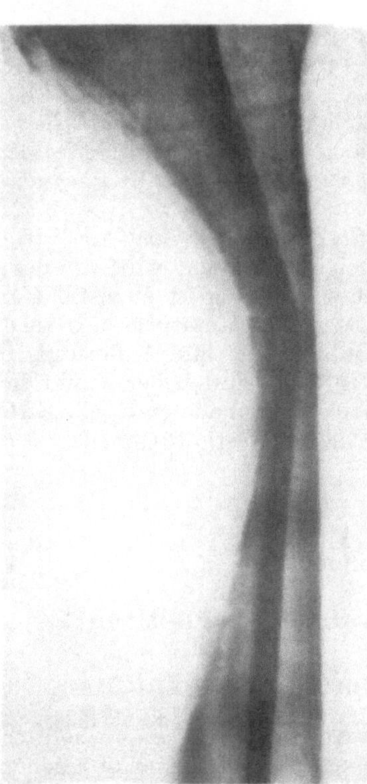

Großer, bis tief in die Markhöhle reichender Knochendefekt der eingebrochenen Tibia.

Extensive bone defect reaching far into the marrow hollow of the invaded tibia.

Series 148.

Bone Regeneration and Independent Auto-Transplantation.

The *regenerating power* of the tibia after growth had ended, was so great that it remedied the extensive chisel defect by creating a thick closed marrow-bone. The auto-plastic, independently planted bone fragments healed and showed bone-creating power by uniting strongly with one another and with the tibia.

2.

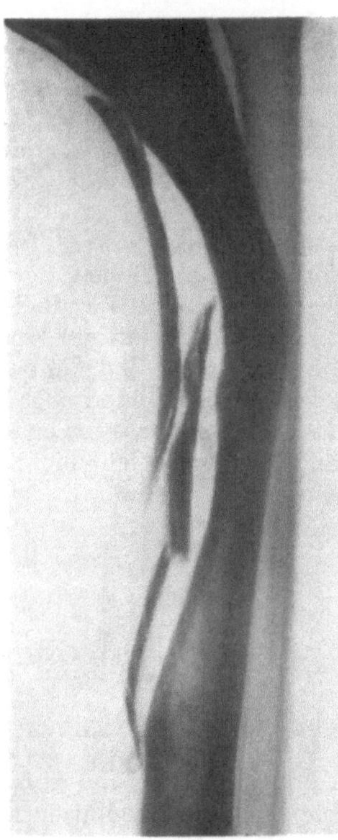

Nach $^1/_2$ Jahr ist eine Regeneration der Tibia schon deutlich; außerdem überbrücken autoplastisch frei verpflanzte Knochenspäne die Lücke.

After six months regeneration of tibia is visible, besides which, the autoplastic independently transplanted bone fragments span the defect.

Serie 148.

3.

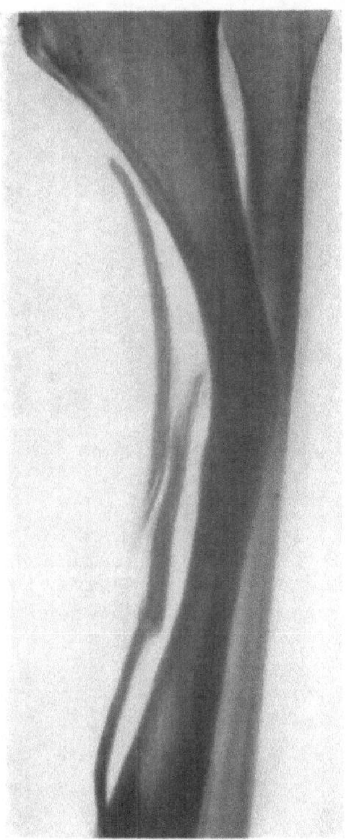

Nach ³/₄ Jahr ist der Befund noch etwa der gleiche.

After nine months the condition is almost unaltered.

4.

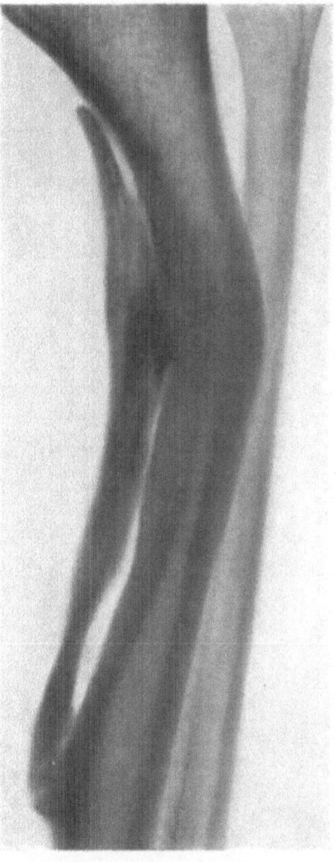

Nach 1¹/₂ Jahren ist die Tibia als ein breiter geschlossener *Röhrenknochen wiederhergestellt.* — Die transplantierten *Knochenspäne* sind miteinander sowie mit der Tibia *verwachsen und* erheblich *breiter* geworden.

After one year and a half the tibia has *again become a wide, closed marrow-bone.* The transplanted bone fragments have united with the tibia and with one another and have become considerably thickened.

5.

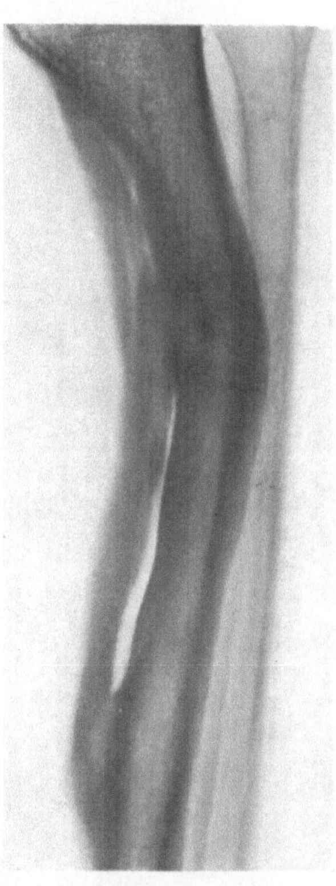

Nach 4 Jahren ist das Transplantat noch breiter geworden und flächenhafter mit der Tibia verwachsen. Im übrigen hat sich der Befund nicht mehr verändert.

After four years the transplanted fragments have become wider and the union more complete. Otherwise the condition is unchanged.

Serie 149.

Freie Autotransplantation (Pseudarthroseoperation).

Neben den angefrischten Bruchenden ist das Knochentransplantat Quelle der — den Bruch heilenden — Knochenwucherung. Sein Periost blieb am Leben und bildete reichlich Knochen (s. Bild 5); die Knochensubstanz aber starb ab und wurde von dem lebenden Periost bzw. dem Bett neu ersetzt.

Series 149.

Independent Autotransplantation (Pseudarthrosis Operation).

The bone growth which healed the fracture is traceable to two causes. 1. The freshly scraped fracture ends. 2. The transplanted bone-fragment. The periosteum flourished and formed bone in abundance (No. 5); the bone-substance died but was renewed by the periosteum.

$^7/_{10}$ n. Gr.   1.   2.

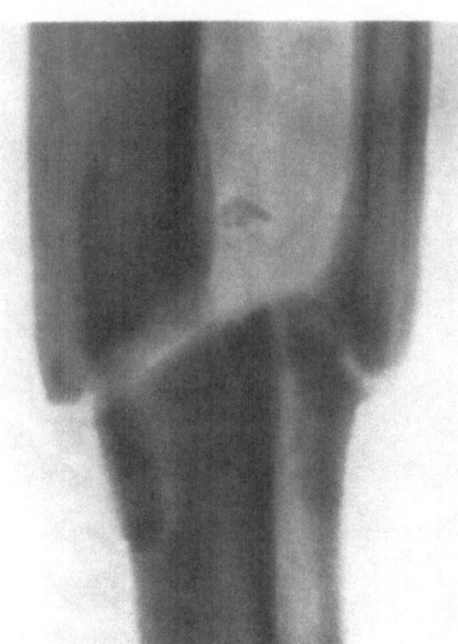

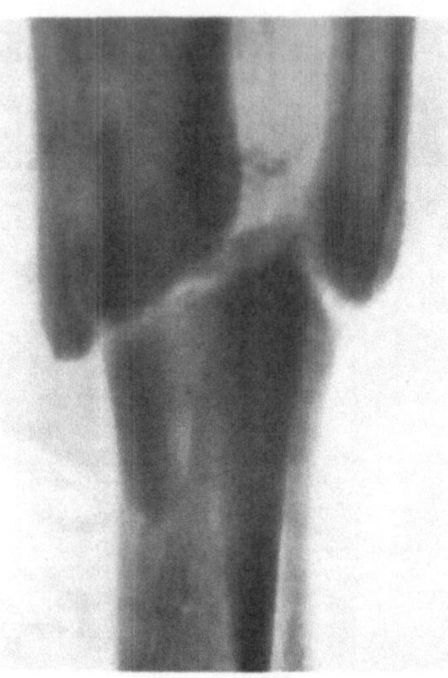

Ein eingekeilter Knochenspan überbrückt die angefrischten Bruchenden. (Befund 2 Tage p. op.)

A bone fragment spans the freshly scraped fracture ends. (Condition two days after operation.)

Nach 3 Wochen hat die knöcherne Verwachsung der frischen Wundflächen schon begonnen.

After three weeks, union of the fresh wound surfaces has commenced.

5.

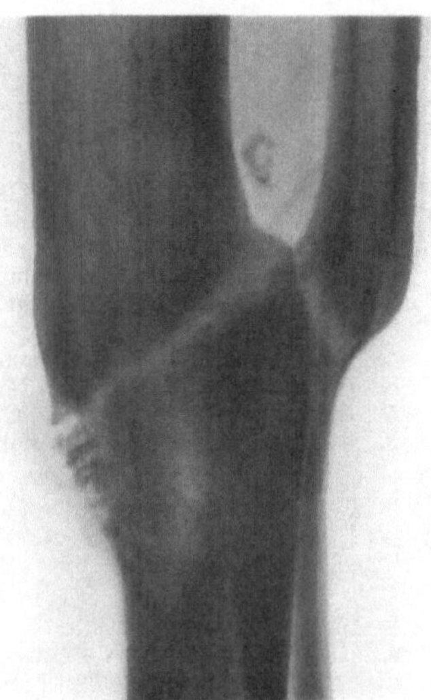

Nach 6½ Monaten hat das Periost des Transplantates deutlich Knochen gebildet; die Knochensubstanz des Spanes ist umgebaut und in der Struktur der Tibia größtenteils aufgenommen.

After six months and a half, the periosteum of the transplanted fragment has plainly generated new bone. The bone substance of the span has been surrounded and almost entirely resorbed into the tibia-structure.

Serie 149.

3.

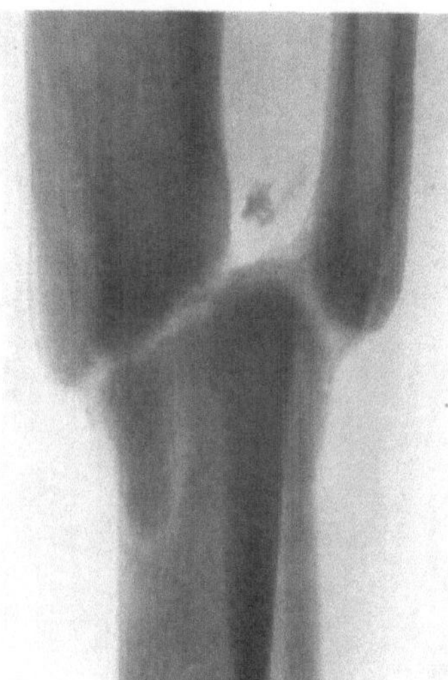

Nach 3 Monaten hat die Knochenbildung nur
wenig zugenommen.

After three months. During this time very little
progress was made.

4.

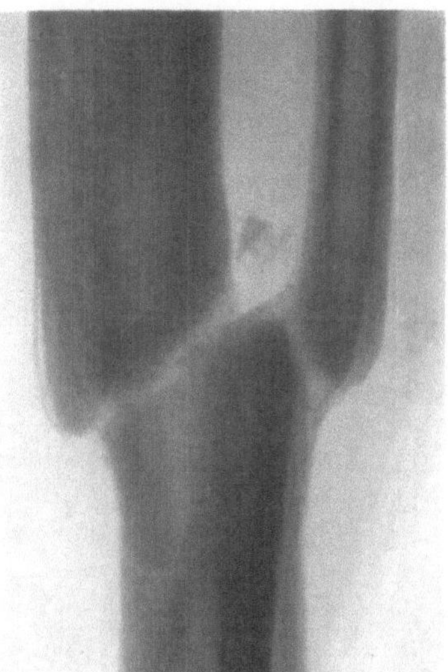

Nach 4 Monaten ist die Knochensubstanz des
Spanes weitgehend resorbiert und ersetzt.

After four months. The bone tissue of the span
has been to a very great extent resorbed
and replaced.

6.

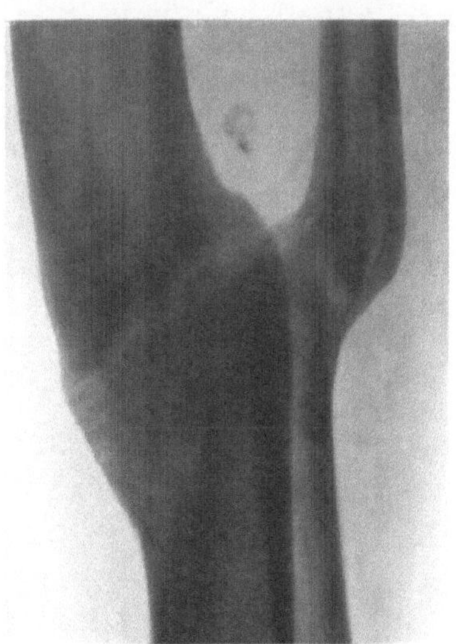

Nach 10 Monaten ist der Bruchspalt zwar noch erkennbar,
doch besteht eine breite knöcherne Verbindung; die äußere
Form der Frakturstelle ist abgerundet.

After ten months, the breach is still recognizable but a
wide ossified connection exists; the outline of the fractured
portion.

Serie 150.

Gestielte Knochenverlagerung.

Im Zusammenhang mit den Weichteilen wurde die Fibula bei dem 4 jährigen Mädchen in den durch fälschliche Resektion der osteomyelitischen Tibiadiaphyse gesetzten Defekt verlagert. Sie heilte ein, begann sehr bald mit periostaler Knochenbildung und wuchs unter der funktionellen Beanspruchung im Laufe der Jahre *erheblich in die Breite, jedoch gar nicht in die Länge.*

Series 150.

Transference of Bone Stem.

The fibula and connecting fleshy parts of a girl of four years were transferred into the defect caused by a faulty resection of the osteomyelitic tibial diaphysis. It healed well and the growth of periosteum soon commenced and continued, during which time the leg was continually used. In the course of years it grew considerably in width but not at all in length.

¹/₂ n. Gr. 1.   2.   3.   4.

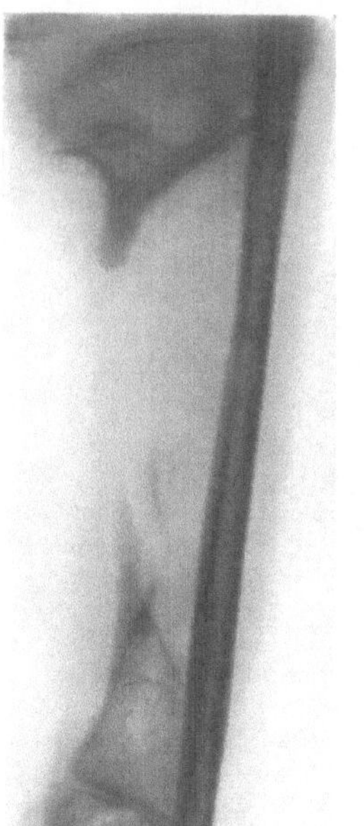

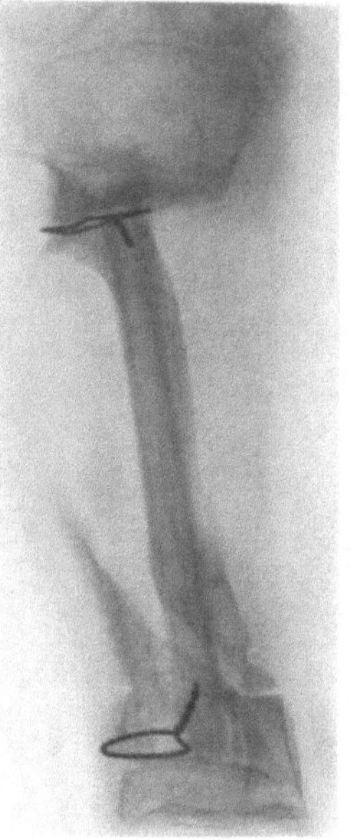

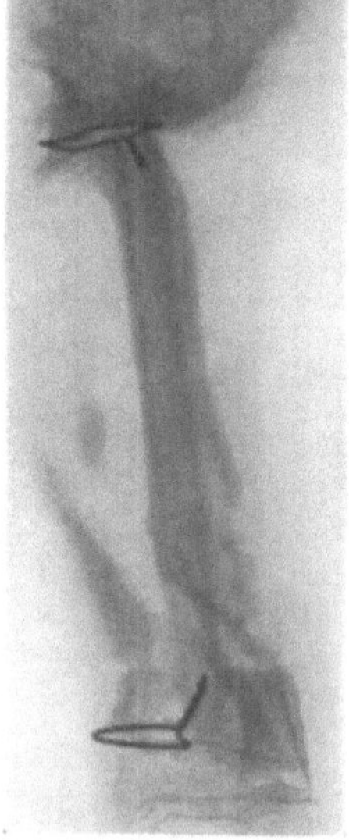

Defekt der Tibiadiaphyse.

Defect of the tibial diaphysis.

Die vor 4 Wochen gestielt verlagerte und durch Drahtnaht fixierte Fibula zeigt bereits periostale Knochenbildung.

Periosteal growth commenced four weeks after the fibula stem had been transplanted and fastened by wire.

Nach 2 und 3 Monaten hat die Knochenbildung des Periostes mehr und mehr zugenommen. (Feinere Vorgänge kommen im Röntgenbild nicht zum Ausdruck.)

After two and three months, the bone growth has increased. (Precise details cannot be seen in X-ray photos.)

Serie 150.

5a.   5b.

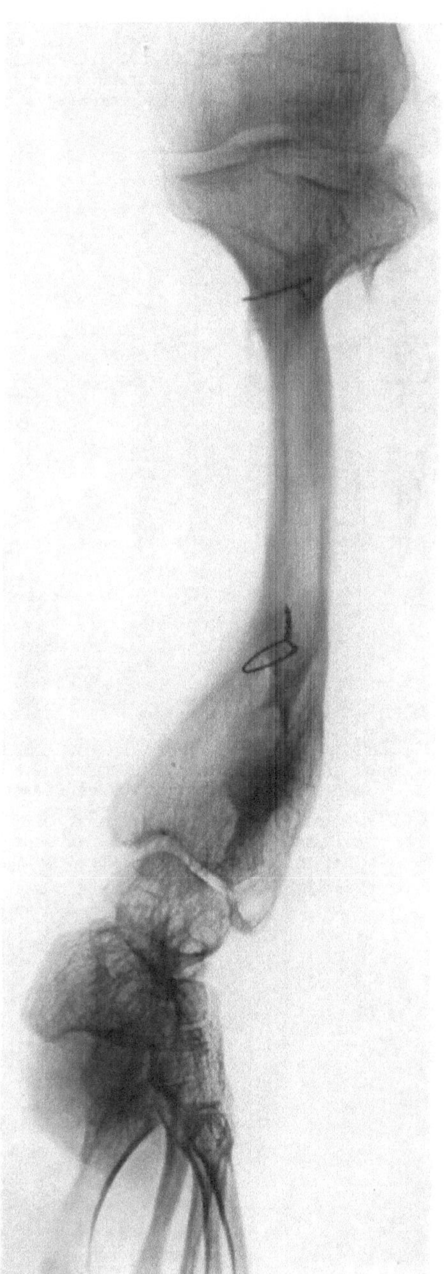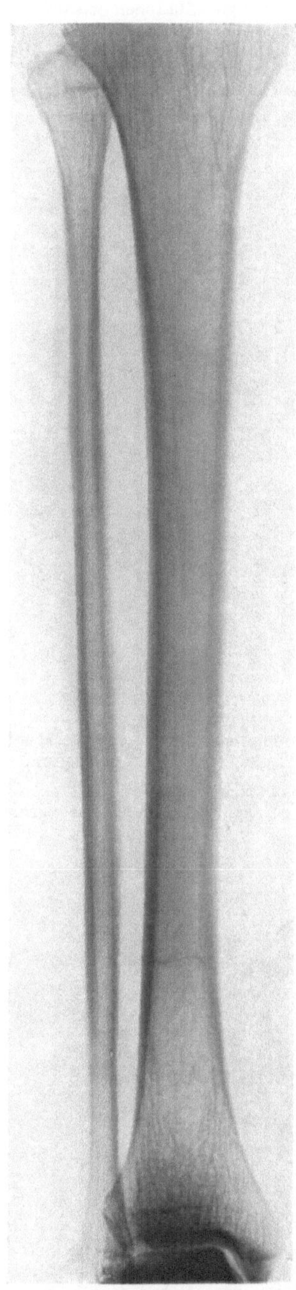

Nach 11 Jahren hat sich die verpflanzte Fibula — wie die Röntgenaufnahme der anderen Seite zeigt — auf mehr als das Doppelte verbreitert, Längenwachstum aber nicht entwickelt.

After eleven years. The transferred fibula, comparing it with the X-ray photo of other leg, has more than doubled its width but has not grown in length at all.

Serie 151.

Hetero-Transplantation.

Dem 18 jährigen Mädchen wurde nach Resektion des tuberkulös erkrankten Oberarmkopfes das proximale Humerusende eines Affen (Macacus rhesus) überpflanzt. Die Einheilung blieb aus, so daß das Transplantat nach $1^1/_2$ Jahren entfernt werden mußte.

$^3/_4$ n. Gr.

Series 151.

Hetero-Transplantation.

A girl of 18, after the resection of the tuberculous head of humerus, had the proximal end of humerus of an ape (macacus rhesus) transplanted. No healing took place, so the transplanted bone had to be removed after a year and a half.

1.

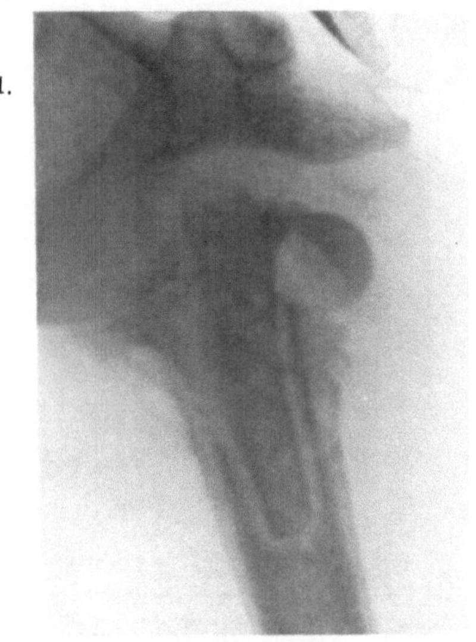

10 Wochen nach der Operation. Der Oberarmkopf des Transplantates ist gelöst und abgeglitten.

10 weeks after the operation: The head of humerus of the transplanted bone has become loose and slipped off.

2.

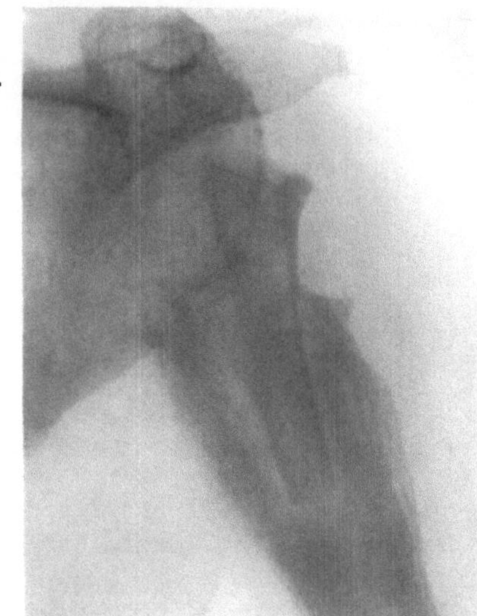

Nach weiteren 6 Monaten ist das Transplantat noch unverändert (kein Umbau oder Resorption, keine Verwachsung mit dem Mutterboden).

6 months later the transplanted bone is still unaltered. (No reconstruction or resorption. No union with original surroundings.)

3.

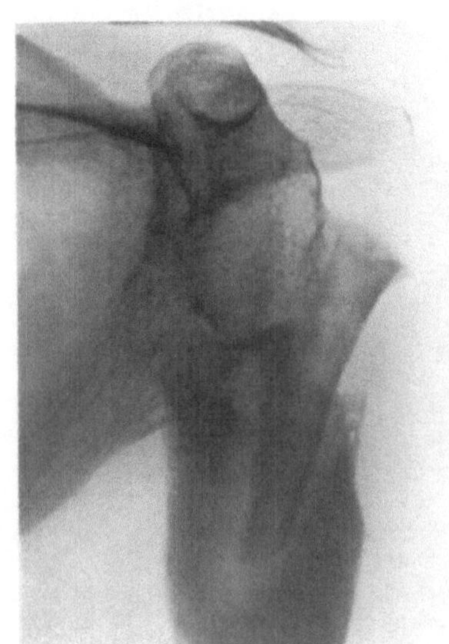

$1^1/_2$ Jahre nach der Einpflanzung besteht noch der gleiche Zustand des toten Fremdkörpers.

Eighteen months after implantation. The implanted humerus is still in the same condition.

B. Gelenkplastik und Nearthrose.

Ein so differenziertes Gewebsgefüge, wie es ein Gelenk darstellt, kann nach seiner Zerstörung anatomisch nur ganz unvollkommen wieder erstehen, das gilt sowohl für die operative Plastik als auch für die spontane Nearthrose. Immerhin kann das dabei vorhandene Ausmaß von Gelenkfunktion praktisch bedeutungsvoll sein. Für jede Art von Gelenkneubildung ist die Funktion von entscheidender Bedeutung. Ein operativ gesägtes Gelenk erfährt (Serie 152) eine lebendige Modellierung durch Resorption und Verdichtung des Knochengewebes. *Es bleibt immer primitiv,* d. h. 2 harte, aber nicht überknorpelte Knochenflächen, die in einem Spaltgewebe gegeneinander beweglich sind. — *Bei spontaner Nearthrosenbildung schleifen sich die gegenüberstehenden Knochenflächen in der gleichen Weise als eine Art Pfanne und Gelenkkopf aus* (Serie 154), während das alte Gelenk abflacht und verödet. Die differenziert angelegte Gelenkpfanne bei angeborener Hüftgelenkluxation aber vertieft und entwickelt sich noch verspätet nach der Einrichtung vollwertig (Serie 155). Entsteht eine flache Pfanne, so wird sogar eine Verlängerung des Pfannendaches durch osteophytäre Randwucherung angestrebt (Serie 156).

B. Joint-Plasty and Nearthrosis.

A tissue which is so greatly differentiated as that which enters into the construction of the joint, can only be very incompletely restored after its decay. This applies both to plastic surgery and to spontaneous nearthrosis. Nevertheless, the joint can still be of great practical use. Function is of decisive significance for every kind of joint rebuilding. A sawn joint (Series 152) is remodelled by the bone tissue becoming absorbed and thickened. The two hard bone surfaces moving against one another, without any cartilage covering, necessarily form a very primitive joint. In a case of spontaneous nearthrosis, the opposing bone surfaces become smooth and mould one another into poor substitutes for socket and joint head (Series 154) and the old joint is destroyed. In a case of congenital dislocation of the hip-joint, the existing joint socket becomes deeper and develops normally after it has been reset. This however, occurs rather late. (Series 155.) Should a flattened socket develop, an attempt to deepen it is made by peripheral osteophytic growth. (Series 156.)

<table>
<tr><td>

Serie 152.
Gelenkplastik.

Das infolge Schußverletzung knöchern versteifte Kniegelenk wurde operativ neu geformt (Aussägen der Gelenkflächen mit Zwischenlagerung von Fascie) und hat sich dann unter dem Einfluß der Funktion geweblich ausdifferenziert und ausgeschliffen, indem dem Stadium der Resorption das der Knochenverdichtung an den Gelenkenden folgte. Der Erfolg war ein voller.

$^6/_{10}$ n. Gr.

</td><td>

Series 152.
Plastic Surgery of Joint.

A knee-joint which was stiffened by ossification following a bullet-wound, was reformed by operation. (Sawing out of the joint surfaces and interposition of fascia.) Under functional influence, the tissues became equalized and smoothed as the stage of resorption was followed by the consolidation of the bone at the joint ends. It was a complete success.

</td></tr>
</table>

1.

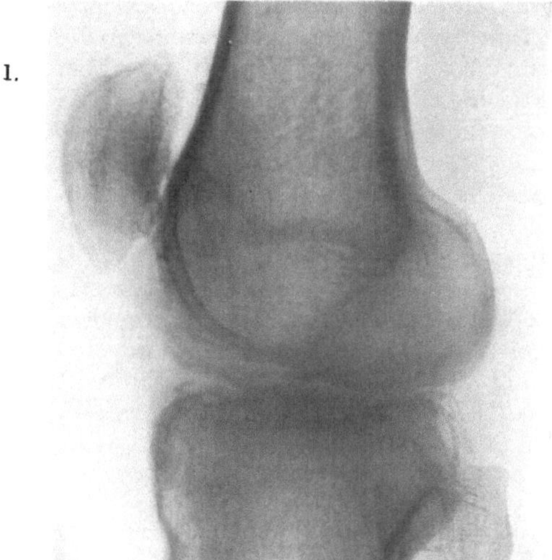

2.

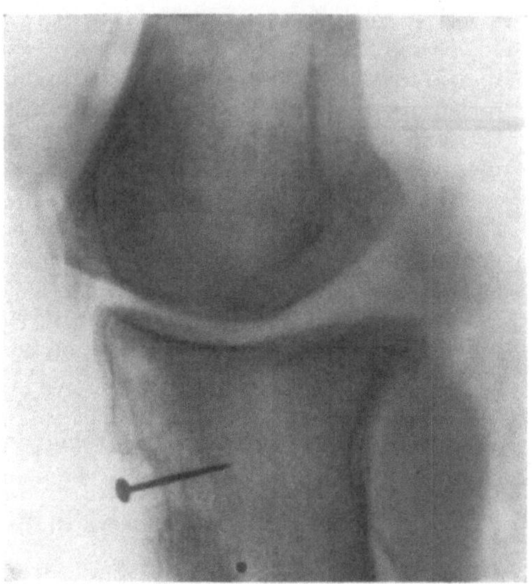

Die knöcherne Ankylose.
The osteo-ankylosis.

Die frisch *ausgesägten Gelenkflächen*.
The *freshly sawn joint surfaces*.

5.

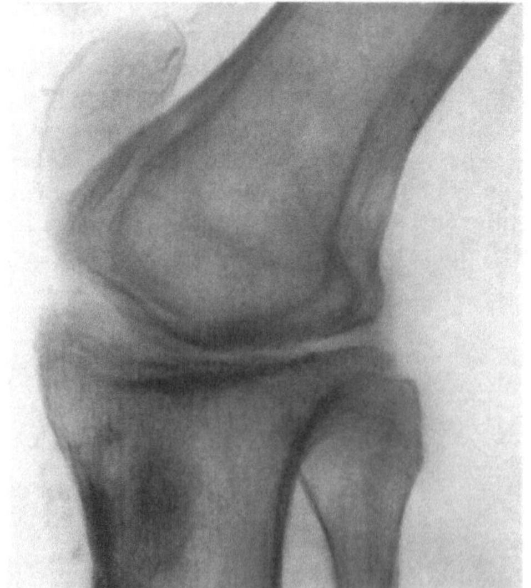

Nach 1$^1/_2$ Jahren ist der *Endzustand fast erreicht* (vgl. Abb. 6): feste Gelenkflächen und ein Gelenkspalt sind ausgebildet.
After one year and a half the *final stage has almost been reached.* (Compare picture No. 6.) Firm joint surfaces and a joint cleft have been formed.

Serie 152.

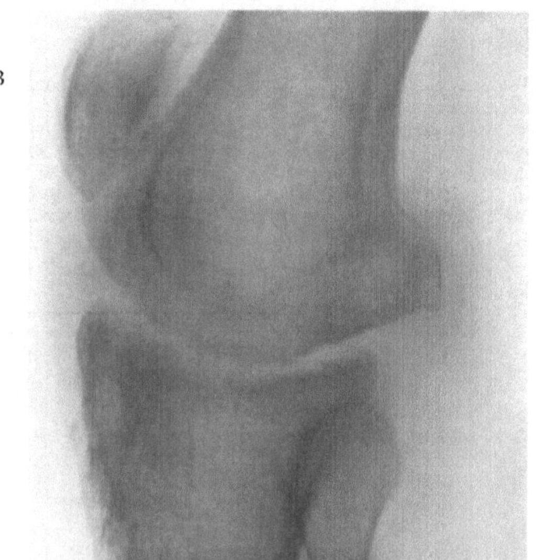

3

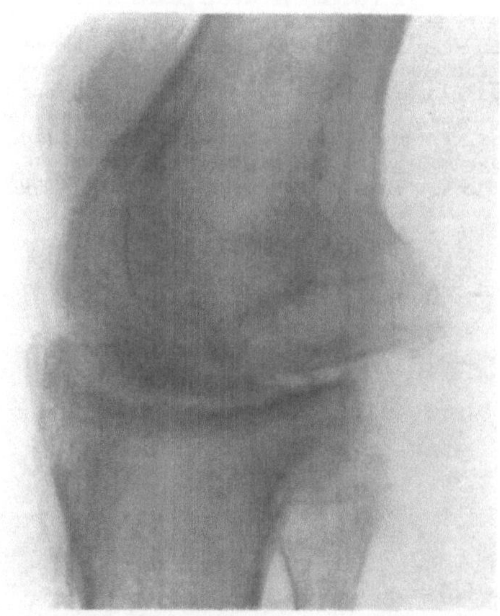

4.

Nach 1 Monat spielen sich an den Sägeflächen
allenthalben *resorptive* Prozesse ab.

After one month, *resorption* processes are visible at
the sawn surfaces.

Nach 2¹/₂ Monaten hat die Resorption den Höhepunkt überschritten und *Knochenapposition*
bereits eine Verdichtung der Gelenkränder
geschaffen.

After two months and a half, resorption has
passed the climax and bone-apposition already
has caused a consolidation of the edges of joint.

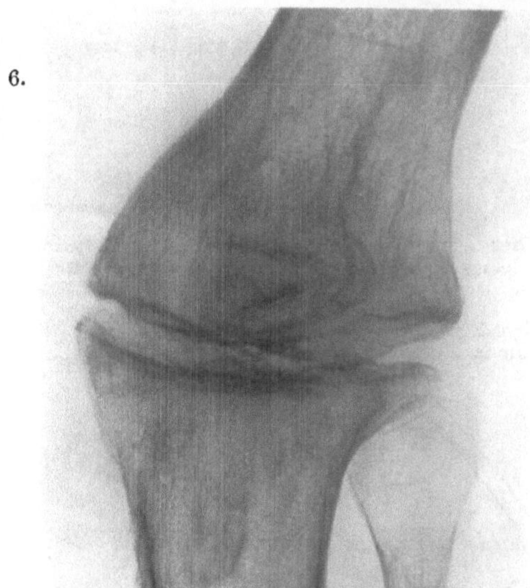

6.

Nach 9 Jahren ist der anatomische Zustand des Gelenkes ungefähr der gleiche wie er schon nach 1¹/₂ Jahren
war; immerhin sind die Ränder noch etwas fester und schärfer; die Knochenatrophie ist ganz behoben.

After nine years the anatomical condition of the joint is about the same as it was at one year and a half,
except that the edges are somewhat firmer and stronger. The bone atrophy has absolutely vanished.

Serie 153.

Pfannendachplastik.

Das eigenartige, am Ende des Wachstums schleichend
einsetzende Hüftleiden führte zu einer Ausweitung
und Abflachung der Gelenkpfanne, somit zur Subluxation des Schenkelkopfes, so daß die Kranke mehr
und mehr hinkte. Die Operation erstrebte, durch freie
Knochentransplantation das Pfannendach zu ver-
größern, und hatte — anatomisch wie funktionell —
vollen Erfolg.

Series 153.

Plastic Surgery of Roof of Acetabulum.

Towards the end of the growth period, a strange slowly
developing hip-disease led to the widening and flattening of the joint socket and to subluxation of femur-
head, causing an ever-increasing lameness. It was
hoped by operation and transplantation of bone to
enlarge the roof of the acetabulum. Both anatomically
and functionally the operation proved successful.

$^1/_2$ n. Gr.   1.   2.

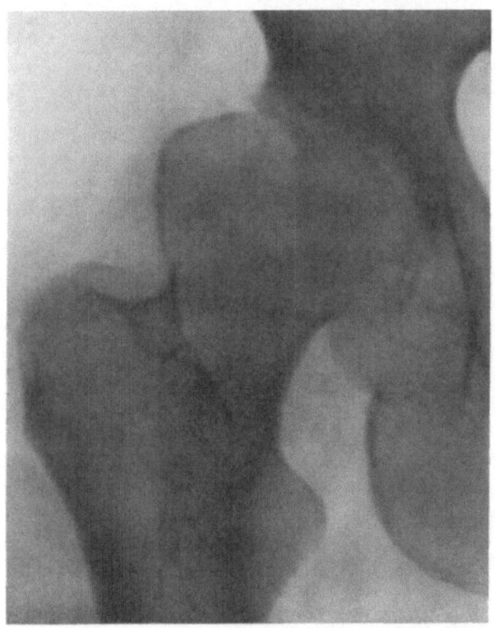
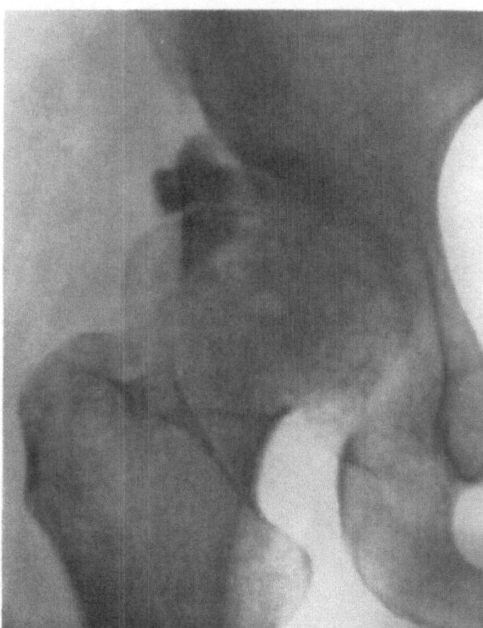

Das Hüftgelenk im Zustand einer „gewanderten"
und abgeflachten Pfanne sowie eines subluxierten
Schenkelkopfes.

The hip joint exists as a misplaced and flattened
socket — the head of the femur is subluxated.

Die Aufnahme nach der Operation zeigt die am
oberen Pfannenrand eingekeilten, frei transplantierten Tibiaspäne.

The photograph after operation shows the transplanted tibial fragment which healed into upper edge
of socket.

Serie 153.

3.

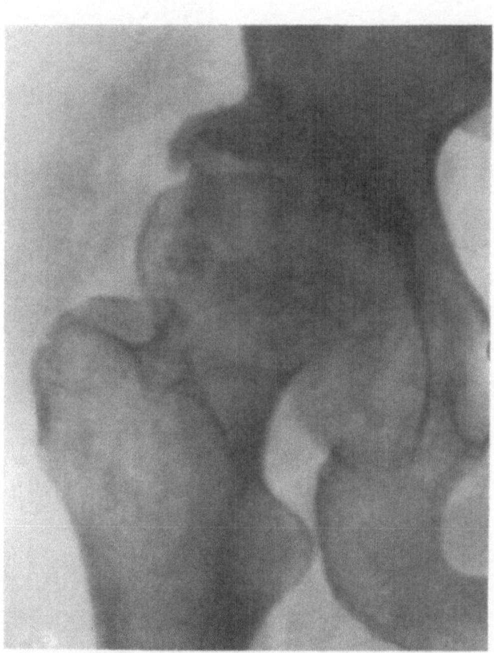

Nach 2 Jahren ist ein festes, organisch eingefügtes Pfannendach aus den frei verpflanzten Knochenstücken gebildet und die Subluxation beseitigt.

After two years a firm organically healed acetabular roof has been formed by the transplanted bone and the subluxation has disappeared.

Serie 154.

Nearthrose.

Die Spontanluxation der Hüfte, welche im Verlaufe einer hämatogenen Osteomyelitis des anderen Oberschenkels aufgetreten war, konnte weder unblutig noch blutig nach Resektion des Schenkelkopfes eingerichtet werden. Im Laufe der Jahre bildete sich aus dem Schenkelhalsstumpf und der gegenüberliegenden Darmbeinfläche ein — freilich deformes — Gelenk.

Series 154.

Nearthrosis.

During a haematogenous osteomyelitis of the other leg, a spontaneous luxation of the hip occured. It was impossible to replace this, either bloodlessly or after resection of the femur head. Subsequently a joint — of course deformed — was fashioned between the stump of the femoral neck and the opposing pelvic bone.

$^1/_2$ n. Gr.   1.   2.

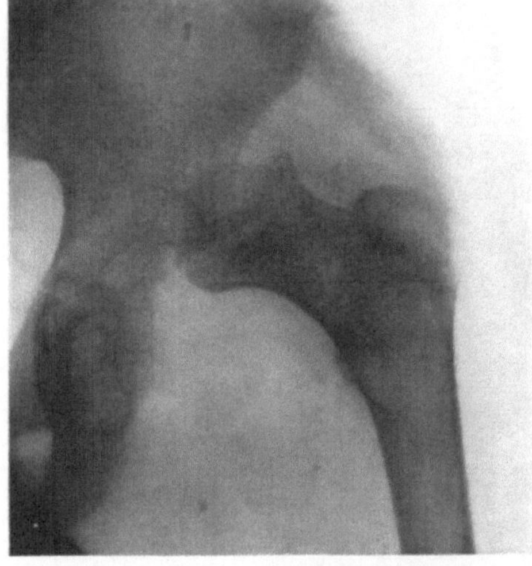

Spontanluxation der Hüfte (9 jähriger Knabe).
Spontaneaous luxation of the hip. (Boy of nine.)

Auch nach Resektion des Kopfes steht der Schenkelhals außerhalb der Gelenkpfanne.
After resection of head, the neck of femur is outside the joint-pan.

3.

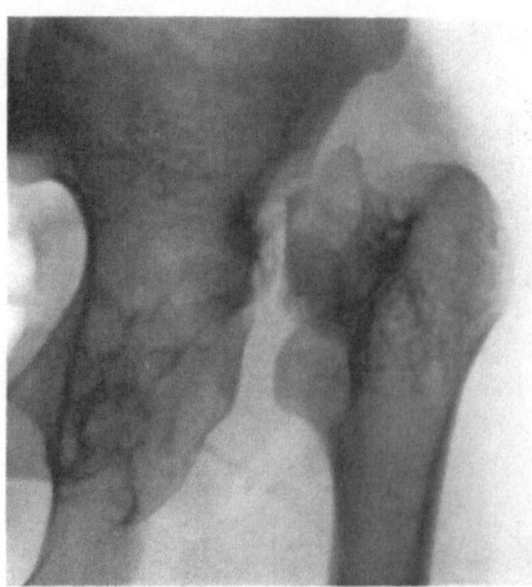

10 Jahre später ist *die normale Hüftpfanne* verödet, oberhalb aber *ein neues Gelenk* — eine pfannenartige Ausdellung des Darmbeines und pilzartige Verbreiterung des Schenkelhalses — entstanden.
Ten years later *the normal* hip socket is destroyed, but *a new joint* — a cup shaped dent of the pelvic bone and a mushroomlike widening of the neck of femur — has appeared.

Serie 155.

Luxatio coxae congenita.

Durch unblutige Einrichtung der angeborenen Hüftverrenkung, welche im 3. Lebensjahr geschah, wurde Beschwerdefreiheit und normaler Gang erreicht; das Gelenk hat sich bis zum 7. Jahr gut entwickelt.

Series 155.

Congenital Luxation of the Hip.

A child was born with a dislocated hip which was set in the third year without bleeding. After this, a normal gait was attained. Until the seventh year the development of the joint has been satisfactory.

$^1/_2$ n. Gr.

1.

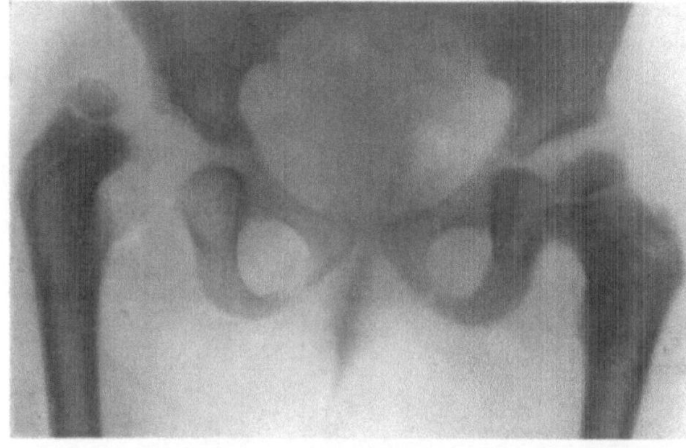

Der linke Hüftkopf steht außerhalb der sehr flachen Pfanne.

The left femoral head stands outside the very shallow socket.

2.

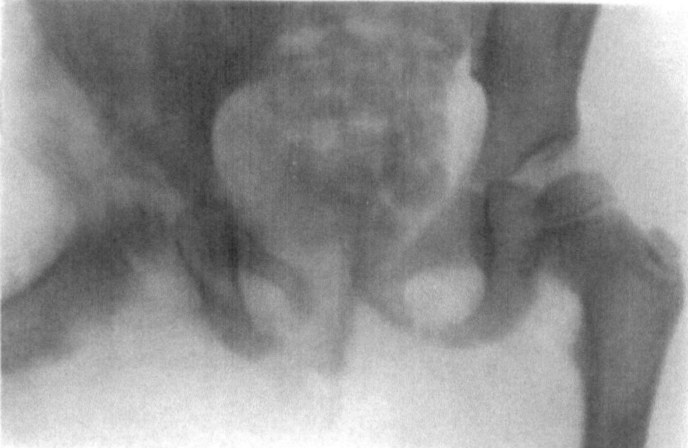

Der eingerenkte Oberschenkelkopf wird durch den Gipsverband in der Gelenkpfanne gehalten.

The replaced femoral head is held firmly in the joint socket by plaster-of-Paris bandages.

3.

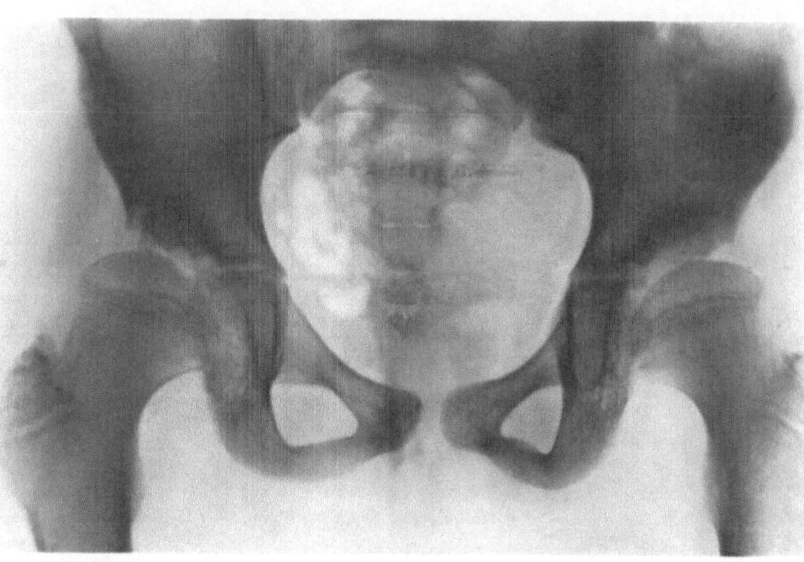

4 Jahre später ist das Hüftgelenk gut ausgebildet, nur die Gelenkpfanne noch ein wenig flacher.

Four years later the hip-joint is well developed but the joint socket is still somewhat shallow.

<table>
<tr><td>

Serie 156.

Luxatio coxae congenita.

Nachdem die angeborene Hüftverrenkung im 2. Lebensjahr unblutig eingerichtet war, wurde schließlich ein völlig normaler Gang erreicht. Seit dem 18. Lebensjahr aber besteht ein leichtes Hinken, das seinen Grund in der Flachheit der Pfanne hat. Im Laufe der folgenden Jahre wurde das Pfannendach durch eine Randwucherung — freilich nur unzureichend — verlängert.

</td><td>

Series 156.

Congenital Luxation of the Hip.

A child was born with a dislocated hip which was not set until it was in its second year, but then so successfully that an absolutely normal gait was achieved. However, after the eighteenth year a slight lameness became noticeable. It was caused by the shallowness of the socket. In the course of the following years, by the exuberant growth of the edge, the roof of socket was deepened, but of course not sufficiently.

</td></tr>
</table>

$^1/_2$ n. Gr.   1.   2.

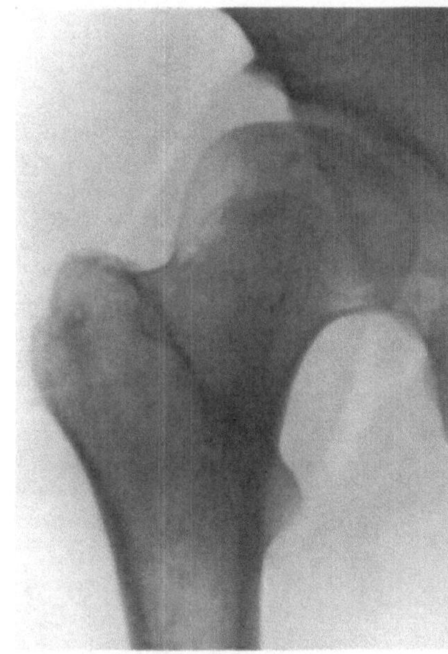

Lebensalter: 18 Jahre. — Flache Hüftpfanne und subluxierter Hüftkopf.

Eighteen years of age. — Shallow acetabulum and subluxated femoral head.

Lebensalter: 29 Jahre. — Die kleine *Randwucherung*, welche schon vor ·10 Jahren angedeutet war, ist größer geworden und hat das Pfannendach ein wenig verlängert (ein Vorbild der Pfannendachplastik).

Twenty-nine years of age. — The edge-growth, which ten years previously had been but slight, has become more exuberant and somewhat deepened the socket. (An example of acetabular plasty.)

Sachverzeichnis.

(Die Ziffern bedeuten die Seriennummern.)

Abstützung, statische
bei Arthropathia tabica 117,
118
Coxa vara adulescentium
86
Osteomyelitis der Wirbel-
säule 7
Spondylitis luetica 56.

Arthritis
deformans 111—116
gonorrhoica 20—22
luetica 54, 55 b u. c.
septische Metastase 25
traumatische 145
tuberculosa 26—41, 47—50
ulcerosa 110
unspezifische akute 23, 24
„   chronische 106
bis 109
Wiederherstellung des Gelenkspaltes 21, 23, 24.

Atrophie
entzündliche, s. Tuberkulose
usw.
nach Distorsion 143.
Gefäßzerreißung 146
Kontusion 144
Luxation 145.

Calcaneus
Gicht 104
Sarkom 62.

Chondrodystrophie 74
Chondromatose 70 a—c.
Coxa vara adulescentium 86, 87.

Ellenbogen
Ankylose 10, 35
Lues 54, 55c
Luxation 141
Tuberkulose 35, 36, 47, 48.

Epiphysenfuge
bei Chondrodystrophie 74
Osteoarthritis deformans
juvenilis coxae 81
Osteomyelitis 4, 11, 12, 17
Rachitis 98—101
Tuberkulose 26, 37
Verletzung 131—134.

Exostose 1, 71—73, 121.

Femur
Fraktur 122, 124, 125
Osteomyelitis 3, 5, 6, 8, 11

Periostitis 19
Sarkom 64, 65.

Fibula
Exostose 71, 73
Sarkom 61
Transplantation 150.

Formangleichung
Fraktur (Callus und Dislokation) 76, 122, 124, 125, 149
Möller-Barlowsche Krankheit
(subperiostales Hämatom)
103
Osteomyelitis (Totenlade) 4.

Funktionelle Anpassung
akute Coxitis 23
Fraktur 76
Gelenkplastik 152
Luxatio coxae congenita 155
Luxationsfraktur 137
Metatarsus 119
Nearthrose 154
progressiver Gelenkrheumatis-
mus 108.

Fußgelenk
Fraktur 137, 138
Osteochondritis dissecans 97
Tuberkulose 30.

Gelenk
Bildung 154, 155, 108
Bruch 135—139
Plastik 152, 153.

Gelenkmaus 113.

Gelenkrheumatismus
deformierender 111—116
primär chronischer 109. 110
progressiver 106, 107, 109
sekundär chronischer 108.

Geschwülste
Carcinom-Metastasen 66—69
Chondro-Sarkom 63
Osteoid-Sarkom 64, 65
Osteoplastisches Carcinom 67
Strukturveränderung 62
Spindelzell-Sarkom 59—62
Spontanfraktur 59, 60. 66, 67.

Gicht 104.

Hämophilie 121.

Handgelenk
Gonorrhöe 22
Lues 55b u. 58
Tuberkulose 40, 41.

Hüftgelenk
akute unspezifische Entzün-
dung 23—24
Arthritis deformans (hyper-
trophische Form) 114
Coxa vara adulescentium 86,
87
Gonorrhöe 20, 21
Luxatio coxae congenita 155,
156
Osteoarthritis deformans juve-
nilis 81—85
Schenkelhalsfraktur 140
septische Metastase 25
Spontanluxation 9
Tuberkulose 31—34

Humerus
Carcinom-Metastasen 66, 67
Fraktur 123, 124 (Anhang)
Lues 52, 54
Ostitis fibrosa 92, 93.

Hypertrophie
Arthritis deformans 114
vicariierende 119, 148, 150.

Ischaemische Muskelkontraktur
147.

Kalkgicht 105

Kallus
normale Bildung 122, 124
verzögerte Bildung 127, 128
bei Osteogenesis imperfecta 75
Osteopsathyrosis 76.

Kiefer 14—16.

Knie
Ankylose 8, 27, 28, 50, 107, 110
Arthritis deformans 111—113
Arthropatia tabica 117—118
Fraktur 136, 139
Osteochondritis dissecans 96
Plastik 152
Tuberkulose 26—29, 50.

Knochenbruch
ausgebliebene Verknöcherung
129, 130
Ausgleich der Dislokation 123
normale Heilung 122
Radius 131, 132
Schenkelhals 140
verzögerte Heilung 128
des wachsenden Knochens 76,
123, 126

Knochenbruch
  der Wachstumsfuge 131, 132,
    133, 134
  Wirbelsäule
  der Gelenke 135—139.
Knochenkerne
  Kretinismus 80
  Myxödem 79
  Rachitis 98, 99.
Köhlersche Krankheit 89.
Kretinismus 80.

Luxation
  kongenitale 155, 156
  pathologische 9, 154
  traumatische 145.

Malum perforans pedis 119
Möller-Barlowsche Krankheit 103.
Myositis ossificans 141, 142.
Myxödem 79.

Ossification (enchondrale)
  Chondrodystrophie 74
  Lues congenita 51
  Rachitis 98—101.
Osteoarthritis deformans juvenilis
  coxae 81—85.
Osteochondritis dissecans 96—97.
Osteogenesis imperfecta 75.
Osteomyelitis
  Ankylose 8, 10
  Dehnungsverrenkung 9
  dentale 14—16
  Epiphysenschädigung 4, 11,
    12, 17
  haematogene 1—13
  Knochenabsceß 13
  Regeneration 1, 2, 3, 4, 8, 17,
    18
  schleichender Umbau 5, 6, 7
  Sequester 2, 3, 4, 10, 14, 15
  Spontanfraktur 2, 8, 14
  Totenlade 2, 3, 4
  traumatische 17 u. 18.
Osteopsathyrosis 76
Ostitis fibrosa
  generalisierte 95
  Humerus 92, 93
  Schädel 94
  Tibia 91

Periostitis
  luetische 51—54
  sekundäre 19

Pseudarthrose
  congenitale 78
  Operation 149
  traumatische 129, 130.

Rachitis
  Spontanfraktur 98
  Umbauzonen 100
  Verkrümmungen 100—102.
Radius
  Fraktur 131, 132
  Lues 58
  Osteomyelitis 4.

Schenkelhals
  Ostitis fibrosa 95
  Sarkom 60
  Schwund bei Fraktur 140.
Schlattersche Krankheit 88.
Schultergelenk
  Hetero-Transplantation 151
  traumatische Arthritis 145
  Tuberkulose 37—39.
Spontanfraktur
  Carcinom-Metastasen 66, 67
  Osteomyelitis 2, 8, 14
  Ostitis fibrosa 91—93
  Rachitis 98
  Sarkom 59, 60.
Spontanluxation
  Osteomyelitis 9, 154
  progressiver Gelenkrheumatis-
    mus 106, 108.
Syphilis
  angeborene 51—53
  erworbene 54—58
  Gumma 55
  Heilung durch Arsen 51, 52
    "   " Hg 58
    "   " Salvarsan 53
    bis 56
  maligne 55
  Mischinfektion 57
  ossale Gelenksyphilis 55 b u. c
  Osteochondritis 51
  Periostitis 51—54
  refraktäres Verhalten 55, 57
  Sequester 57
  Spondylitis 56

Tabische Arthropatie 117—120.
Tibia
  Exostose 71, 72
  Fraktur 127, 129

Gumma 55a
  Osteomyelitis 1, 2
  Periostitis luetica 51, 52
  Sarkom 59
Transplantation
  freie 148, 149
  gestielte 150
  Hetera- 151.
Tuberkulose
  Defektheilung 27, 28, 31, 33, 35,
    38, 42
  Ellenbogen 35, 36, 47, 48
  fortschreitende Zerstörung 39
  Fußgelenk 30
  Gibbus 43—45
  Handgelenk 40, 41
  Hüftgelenk 31—34, 49
  Kniegelenk 26—29, 50
  operative Heilung 29, 36, 40, 41
  ossale Gelenktuberkulose 31,
    32, 35—37
  Pfannenwanderung 31, 32, 33
  Restitutio ad integrum 26, 27
  Schambein 46
  Schulter 37—39
  Spina ventosa 42
  synoviale Gelenktuberkulose
    27, 30, 34, 36, 41
  Wirbelsäule 43—45.

Ulna
  Lues 55 b
  Tuberkulose 40
Unterarmfraktur 128, 130.

Verkalkung
  Hämatom 73, 103
  Myositis ossificans 141, 142.

Wirbelsäule
  Carcinom-Metastase 68
  Fraktur 126
  Lues 56
  Osteomyelitis 7
  Spondylitis deformans 115
  Spondylitis tabica 120
  Tuberkulose 43—45
  Wachstumsstörung 90.

Zahn
  dentale Osteomyelitis 14—16
  sequestrierende Zahnkeiment-
    zündung 15.

VERLAG VON JULIUS SPRINGER / BERLIN UND WIEN

Pathologische Anatomie und Histologie der Knochen, Muskeln, Sehnen, Sehnenscheiden, Schleimbeutel. (Bildet Band IX vom „Hand-buch der speziellen pathologischen Anatomie und Histologie".)

Erster Teil: Mit 195 zum Teil farbigen Abbildungen. VIII, 678 Seiten. 1929.
RM 146.—; gebunden RM 149.80

Inhaltsübersicht: 1. Rhachitis und Osteomalazie. Von Geh. Hofrat Professor Dr. M. B. Schmidt-Würzburg. — 2. Die Entwicklungsstörungen der Knochen. Von Professor Dr. A. Dietrich-Tübingen. — 3. Infantiler Skorbut (Möller-Barlowsche Krankheit). Von Professor Dr. E. Fraenkel †-Hamburg, unter Hinzufügung einiger Ergänzungen von Professor Dr. Fr. Wohlwill-Hamburg. — 4. Angeborene Knochensyphilis. Von Professor Dr. L. Pick-Berlin. — 5. Die quergestreifte Muskulatur. Von Professor Dr. H. v. Meyenburg-Zürich. — 6. Spezielle Pathologie der Sehnen, Sehnenscheiden und Schleimbeutel. Von Dr. A. v. Albertini-Zürich. — Namenverzeichnis. — Sachverzeichnis.

Zweiter Teil: In Vorbereitung.

Inhaltsübersicht: Entzündungen. Spezifische Infektion (außer angeborener Syphilis). — Geschwülste. — Gelenke. Von Professor Dr. W. Ceelen-Bonn. — Kreislauf- und Ernährungsstörungen des Knochens. Von Professor Dr. G. Axhausen-Berlin. — Belastungsverunstaltungen. Von Dr. W. Putschar-Göttingen.

Die Abnahme eines Teiles des Bandes verpflichtet zum Kauf des ganzen Bandes.

Mikroskopische Anatomie der Gewebe. (Bildet Band II vom „Handbuch der mikroskopischen Anatomie des Menschen".)

Erster Teil: **Epithel- und Drüsengewebe. Bindegewebe und blutbildende Ge-webe. Blut.** Mit 305 zum Teil farbigen Abbildungen und 1 Tafel. X, 703 Seiten. 1927.
RM 135.—; gebunden RM 141.—

Inhaltsübersicht: Das Epithelgewebe. Von Professor Dr. J. Schaffer-Wien. — Bindegewebe und blutbildende Gewebe. Von Professor Dr. A. Maximow-Chicago. — Blut. Von Professor Dr. J. Brodersen-Hamburg. — Namen- und Sachverzeichnis.

Zweiter Teil: **Stützgewebe. Knochengewebe. Skeletsystem.** Mit 521 zum Teil farbigen Abbildungen. VII, 699 Seiten. 1930. RM 168.—; gebunden RM 176.—

Inhaltsübersicht: Die Stützgewebe. Von Professor Dr. J. Schaffer-Wien. — Das Knochengewebe. Von Professor Dr. F. Weidenreich-Frankfurt a. M. — Die Organe des Skeletsystems. Von Professor Dr. H. Petersen-Würz-burg. — Namen- und Sachverzeichnis.

Dritter Teil: In Vorbereitung.

Inhaltsübersicht: Muskelgewebe. Von Professor Dr. G. Häggqvist-Stockholm.

Die Abnahme eines Teiles des Bandes verpflichtet zum Kauf des ganzen Bandes.

Die Tuberkulose der Knochen und Gelenke. Ihre Pathologie, Diagnostik, Therapie und soziale Bedeutung. Von Dr. **Wilh. Kremer,** Dirig. Arzt an den Heilstätten Beelitz (Mark), und Dr. **Otto Wiese,** Chefarzt der Kaiser Wilhelm-Tuberkulose-Kinderklinik bei Landeshut (Rgb.). (Bildet Band VIII der Sammlung „Die Tuberkulose und ihre Grenz-gebiete in Einzeldarstellungen".) Mit 197 Abbildungen. VI, 358 Seiten. 1930.

RM 46.—; gebunden RM 49.—

Die Abonnenten der „Beiträge zur Klinik der Tuberkulose" sowie des „Zentralblattes für die gesamte Tuberkulose-forschung" erhalten einen Nachlaß von 10%.

Die Lebensvorgänge im normalen Knorpel und seine Wucherung bei Akromegalie. Von Professor Dr. **J. Erdheim,** Wien. (Bildet Band III der Samm-lung „Pathologie und Klinik in Einzeldarstellungen".) Mit etwa 31 Abbildungen. Etwa 165 Seiten.

Erscheint im Frühjahr 1931

Bernhard Heine's Versuche über Knochenregeneration. Sein Leben und seine Zeit. Von der Deutschen Gesellschaft für Chirurgie anläßlich ihrer 50. Tagung den Fachgenossen unterbreitet. Herausgegeben von der Anatomischen Anstalt der Uni-versität Würzburg (Direktor Professor Dr. H. Petersen), der Chirurgischen Uni-versitätsklinik Würzburg (Direktor Professor Dr. F. König), der Chirurgischen Universitätsklinik Berlin (Direktor Professor Dr. A. Bier). Bearbeitet durch Dr. K. Vogeler, Assistent der Chirurgischen Klinik, Würzburg, Dr. E. Redenz, Prosektor der Anatomischen Anstalt, Würzburg, Dr. H. Walter, Assistent der Chirurgischen Klinik, Würzburg, Professor Dr. B. Martin, Assistent der Chirurgischen Klinik, Berlin. Mit einem Vorwort von Professor Dr. A. Bier. Mit 105 Textabbildungen und einem Porträt. VIII, 224 Seiten. 1926. RM 7.50

Konstitutionspathologie in der Orthopädie. Erbbiologie des peripheren Be-wegungsapparates. Von Dr. **Berta Aschner,** Wien, und Dr. **Guido Engelmann,** Privat-dozent in Wien. („Konstitutionspathologie in den medizinischen Spezialwissenschaften", herausgegeben von Julius Bauer, Wien, 3. Heft.) Mit 80 Abbildungen. VII, 312 Seiten. 1928.
RM 28.—